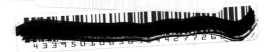

Handbook of Gynaecology Management

Handbook of Gynaecology Management

SYLVIA K. ROSEVEAR
MD, FRCOG
Consultant Obstetrician and Gynaecologist

Blackwell
Science

© 2002 by
Blackwell Science Ltd
Editorial Offices:
Osney Mead, Oxford OX2 0EL
25 John Street, London WC1N 2BS
23 Ainslie Place, Edinburgh EH3 6AJ
350 Main Street, Malden
  MA 02148 5018, USA
54 University Street, Carlton
  Victoria 3053, Australia
10, rue Casimir Delavigne
  75006 Paris, France

Other Editorial Offices:

Blackwell Wissenschafts-Verlag GmbH
Kurfürstendamm 57
10707 Berlin, Germany

Blackwell Science KK
MG Kodenmacho Building
7–10 Kodenmacho Nihombashi
Chuo-ku, Tokyo 104, Japan

Iowa State University Press
A Blackwell Science Company
2121 S. State Avenue
Ames, Iowa 50014-8300, USA

The right of the Author to be identified as the Author of this Work has been asserted in accordance with the Copyright, Designs and Patents Act 1988.

All rights reserved. No part of this publication may be reproduced, stored in a retrieval system, or transmitted, in any form or by any means, electronic, mechanical, photocopying, recording or otherwise, except as permitted by the UK Copyright, Designs and Patents Act 1988, without the prior permission of the publisher.

First published 2002

Set in 8 pt Trump Medaevil
by SNP Best-set Typesetters Ltd., Hong Kong
Printed and bound in Great Britain by
MPG Books Ltd, Bodwin, Cornwall

The Blackwell Science logo is a trade mark of Blackwell Science Ltd, registered at the United Kingdom Trade Marks Registry

DISTRIBUTORS

Marston Book Services Ltd
PO Box 269
Abingdon
Oxon OX14 4YN
(*Orders:* Tel: 01235 465500
         Fax: 01235 465555)

USA
Blackwell Science, Inc.
Commerce Place
350 Main Street
Malden, MA 02148 5018
(*Orders:* Tel: 800 759 6102
                781 388 8250
         Fax: 781 388 8255)

Canada
Login Brothers Book Company
324 Saulteaux Crescent
Winnipeg, Manitoba R3J 3T2
(*Orders:* Tel: 204 837-2987
         Fax: 204 837-3116)

Australia
Blackwell Science Pty Ltd
54 University Street
Carlton, Victoria 3053
(*Orders:* Tel: 03 9347 0300
         Fax: 03 9347 5001)

A catalogue record for this title is available from the British Library

ISBN 0-632-05588-X

Library of Congress
Cataloging-in-Publication Data

Handbook of gynaecology management/ [edited by] Sylvia K. Rosevear.
    p. cm.
  Includes bibliographical references and index. [ADJUST 008?]
  ISBN 0-632-05588-X (alk. paper)
  1. Gynecology. 2. Gynecologic nursing.
  3. Women—Diseases. I. Rosevear, Sylvia K.
  [DNLM: 1. Genital Diseases, Female—nursing—Nurses' Instruction. WY 156.7
  H236 2002]
  RG105 .H35 2002
  618.1—dc21   2001043481

For further information on Blackwell Science, visit our website:
www.blackwell-science.com

Contents

CONTRIBUTORS, xi

PREFACE, xiii

ACKNOWLEDGEMENTS, xv

ABBREVIATIONS, xvii

1 HORMONAL CONTRACEPTION AND
STERILISATION, 1
The oral contraceptive pill, 1
Types of injectable contraception, 23
Intrauterine devices, 25
Barrier methods of contraception, 29
Sterilisation, 30
Vasectomy, 30
Stopping contraception, 32
Hormone replacement therapy and contraception, 32
The premenstrual syndrome, 32

2 EARLY PREGNANCY, 37
Diagnosing pregnancy, 37
Bleeding in early pregnancy (threatened miscarriage or
missed miscarriage), 39
First trimester miscarriage, 39
Second trimester miscarriage, 50
Ectopic pregnancy, 56
Termination of pregnancy, 63
Gestational trophoblastic disease, 69

3 CERVICAL SCREENING AND PREMALIGNANT
DISEASE OF THE CERVIX, 80
Prevention, 80
Screening for cervical cancer, 80
Diagnoses, 84

4 GYNAECOLOGICAL ENDOCRINOLOGY, 94
Polycystic ovary syndrome, 94
Hirsutism, 96

Ovulation induction in anovulatory women with PCOS, 100
Amenorrhoea, 101
Premature ovarian failure, 102
Anorexia nervosa, 104
Hyperprolactinaemia, 105

5   INFERTILITY AND ASSISTED REPRODUCTIVE
    TECHNIQUES, 118
    Fecundity, 118
    Treatment of male infertility, 130
    Ovulation disorders and ovulation induction, 136
    In vitro fertilisation, 146
    Tubal surgery, 151

6   ULTRASOUND AND THE USE OF IMAGING
    IN GYNAECOLOGY, 155
    Wendy Hadden
    Pelvic ultrasound, 155
    Early pregnancy – first trimester ultrasound, 167
    Uterine pathology, 173
    Ultrasound assessment of the endometrium, 177
    The adnexa – ovarian lesion, 188
    Polycystic ovaries, 196
    Adnexal abnormalities, 200
    Fallopian tube pathology, 203
    Pelvic pain, 204
    Mimics of gynaecological disease, 206
    Paediatric age group, 206
    Fertility, 208
    Cervical abnormalities, 209
    Urogynaecological ultrasound, 210
    Ultrasound and the diagnosis of breast disease, 211
    Conclusion, 217

7   MENORRHAGIA, 221
    Dysfunctional uterine bleeding, 223
    Medical management of menorrhagia, 228
    Surgical treatment for menorrhagia, 237

8   THE MENOPAUSE AND HORMONE
    REPLACEMENT THERAPY, 245
    The menopause, 245
    Effects of oestrogen deficiency, 247

History taking prior to commencing HRT, 249
Effects of oestrogens, 250
Types of oral oestrogen, 253
Non-oral administration of oestrogen, 255
Progestogens, 258
Oestrogen and progestogen regimens, 261
Side effects of HRT, 265
Endogenous ovarian activity and exogenous
    hormone treatment, 268
The theoretical benefits of HRT, 270
Osteoporosis, 271
Cardiovascular disease and oestrogen replacement therapy:
    mechanisms of protection, 278
HRT and the risk of breast cancer, 281
HRT and those with established breast cancer, 283
Oestrogen replacement therapy and venous
    thromboembolism, 283
Oestrogen replacement therapy and fatal colorectal cancer, 285
Dementia, 285
Androgen replacement, 286
Other effects of oestrogen, 286
Oestrogens and diet, 286
HRT and diabetes, 287
Hyperlipidaemia, 287
HRT and endometrial cancer, 288
Summary of use of HRT, 289

9 UROGYNAECOLOGY, 292
    Rose Elder and Cornelius Kelleher
    Urinary incontinence, 292
    History, 297
    Quality of life, 299
    Examination, 299
    Investigations, 301
    Genuine stress incontinence, 305
    Detrusor instability, 313
    Overflow incontinence/difficulty voiding, 316

10 SEXUAL HEALTH AND DISEASE, 321
    Janet Say
    Sexual health, 321
    Sexually transmitted infections, 324

Lower genital tract bacterial infections, 330
Upper genital tract bacterial sexually transmitted infections –
    pelvic inflammatory disease, 335
STIs and sexual assault, 338
Syphilis (*Treponema pallidum*), 338
Genital herpes – herpes simplex types 1 and 2, 339
Genital warts – human papillomavirus, 343
Hepatitides, 348
Human immunodeficiency virus (HIV 1 and 2), 348
Other conditions affecting the external genital area, 349

11 ENDOMETRIOSIS AND CHRONIC PELVIC
    PAIN, 355
Definition of endometriosis, 355
Symptoms of endometriosis and diagnosis, 356
Clinical findings, 357
Investigation, 358
Aims of management, 358
Visual features of endometriotic lesions at
    laparoscopy, 359
Classification of endometriosis, 362
Treatment, 362
Medical therapy for endometriosis, 363
Surgical treatment, 370
Pelvic pain – irritable bowel syndrome, 375
Bladder-related pain, 377
Musculoskeletal pain, 377
Nerve-related pain, 378

12 VULVAL DISEASE AND GYNAECOLOGICAL
    DERMATOLOGY, 380
Vulval disease, 380
Dermatological vulval conditions, 386
Topical steroids and vulval disease, 389
Creams and emollients, 391
Management of Bartholin's swelling, 393
Extramammary Paget's disease, 393
Squamous hyperplasia, 394
Vulval intraepithelial neoplasia, 394
Vulval carcinoma, 397

13 GYNAECOLOGICAL SURGERY, 402
Consent for surgery, 402
Operating theatre set-up, 402
Anatomical considerations in gynaecological surgery, 402
Principles of laparoscopic surgery, 408
Hysterectomy, 424
Vaginal hysterectomy, 425
Prophylactic oophorectomy, 426
Laparoscopic hysterectomy, 428
Laparoscopic oophorectomy, 429
Supracervical hysterectomy, 430
Genital prolapse, 431
Operating for gynaecological cancer, 443

14 GYNAECOLOGICAL ONCOLOGY, 452
Cheryl Wright
Cervical malignancies, 452
Ovarian malignancies, 462
Fallopian tube malignancies, 475
Endometrial carcinomas, 475
Uterine sarcomas, 484
Vulval malignancies, 486
Vaginal malignancies, 494

INDEX, 505

Contributors

Rose Elder, FRANZCOG
Consultant Obstetrician and Gynaecologist
National Women's Hospital
Auckland
New Zealand

Wendy E. Hadden, MB ChB FRANZCR
Radiologist
National Women's Hospital
Epsom
Auckland
New Zealand

Cornelius Kelleher, MB BS BSc MD
Consultant Obstetrician and Gynaecologist
St Thomas' Hospital
London
UK

P. Janet Say, MBBS FRCPath FACSHP DipVen
Sexual Health Physician
Auckland Sexual Health Service
Auckland Hospital
Auckland
New Zealand

Cheryl L. Wright, MD FRCP(C)
Consultant Pathologist
Surgical Pathology Unit
North Shore Hospital
Auckland
New Zealand

Preface

In the information age, one wonders if a handbook such as this is an anachronism. Information is prolific, judgement is often elusive. Information needs collating and needs both evidence and understanding. This book provides an 'anthology' of information from a clinical perspective. It acknowledges the arguments for evidence-based medicine, recognising level of evidence according to the Royal College of Obstetricians and Gynaecologists' definition:

(1) based on randomised controlled trial (RCT)

(2) based on other robust experimental or observational studies

(3) based on more limited evidence but relying on expert opinion with the endorsement of respected authorities.

The Cochrane levels of evidence are defined as follows:

Ia Evidence obtained from a meta-analysis of RCTs

Ib Evidence obtained from at least one RCT

IIa Evidence obtained from at least one well-designed, controlled study without randomisation

IIb Evidence obtained from at least one other type of well-designed quasi-experimental study

III Evidence obtained from well-designed, non-experimental, descriptive studies, such as comparative studies, correlation studies and case-control studies

IV Evidence obtained from expert committee reports or opinions and/or clinical experience of respected authorities.

This book provides information as contextual guidelines. It seeks to provide knowledge and inspiration and application of interest to the expert care of women patients. As well as providing information, it aims at heightening the awareness of the breadth of conditions and their treatment.

The internet is a profound source of specific information. Information regarding randomised controlled trials may be accessed from the Cochrane Database, www.cochrane.de. National societies have their own websites, e.g. www.rcog.org.uk/guidelines/c_guidelines. html, www.figo.org, www.acog.org, sogc.medical.org/SOGC-net/sogc_docs/common/guide/library_e.shtml, www.nvog.nl.

Sylvia Rosevear
MD, FRCOG

Acknowledgements

Professor Victor Barley, Consultant Clinical Oncologist, Bristol Haematology and Oncology Centre, UK.

Dr David Downey, Consultant Dermatologist, Auckland, New Zealand.

Dr Patrick Frengley, Consultant Endocrinologist, National Women's Hospital, Auckland, New Zealand.

Dr Freddie Graham, Consultant Gynaecologist, Ascot Hospital, Auckland, New Zealand.

Dr G. Mark Insull, Consultant Gyanaecologist, Auckland, New Zealand.

Mr Ron Jones, Consultant Gynaecologist, National Women's Hospital, Auckland, New Zealand.

Dr Andrew Mackintosh, Consultant Gynaecologist, Ascot Hospital, Auckland, New Zealand.

Mr Misch Neill, Consultant Colorectal Surgeon, Auckland, New Zealand.

Professor Ed Newlands, Professor of Cancer Medicine, Trophoblastic Tumour Screening and Treatments Centre, Dept of Medical Oncology, Charing Cross Hospital, London.

Dr David Peddie, Consultant Obstetrician and Gynaecologist, Christchurch Women's Hospital, New Zealand.

Dr Fiona Stewart, Consultant Physician, National Women's Hospital, Auckland, New Zealand.

Dr John Whittaker, Consultant Obstetrician and Gynaecologist, National Women's Hospital, Auckland, New Zealand.

Abbreviations

ACA	anticardiolipin antibodies
ACTH	adrenocorticotrophic hormone
αFP	α-fetoprotein
AGCT	adult granulosa cell tumours
AGUS	atypical glandular cells of undetermined significance
AIDS	acquired immune deficiency
AIS	adenocarcinoma in situ
ANA	antinuclear antibodies
AP	anteroposterior
APA	antiphospholipid antibodies
APTT	activated partial thromboplastin time
ART	assisted reproductive techniques
ASCUS	atypical squamous cells of undetermined significance
ATP	adenosine triphosphate
b.i.d.	*bis in die* (twice a day)
BCC	basal cell carcinoma
BMI	body mass index
BPL	Bio Products Laboratory
BSO	bilateral salpingo-oophorectomy
BV	bacterial vaginosis
CA125	cancer cell surface antigen 125
CDC	Centers for Disease Control
CEE	conjugated equine oestrogen
CHD	coronary heart disease
CI	confidence interval
CIGN	cervical intraepithelial glandular neoplasia
CIN	cervical intraepithelial neoplasia
CIS	carcinoma in situ
CISH	classic interstitial Semm hysterectomy
CLSI	capillary/lymphatic space invasion
CNS	central nervous system
CO_2	carbon dioxide

COC	combined oral contraceptive
CPP	chronic pelvic pain
CRL	crown rump length
CT	computerised tomography
Cu	copper
CURT	calibrated uterine resection tool
CVP	central venous pressure
D&C	dilatation and curettage
DBCP	dibromochloropropane
DCIS	ductal carcinoma in situ
DDAVP	1-desamino-8-D-arginine vasopressin
DES	diethylstilbestrol
DEXA	double X-ray absorptiometry
DGI	disseminated gonococcal infection
DHT	dihydrotestosterone
DI	detrusor instability
DMPA	depo-medroxyprogesterone acetate
DNA	deoxyribonucleic acid
DRVTT	dilute Russell's viper venom time
DUB	dysfunctional uterine bleeding
DVT	deep vein thrombosis
DXA	double X-ray absorptiometry
EBRT	external beam radiation therapy
ECC	endocervical curettage
EDRF	endothelial-derived relaxing factor
ELISA	enzyme-linked immunosorbent assay
EMA-CO	etoposide, methotrexate, actinomycin D, cyclophosphamide, vincristine
EMBT	endocervical-like mucinous borderline tumour
ENA	extractable nuclear antigen
ESR	erythrocyte sedimentation rate
ESS	endometrial stromal sarcoma
EUA	examination under anaesthesia
FBC	full blood count
FIGO	International Federation of Gynecology and Obstetrics
FMH	fetal maternal haemorrhage
FPA	Family Planning Association

FSH	follicle-stimulating hormone
FTA abs	fluorescent treponemal antibody (absorbed)
GnRH	gonadotrophin-releasing hormone
GnRHa	gonadotrophin-releasing hormone agonist
GSI	genuine stress incontinence
GTD	gestational trophoblastic disease
H_2O_2	hydrogen peroxide
Hb	haemoglobin
hCG	human chorionic gonadotrophin
HDL	high density lipoprotein
HERS	Heart and Estrogen/Progestin Replacement Study
HIV	human immunodeficiency virus
HLA	human leukocyte antigen
hMG	human menopausal gonadotrophins
HNPCC	hereditary non-polyposis colorectal cancer
HPV	human papillomavirus
HRT	hormone replacement therapy
HSG	hysterosalpingogram
HSIL	high grade squamous intraepithelial lesion
HSV	herpes simplex virus
HTF	Human tubal fluid
HVS	High vaginal swab
i.m.	intramuscularly
i.n.	intranasally
i.v.	intravenously
IBS	irritable bowel syndrome
ICS	International Continence Society
ICSI	intracytoplasmic sperm injection
Ig	immunoglobulin
IGF	insulin-like growth factor
IMBT	intestinal-type mucinous borderline tumour
INS-VNTR	insulin variable number of tandem repeats
ISGP	International Society of Gynaecological Pathologists
ISSVD	International Society for the Study of Vulval Disease
IUD	intrauterine device
IUI	intrauterine insemination
IUS	intrauterine system

IVF	*in vitro* fertilisation
IVF-ET	*in vitro* fertilisation and embryo transfer
IVP	intravenous pyelogram
JGCT	juvenile granulosa cell tumours
LA	lupus anticoagulant
LAVH	laparoscopically assisted vaginal hysterectomy
LCR	ligase chain reaction
LDH	lactate dehydrogenase
LDL	low density lipoprotein
LEEP	loop electrosurgical excision procedure
LFT	liver function test
LH	laparoscopic hysterectomy
LH	luteinising hormone
LHRH	luteinising hormone-releasing hormone
LLETZ	large loop excision of the transformation zone
LMP	last menstrual period
LMWH	low molecular weight heparins
LNG	levonorgestrel
LNG-IUS	levonorgestrel intrauterine releasing system
LSIL	low grade squamous intraepithelial lesion
LVSI	lymphatic/vascular space invasion
MAC	methotrexate, actinomycin D, cyclophosphamide
MBL	menstrual blood loss
MI	myocardial infarction
MIF	microimmunofluorescent
MISTLETOE	minimally invasive surgical techniques – laser, endothermal or endoresection survey
MMK	Marshall Marchetti Krantz
MMMT	malignant mixed Müllerian tumour
MPA	medroxyprogesterone acetate
MRI	magnetic resonance imaging
MRSA	methicillin-resistant *Staphylococcus aureus*
MSU	mid-stream urinalysis
Nd:YAG	neodymium:yttrium–aluminium–garnet laser
NET-EN	norethidrone enanthate

NETA	norethisterone acetate
NORG	norgestrel
NSAID	non-steroidal anti-inflammatories
NT	nuchal translucency
OAB	overactive bladder
OHSS	ovarian hyperstimulation syndrome
p.o.	per os
p.r.	per rectum
p.r.n.	*pro re nata* (when required)
PCB	polychlorinated biphenyls
PCOS	polycystic ovary syndrome
PCR	polymerase chain reaction
PE	pulmonary embolism
PEPI	Postmenopausal Estrogen/Progestin Interventions Trial
PFL	Plasma Fractionation Laboratory
PG	prostaglandin
PI	pulsatility index
PID	pelvic inflammatory disease
PIF	prolactin inhibitor factor
PMS	premenstrual syndrome
POF	premature ovarian failure
POP	progestogen-only pill
POPQ	pelvic organ prolapse quantification
PSTT	placental site trophoblastic tumour
q.i.d.	*quater in die* (four times a day)
QCT	quantitative computerised tomography
QoL	quality of life
rAFS	(revised) American Fertility Society
RCT	randomised controlled trial
RI	resistive index
RIF	right iliac fossa
RLE	radical local excision
RNA	ribonucleic acid
RPR	rapid reagin test
RR	relative risk

s.c.	subcutaneously
SCC	squamous cell carcinoma
SD	standard deviation
SD	systolic diastolic ratio
SERM	selective oestrogen receptor modulator
SGO	Society of Gynecologic Oncology
SHBG	sex hormone-binding globulin
SIL	squamous intraepithelial lesion
SIS	saline infusion sonography
SLE	systemic lupus erythematosus
SSRI	selective serotonin reuptake inhibitor
stat	*statim* (immediately)
STD	sexually transmitted disease
STI	sexually transmitted infection
SXA	single X-ray absorptiometry
t.d.s.	*ter die sumendum* (three times a day)
T_3	triiodothyronine
T_4	thyroxine
TA	transabdominal
TAH	total abdominal hysterectomy
TED	thromboembolic disease
TENS	transcutaneous electrical nerve stimulation
TEWL	transepidermal water loss
TOP	termination of pregnancy
TPHA	*Treponema pallidum* haemagglutination
TRH	thyrotrophin-releasing hormone
TSH	thyroid-stimulating hormone
TV	transvaginal
TVS	transvaginal ultrasound
TVT	tension-free vaginal tape
U&E	urea and electrolytes
UI	urinary incontinence
UTI	urinary tract infection
VAIN	vaginal intraepithelial neoplasia
VDRL	Venereal Disease Reference Laboratory
VEGF	vascular endothelial growth factor
VH	vaginal hysterectomy

VIN	vulval intraepithelial neoplasia
VLDL	very low density lipoprotein
VTE	venous thromboembolus
vWD	von Willebrand's disease
vWF	von Willebrand's factor
WBC	white blood cell
WHO	World Health Organisation
WISDOM	Women's International Study of Long Duration Oestrogen After Menopause
WLE	wide local excision

1 Hormonal Contraception and Sterilisation

Fluctuations of oestrogen and progesterone in the normal ovulatory menstrual cycle may be seen in Fig. 1.1 [1] together with the concomitant follicle-stimulating hormone (FSH) and luteinising hormone (LH) levels. Natural regulation of fertility requires the avoidance of sexual intercourse during the fertile phase of the cycle to avoid pregnancy. The woman is aware of her fertile period by observing factors indicating fertility, such as the increased 'slipperiness' of cervical mucus in the fertile period, the 1° rise in basal body temperature and calendar calculations based on the length of previous cycles.

THE ORAL CONTRACEPTIVE PILL

Contraceptive steroids prevent ovulation mainly by interfering with the release of gonadotropin-releasing hormone (GnRH) from the hypothalamus.

Pharmacology

The oral contraceptive pill consists of either:
- A fixed-dose combination usually with 30 μg of ethinyloestradiol
- A combination of oestrogen and progestogen in a phasic form given daily for 3 weeks.
- Progestogen-only pills (Table 1.1).

Uterine bleeding occurs in the week when the steroid component of the pill is not taken. Menstrual bleeding lasts 3–4 days and the average blood loss is 25 ml (mean of 35 ml for normal ovulatory menstrual cycles).

Phasic formulations (biphasic or triphasic) contain two or three different amounts of the same oestrogen and progestogen. This is thought to result in a lower total dose of steroid without a concomitant incidence in breakthrough uterine bleeding. There is no evidence for fewer adverse effects compared to fixed-dose combined oral contraceptives (COCs). COCs do not contain natural oestrogens

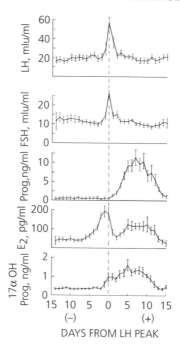

Fig. 1.1 Mean values of LH, FSH, progesterone, oestradiol and 17-hydroxyprogesterone in daily serum samples of nine women during ovulatory menstrual cycles. Data from different cycles combined with the use of the day of the mid-cycle LH peak as the reference day (Day 0). (Reproduced with permission from Thorneycroft, I.H., Mishell, D.R., Stone, S.C., Kharma, K.M. & Nakamura, R.M. (1971) The relation of serum 17-hydroxyprogesterone and estradiol-17β levels during the human menstrual cycle. *American Journal of Obstetrics & Gynecology,* **111**, p. 950.

Table 1.1 Types of progesterone-only pills.

Femulen	Ethynodiol diacetate	500 μg
Micronor/Noriday	Norethisterone	350 μg
Microval/Norgeston	Levonorgestrel	30 μg
Neogest	Norgestrel	75 μg

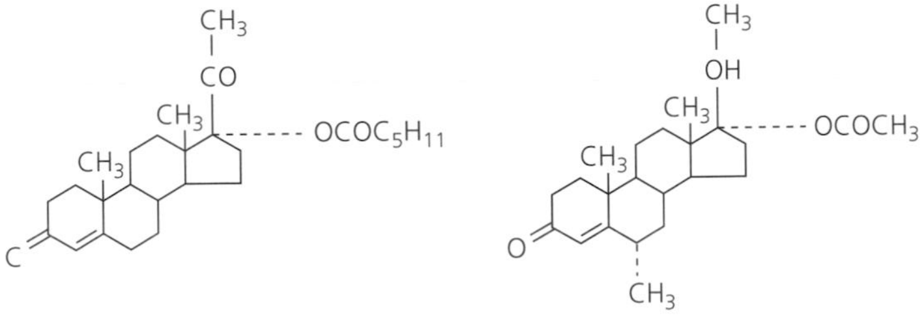

17α-hydroxyprogesterone caproate
PRIMOLUT DEPOT

Medroxyprogesterone acetate
PROVERA

Fig. 1.2 Chemical structure of the 17-hydroxyprogestogens.

or progestogens. Progestogen-only contraception should be taken daily continuously.

Types of progestogens

Derivatives of:
- 19-nortestosterone progestogens resemble testosterone more closely than C21 acetoxyprogestogens. This accounts for the androgen activity in the COC.
- 17α-acetoxyprogesterone, which include C21 progestogens (Fig. 1.2).
- DL-Norgestrel consisting of two isomers, dextro (D) and levo (L). Only the levo form is biologically active.
- Desogestrel, gestodene and norgestimate are less androgenic derivatives of levonorgestrel.

First generation COCs

All of the older higher dosage COC formulations contained the oestrogen mestranol which is still part of some 50 µg formulations. COCs containing less than 50 µg oestrogen contain ethinyloestradiol (Fig. 1.3).

Second generation COCs

These contain 20–35 µg of ethinyloestradiol with a balanced dose of a progestogen, except for the three newest levonorgestrel derivatives, i.e. desogestrel, gestodene or norgestimate.

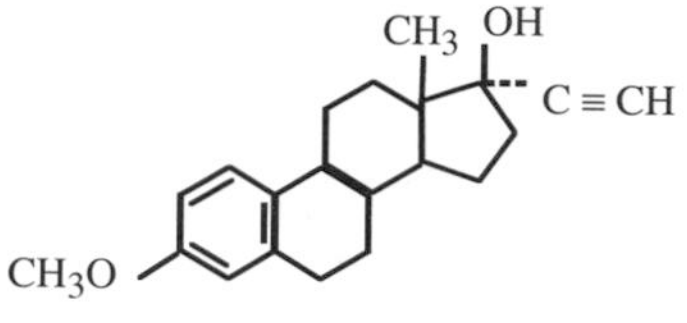

Fig. 1.3 Structure of the two oestrogens in COCs.

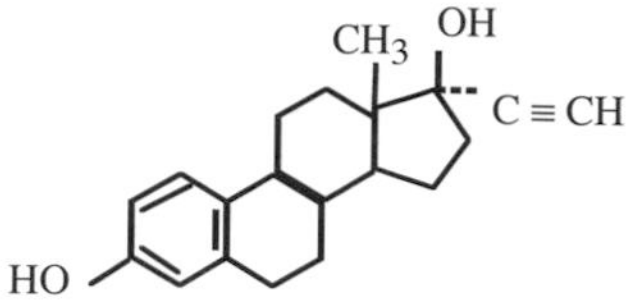

Third generation COCs

These contain ethinyloestradiol plus desogestrel, gestodene or norgestimate (Fig. 1.4).

There has been an evolution in the types of progesterone in the oral contraceptive pill. In the 1960s and 1970s the progestogens were related to norethisterone. Levonorgestrel came into use during the latter half of the 1970s. In 1981 desogestrel was the first of a new series of progestogens. It differs from levonorgestrel and norethisterone by combining high progestational potency with low androgenicity. Desogestrel formulations are associated with a lower incidence of androgenic side effects such as hirsutism and acne, partly due to the inability of these progesterones to oppose the oestrogen-induced increase in sex hormone-binding globulin, higher levels of which reduce levels of free testosterone. High density lipoprotein (HDL) levels are also increased.

Gestodene and norgestimate are similar. They were widely marketed as being protective from arterial disease on the basis of a 10–15 per cent increase in serum HDL levels, resulting from the weak ability of these progestogens to oppose the oestrogen-induced increase in HDL. Women with high HDL levels are less likely to suffer from myocardial infarction than those with low levels, due to the anti-atherogenic potential of this lipoprotein.

All of the synthetic oestrogens and progestogens in COCs have an ethinyl group at division 17. This prevents rapid metabolism through the intestinal mucosa and liver, via the portal system. This means that the synthetic ethinyloestradiol has approximately 100 times the potency of an equivalent weight of conjugated equine oestrogen or oestrone sulphate for stimulating synthesis of various hepatic

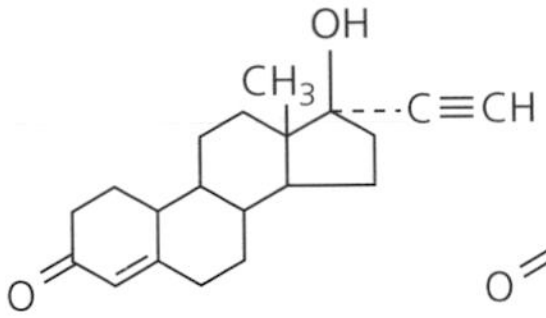

NORETHISTERONE
(17α-ethinyl-19-nor testosterone)
Primolut N
Norethindrone

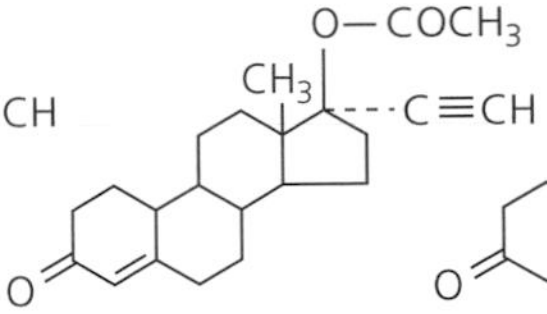

NORETHISTERONE ACETATE

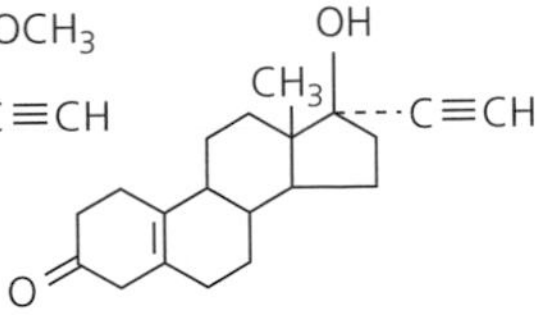

NORETHYNODREL
(17α-ethinyl-5(10)-oestrone 17β-ol-3-one)

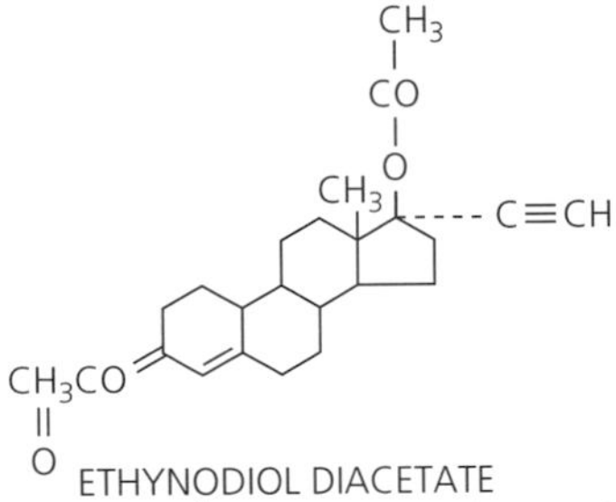

ETHYNODIOL DIACETATE
(17α-ethinyl-Δ^4-oestrone 3,17-diacetate)

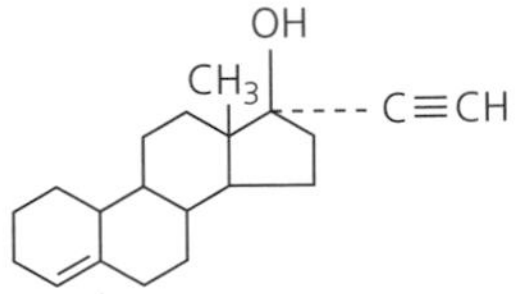

LYNOESTRENOL
(17α-ethinyl-Δ^4-oestrone 17β-ol)

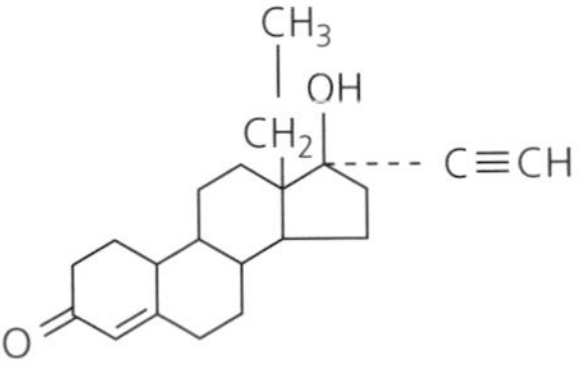

NORGESTREL
(DL-13β-ethyl-17α-ethinyl-17-hydroxy-gon-4-en-3-one)

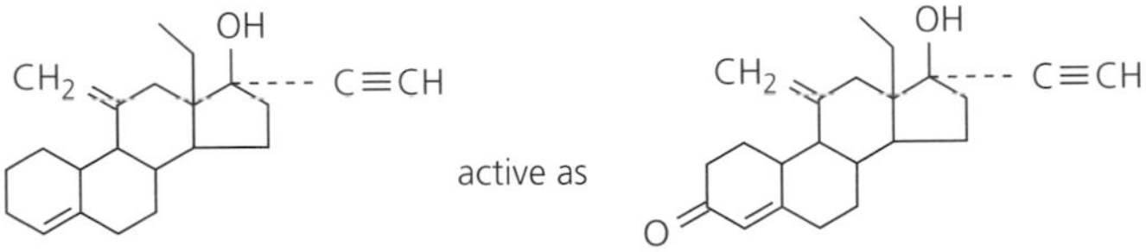

DESOGESTREL

3-KETO METABOLITE

Fig. 1.4 Chemical structure of the 19-nortestosterone progestogens.

Table 1.2 A few examples of combined oral contraceptive pills and their constituents.

Microgynon/Ovranette	30 µg ethinyloestradiol + 150 µg levonorgestrel
Ovysmen/Brevinor	35 µg ethinyloestradiol + 500 µg norethisterone

Of these two formulations, Microgynon/Ovranette gives better cycle control, but is more progestogenic, i.e. there are more likely to be problems with acne or unwanted hair. Ovysmen/Brevinor is much less progestogenic, and is therefore good for acne, but often gives problems with breakthrough bleeding. In that case, Norimin or Trinovum might be tried.

Cilest	35 µg ethinyloestradiol (oestrogen) + 250 µg norgestimate
Minulet/Femodene	30 µg ethinyloestradiol + 75 µg of gestodene
Marvelon	30 µg ethinyloestradiol + 150 µg desogestrel
Mercilon	20 µg ethinyloestradiol + 150 µg desogestrel

Second generation COCs: oestrogen-dominant

Ovysmen/Brevinor	35 µg ethinyloestradiol + 500 µg norethisterone
Norimin	35 µg ethinyloestradiol + 1 mg norethisterone

Second generation COCs: progestogen-dominant

Loestrin 30	30 µg ethinyloestradiol + 1.5 mg norethisterone
Microgynon/Ovranette	30 µg ethinyloestradiol + 150 µg levonorgestrel
Loestrin 20	20 µg ethinyloestradiol + 1 mg norethisterone acetate

Triphasics: oestrogen-dominant

TriNovum	21 tablets of 35 µg ethinyloestradiol + 500 µg, 750 µg and 1 mg norethisterone (7 tablets of each)

Triphasics: progestogen-dominant

Trinordiol/Logynon	6 tablets containing 30 µg ethinyloestradiol + 50 µg levonorgestrel, 5 tablets containing 40 µg ethinyloestradiol + 75 µg levonorgestrel, and 10 tablets containing 30 µg ethinyloestradiol + 125 µg levonorgestrel

globulins. An important consideration in the efficacy of the COC is not just the amount of steroid present but the biological activity. Norgestrel is more potent than norethindrone. Norethindrone acetate and ethynodiol diacetate are metabolised to norethindrone. Levonorgestrel is 10–20 times more potent (Table 1.2).

Mechanism of action of the oral contraceptives

The COC inhibits the mid-cycle gonadotropin (LH) surge preventing ovulation. Progestogen-only formulations do not consistently inhibit ovulation.

Other effects of the COC that decrease conception are:
- Alteration of cervical mucus making it thick, viscous and scanty, thus not enabling optimal penetration of sperm
- Alteration of the uterus and oviduct impairing transport of both ova and sperm
- Decrease in glycogen production in the endometrium, thus reducing the ability of the blastocyst to survive in the uterine cavity

Table 1.2 *Continued*

Third generation triphasics	
Tri-Minulet/Triadene	6 tablets containing 50 µg gestodene + 30 µg ethinyloestradiol, 5 tablets containing 70 µg gestodene + 40 µg ethinyloestradiol, and 10 tablets containing 100 µg gestodene + 30 µg ethinyloestradiol

Among the newest pills, none exhibits real progestogenic side effects, but all vary in their oestrogen dominance and control of bleeding. In descending order of oestrogen dominance they are:
- Cilest/Marvelon
- Minulet/Femodene
- Mercilon

Best cycle control is given by Minulet/Femodene; Cilest is next in order and then Marvelon and Mercilon.

Table 1.3 Starting routines for the combined pill.

	When to start	Extra precautions needed?
Starting pill for first time or after a break	First to third day of period	No
	On or after fourth day	Yes, for 7 days
Changing to COC of same or higher dose	After normal 7-day break	No
Changing to lower dose COC	Straight after last pill of previous packet, i.e. no 7-day break	No
	If normal 7-day break	Yes, for 7 days
From POP to COC	First day of period (no break)	No
From POP to COC when there are no periods on POP	Anytime (no break)	No
After a TOP or miscarriage	Same or next day	No
After childbirth (if not breastfeeding)	On 21st day after delivery	No
	After 21st day	Yes, for 7 days

POP, progestogen-only pill; TOP, termination of pregnancy.

• Alteration in ovarian responsiveness to gonadotropin stimulation. Gonadotropin production and ovarian steroidogenesis are not completely abolished.

There is no significant difference in the clinical efficacy of the various COC formulations. As long as no tablets are forgotten, the pregnancy rate is less than 0.2 per cent per year. Progestogen-only tablets need to be taken consistently at the same time to make sure that blood levels of the progestogen do not fall below the effective contraceptive level. A missed pill is one that is taken more than 3 hours later than the time taken the previous day (see Table 1.3 for when to start taking the COC [2]).

Metabolic effects of the COC

Oestrogen
• Nausea (central nervous effect)
• Breast tenderness

- Fluid retention due to decreased sodium excretion
- Chloasma (pigmentation of the malar eminences predominantly). These side effects are related to dosage.

1

Progestogen

Effects include increase in depression, irritability, tension and fatigue.

Because progestogens are structurally related to testosterone they can produce predominantly adverse androgenic effects: weight gain (anabolic effect), acne, nervousness. Women who have acne should have a pill formulation with a low progestogen/oestrogen ratio. Amenorrhoea may occur due to the decrease in synthesis of oestrogen receptors in the endometrium induced by progestogens.

It is not essential, medically, to have a withdrawal bleed, but some women prefer a withdrawal bleed as an indicator of the absence of pregnancy. Breakthrough bleeding usually indicates insufficient oestrogen or excess progestogen or a combination of both.

An increase in the frequency of headaches is a common complaint in women taking COCs. The exact mechanism is not understood. Synthetic oestrogen increases the hepatic production of sex hormone-binding globulin (SHBG). SHBG is inhibited by androgens. Ethinyloestradiol increases factors V, VIII and X and fibrinogen, thus enhancing the risk of thrombosis. Angiotensinogen may be converted to angiotensin causing an increase in blood pressure. SHBG is increased most of all in COCs containing cyproterone acetate, as SHBG binds endogenous testosterone and prevents it from acting on the target tissue. COCs causing the greatest increase in SHBG are associated with fewer androgenic effects.

Carbohydrate metabolism

Generally, the higher the dose and potency of the progestogen, the greater magnitude of impaired glucose metabolism.

Formulations with a low dose of progestogen (including levonorgestrel) do not significantly alter glucose, insulin or glycogen levels after a glucose load in healthy women or in women with a history of gestational diabetes. Multiphasic COCs (norgestrel but not norethindrone) produce some deterioration in glucose tolerance in normal women and women with a history of gestational diabetes, therefore a low-dose COC with norethindrone-type progesterone is indicated when prescribing the COC for women with a history of glucose intolerance.

There is no increased risk of diabetes mellitus amongst current COC users or former COC users, even with a history of a decade or more of use.

Lipids

The oestrogen component of the COC increases levels of HDL cholesterol, decreases levels of low density lipoprotein (LDL) cholesterol and increases total cholesterol and triglyceride levels. The progestogen component decreases HDL cholesterol levels, increases LDL cholesterol levels and decreases total cholesterol and triglyceride levels. Phasic COCs containing levonorgestrel and norethindrone have a significant increase in triglyceride levels but little change in HDL, LDL or total cholesterol levels [3]. The three newer, less androgenic progestogens are associated with a significant increase in HDL cholesterol levels, a significant decrease in LDL cholesterol levels and little change in total cholesterol levels, and a substantial increase in triglyceride levels. The long-term effect of these changes in lipid profiles clinically is not substantiated.

Coagulation profile

The oestrogen component of the COC increases the synthesis of some coagulation factors with enhanced risk of thrombosis in a dose-dependent manner.

If a woman has an inherited coagulation disorder, protein C, protein S or antithrombin 3 deficiency or factor V Leiden, the risk of developing thrombosis is increased several-fold. These factors should be screened for in those at risk. The annual incidence of deep vein thrombosis (DVT) in the reproductive age group for women with activated protein C resistance is 6 per 10000 in non-COC users, and up to 30 per 10000 in COC users. Screening for coagulation deficiencies is not recommended before prescribing the COC unless the woman has a personal family history of thrombotic events.

Venous thromboembolus (VTE)

In 1995 and early 1996 results of four *observational* studies reported the risk of VTE among women using low-dose oestrogen formulations, following in 1989 the German Federal Health Office's warning that gestodene formulations were overrepresented in the adverse drug interactions reports of venous thromboembolism in young women. In those taking low-dose oestrogen COCs containing *desogestrel* or *gestodene*, the risk was increased 1.5–2.5 times relative to the risk for women using COCs containing less than 50 µg of oestrogen and *levonorgestrel*. None of the studies involved a prospective clinical trial and the causal relation of the third generation pills to an increased risk of VTE has not been established. Even if there is an increased risk, it is small (Tables 1.4 and 1.5), and there is

Table 1.4 Risk of developing venous thromboembolism yearly.

	Number of cases per 100 000 women
Women not taking any hormones	5–11
Women taking levonorgestrel/norethisterone (second generation) COCs	15
Women taking gestogene/desogestrel (third generation) COCs	30
Pregnant women	60
Studies performed in the early 1980s: women taking levonorgestrel/norethisterone, i.e. second generation progestogen COCs	30

Table 1.5 Deaths per million women aged 15–44 from various causes in 1992, England and Wales.

Cause of death	Deaths per million
Acute myocardial infarction	39
Strokes	8
Venous thromboembolism (VTE)	14
Ovarian cancer	48
Pregnancy	60
Home accidents	40
Road deaths	80
Smoking-related disease for women aged 35	1670
Related to pill use	10 (approx.)
Family history of DVT in an oral contraceptive user	6.7
Those with protein C resistance	18
Oral contraceptive use, protein C, protein S or antithrombin 3 deficiency	43.3

evidence in the literature for 'prescriber bias'. Women prescribed des-ogestrel formulations tended to be heavier and were more likely to smoke cigarettes. These formulations were perceived as being the best option for women at risk of cardiovascular disease, raising the possibility that increased venous thromboembolism risks might reflect selective prescribing to women who were destined to develop the disease.

The risk of VTE in a woman taking a low-oestrogen COC results in a 50 per cent reduction in the incidence of VTE compared with the risk associated with pregnant or recently postpartum women.

Myocardial infarction

Nearly all published epidemiological studies of former users of the COC show no increased risk of myocardial infarction (MI). The oestrogen component of the COC has a direct protective effect on coronary arteries, reducing the extent of atherosclerosis that would otherwise be accelerated by a decreased level of HDL cholesterol. Smoking is a significant risk factor for myocardial infarction and in those women who smoke at least 25 cigarettes per day using the COC, the increased risk of MI is 30-fold. Smoking alone (without the use of the COC) increases the risk of myocardial infarction approximately nine-fold.

It is thought that smokers using the COC have a significantly greater decrease in levels of endogenous coagulation inhibitors, mostly antithrombin III, and smoking alters the usual balance of prostacyclin and thromboxane, producing a relative excess of thromboxane.

Reproductive effects

There may be an initial reduction in pregnancy rates with dis-continuation of the oral contraceptive but at two years cumula-tively the delay is negligible. There is no difference in the pregnancy incidence.

Breast cancer

In five cohort studies in users of the COC at some point in their life there is no increased risk in the development of breast cancer. In eight case controls in one cohort study investigating the relative risk of breast cancer in COC users who did or did not have a family history of breast cancer, none of the studies showed a significant difference in the risk of breast cancer. Thirteen case control studies have investigated the relative risk of diagnoses of breast cancer prior to the age of 45 associated with COC use. In those under the age of 45, the relative risk for diagnosis of breast cancer was 1.16, indicating a slight clinically significant increase. The relative risk was 1.42 in those who had used the COC long-term.

There is no adverse effect on the risk of diagnosis of breast cancer between the ages of 45 and 60. The conclusion is that COC use increases the risk of breast cancer diagnosis at a younger age but has no significant effect on lifetime risk of breast cancer and it is possibly associated with a decreased risk during the perimenopausal years, when the disease is usually most common. The Collaborative Group on Hormonal Factors in Breast Cancer analysed individual data on 53 297 women with breast cancer and 100 239 women without breast cancer from 54 epidemiological studies [4]. The meta-analysis from this indicated those on COCs had a slightly increased risk of breast cancer being diagnosed with a relative risk (RR) of 1.24 (confidence internal (CI) 1.15–1.30). The magnitude of this risk steadily declined after COC use was stopped. Ten or more years after COC use was stopped, subject women no longer had a significantly increased risk. The cancers diagnosed in women taking the COC were less advanced clinically than those observed in non-users. The risk of having breast cancer that had spread beyond the breast, compared with the risk of having a localised tumour, was significantly reduced (RR 0.88; CI 0.81–0.95) in COC users compared with non-users. It therefore may be concluded that in this group the results could be explained by the fact that the breast cancer was diagnosed earlier in COC users than in non-users, rather than a biological effect of the COC. There is no relationship between the dose or duration of use of oestrogen. Therefore the COC is unlikely to initiate breast cancer.

The conclusions of the analysis were that current COC use, or within 5 years, is associated with an increased (25 per cent) risk of breast cancer diagnosis. The increased risk of breast cancer in current COC users is limited to localised disease. COC users have a significantly reduced incidence of disease that is spread beyond the breast. A decreased risk of advanced disease is also found in older women. The overall data regarding COC use and the incidence of breast cancer risk is very reassuring.

Cervical cancer

Fourteen studies of more than 3800 women with invasive cervical cancer showed a significant increased risk of the disease associated with (not caused by) increased duration of COC use, increasing from 1.37 to 1.6 to 1.77 for 4, 8 and 12 years of COC use respectively. This is supported by two prospective studies and two or three recent case control studies reporting the risk of invasive cervical cancer to be increased with long-term COC use, with a relative risk of between 1.5 and 2.5.

Adenocarcinoma of the cervix is also significantly increased by approximately two-fold amongst COC users compared with non-users and the incidence is related to duration. There is no change in the incidence of cervical intraepithelial neoplasia associated with COC use. Therefore it may be concluded that as invasive epithelial cervical cancer is usually preceded by dysplasia, the relationship between COC use and epithelial cervical cancer is unlikely to be causal.

Endometrial cancer

The COC protects against the risk of endometrial cancer. Women who have used the COC for at least 1 year have an age-adjusted relative risk of 0.5 for development of endometrial cancer between the ages of 40 and 55, as compared with non-users. There is a 20, 40 and 60 per cent reduction in the incidence of endometrial cancer with 1, 2 and 4 years of COC use respectively [5]. This protective effect appeared within 10 years of initial use and persisted for at least 15 years after COC use was terminated. The greatest protective effect is in nulliparous women (RR 0.2) or women of low parity, who are at greater risk of acquiring the disease.

Ovarian cancer

COC use at some time in women's lives results in a 36 per cent reduction in the incidence of epithelial ovarian cancer [6]. The magnitude of the decrease is directly related to the duration of COC use, increasing from approximately 40 per cent reduction with 4 years of use, to 53 per cent with 8 years, and 60 per cent reduction with 12 years of use. Even with just 1 year's use the ovarian cancer risk is reduced by approximately 11 per cent for each of the first 5 years of use. The protective effect begins within 10 years of first use and continues for at least 20 years after COC use stops. The protective effect is limited to women of low parity (≤4), who are at greatest risk of ovarian cancer.

Liver adenoma and cancer

The World Health Organisation has found no increased risk of liver cancer associated with COC users in countries with a high prevalence of this cancer. There is no change in the risk with increasing duration of use or time since first or last use.

Pituitary adenoma

COCs will mask the predominant symptom of a prolactinoma, amenorrhoea and galactorrhoea. There are no data to support the possibility of an increased incidence of pituitary adenoma amongst users of COCs.

Malignant melanoma

COC use does not increase the risk of malignant melanoma.

Overall mortality

Mortality among COC users and non-users was reported from the Oxford Family Planning Association Cohort Study between 1968 and 1974 [7]. There were 238 deaths in a 20-year follow-up amongst 17032 women. The results were corroborated in 1994 by Colditz, who reported mortality rates among the 166755 women enrolled in a nurses' health study in 1976, followed through to 1980 [8]. There were 2879 deaths. There was no change in the risk of death due to cardiovascular disease or cancer. Overall, there was a beneficial effect on mortality with COC use.

Contraindications to the use of the COC

- History of vascular disease, including thromboembolism, thrombophlebitis, atherosclerosis/systemic disease affecting the vascular system.
- Systemic lupus erythematosus (SLE) or diabetes with retinopathy or nephropathy.
- Cigarette smoking by COC users over the age of 35.
- Uncontrolled hypertension, cancer of the breast and endometrium are relative contraindications.
- Pregnant women should not take COCs as 19-norprogestogens may have a masculinising effect on external genitalia of the female

fetus. There is no other documentation of a causal effect of terato-
genicity from the COC.

- Women with functional heart disease should not have the COC
because of fluid retention which could result in congestive heart
failure.
- Mitral valve prolapse is not an absolute contraindication to the use
of the COC.
- With acute liver disease, check normal liver function tests before
resuming COC.

Relative contraindications

- Heavy cigarette smoking under the age of 35
- Migraine headaches
- Undiagnosed aetiology of amenorrhoea
- Depression
- BMI > 30

Approximately 20 per cent of women who have migraine headaches
can have an increase in both the frequency and severity by COC use.
There is no evidence that the risk of stroke is significantly increased
in women with migraine headaches who use the COC compared
with non-users, unless the women have peripheral neurological
symptoms with the migraine headaches. If hypercoagulable effects
occur such as fainting, temporary loss of vision or speech or paraes-
thesiae develop in a COC user, the COC should be stopped because
of the hypercoagulable effect.

In amenorrhoeic women, exclude a prolactin-secreting adenoma
before starting the COC. If galactorrhoea develops, stop the COC
and 2 weeks later measure the serum prolactin level. If it is elevated
the presence of a prolactin-secreting macroadenoma should be
excluded. A microadenoma is not a contraindication for COC use.
The COC does not cause enlargement of prolactin-secreting
pituitary microadenomas or worsen functional prolactinomas.

Gestational diabetes or insulin-dependent diabetes without
vascular disease is not a contraindication for the use of the low-
dose COC.

Adolescents

Regular menstrual cycles indicate probable ovulation and therefore
maturity of the hypothalamic–pituitary–ovarian axis. The COC

will not accelerate epiphyseal closure in the postmenarchal female, because endogenous oestrogens will have initiated the process a few years before menarche.

Use of COCs after pregnancy

The first episode of menstrual bleeding is usually preceded by ovulation. Therefore the COC should be started immediately after the pregnancy. After a term delivery the first episode of bleeding is usually, but not always, anovulatory. Ovulation after a term delivery occurs usually after 6 weeks, but may occur as early as 4 weeks, especially in a woman who is not breastfeeding. After a miscarriage or termination, ovulation occurs at 2–4 weeks.

Oestrogen inhibits the action of prolactin in breast tissue and may affect composition of breast milk. The use of COCs decreases the amount of milk produced by COC users who breastfeed and therefore is contraindicated. Breastfeeding is contraceptive as long as it is occurring every 4 hours, including during the night. Ovulation then does not occur until at least 10 weeks after delivery. Contraceptive steroid is also excreted in breast milk. Any steroids are probably best avoided during the first 6 weeks postpartum. However, because a small percentage of breastfeeding women will ovulate as they continue fully breastfeeding and remain amenorrhoeic, then a barrier method or progesterone-only oral contraceptive can be used until menses resumes. When menses returns, another contraceptive is necessary. If menses has not returned but supplementation is taking place or long periods occur without breastfeeding, additional contraception is necessary. The incidence of pregnancy with lactational amenorrhoea is 2 per cent. Once supplementary feeding is introduced, ovulation resumes promptly and more effective contraception is needed. Progestogens do not diminish the amount of breast milk and are effective.

Before prescribing the COC

Take a history and exclude contraindications, check blood pressure, body weight and physically examine breast, abdomen and pelvis, with cervical cytology if sexually active. With a family history of vascular disease, such as myocardial infarction in a family member prior to the age of 50, screen lipids for hypertriglyceridaemia. With a family history of diabetes or gestational diabetes, a 2-hour postprandial blood glucose should be done before the COC is started. If the blood glucose is elevated obtain a glucose tolerance test. With a history of liver disease ensure liver function tests are normal before COCs begin.

Drug interactions

Some drugs can interfere clinically with the action of COCs by inducing liver enzymes that convert them to more polar and less biologically active metabolites. Drugs that accelerate the biotransformation of steroids include barbiturates, sulphonamides, cyclophosphamide and rifampicin. There is a relatively high incidence of COC failure in women taking rifampicin. Clinical data concerning COC failure in users of antibiotics, e.g. penicillin, ampicillin, sulphonamides, analgesics, phenytoin and barbiturates are less clear.

Women with epilepsy should be treated with COCs containing 50 µg oestrogen because of liver enzyme induction of the antiepileptic medication which renders the COC less effective.

Summary of benefits from the COC in addition to contraception

- Anti-oestrogen action of progestogens
- Reduction in the amount of blood loss at that time of menstruation from 35 ml to 20 ml
- Fifty per cent reduction in iron deficiency anaemia
- Fewer incidents of menorrhagia, irregular menstruation or intermenstrual bleeding
- Because progestogens inhibit the proliferative effect of oestrogens on the endometrium, adenocarcinoma of the endometrium is significantly less likely to develop in women taking COCs
- Progestogens inhibit the synthesis of oestrogen receptors in the breast, reducing the incidence of benign breast disease, with an 85 per cent reduction in the incidence of fibroadenomas and a 50 per cent reduction in both chronic cystic disease and non-biopsy breast lumps, as compared with controls using other forms of contraception.

Benefits from inhibition of ovulation

- Reduction in dysmenorrhoea (63 per cent) and premenstrual tension (29 per cent) compared to controls

- Fewer incidents of functional ovarian, hyperfollicular and luteal cysts that frequently require surgical management
- A 50 per cent reduction in the incidence of rheumatoid arthritis
- A 50 per cent reduction in the incidence of pelvic inflammatory disease (PID) after proven cervical gonococcal infection
- The incidence of *Chlamydia* in COC users is 50 per cent that of controls
- Ectopic pregnancy is reduced by 90 per cent in current users and may reduce the incidence in former users by decreasing their chances of developing PID.

'Side effects' of not being on the pill

- Symptomatic fibroids
- Endometrial cancer and ovarian cancer
- Endometriosis
- Dysmenorrhoea.

The COC should be changed to hormone replacement therapy at about the age of 50. It may be discontinued when ovulation is no longer taking place as indicated by FSH and oestradiol levels taken on the last day of the pill-free interval, that will give information about ovarian follicular activity. If the FSH is elevated and the oestradiol level low, the COC should be discontinued and oestrogen hormone replacement therapy begun if required.

Breakthrough bleeding

If there is breakthrough bleeding in the first week of pill use, try shortening the pill-free week from 7 days to 4. If breakthrough bleeding occurs with:

- Mercilon, Marvelon or Cilest, change to Minulet/Femodene; alternatively Microgynon/Ovranette in the first instance and then to Norimin or Loestrin 30.
- Ovysmen/Brevinor, contain 35 µg oestrogen plus 500 µg norethisterone – breakthrough bleeding is common as well as missing of withdrawal bleeds because it is very oestrogenically biased – change to Marvelon or Cilest. Microgynon/Ovranette contain 30 µg oestrogen plus 150 µg of levonorgestrel. Breakthrough bleeding is unusual, but if it occurs try Minulet/Femodene first. If that does

not work try Loestrin 30 or a new triphasic. Otherwise try a higher dose pill.

- Trinordiol/Logynon/TriNovum, try Minulet/Femodene or Loestrin 30.
- Norimin (35 µg oestrogen plus 1 mg norethisterone acetate) or Loestrin 30 (30 µg oestrogen + 1.5 mg norethisterone acetate), try Minulet/Femodene.
- Loestrin 20 (20 µg of oestrogen + 1 mg norethisterone acetate) – breakthrough bleeding almost universally occurs on this pill; it may be sufficient to change to Mercilon and work up from there. The 20 µg pill with 100 µg levonorgestrel with a progesterone (Microgynon 20) may give better cycle control.

Definition of a missed pill

It is the levonorgestrel that lasts for 3 or 4 days after the last active steroid pill has been taken. That suppresses gonadotropin release during the 1-week steroid-free interval, thus follicle maturation does not occur in the pill-free week. This accounts for the fact that it is very important that the pill-free interval is only 7 days. The most important pill is the first one of each cycle.

If a pill is taken less than 12 hours late, the forgotten one should be taken and the packet continued as usual, with the next pill being taken at the normal time. No other precautions are necessary. If the pill is more than 12 hours late, the pill forgotten should be taken immediately and the next one at the usual time, but extra precautions are needed for the next 7 days. If this occurs when there are less than seven pills remaining in the packet, then as soon as the packet is finished the next packet should be commenced on the following day with no pill-free interval at all.

If a pill is missed through vomiting and diarrhoea, extra precautions are taken for as long as the illness lasts and for 7 days afterwards. Again, if there are less than seven active pills left the new packet should be commenced with no pill-free week.

The first-time user should start with a COC that contains 20 or 30 µg oestrogen with the lowest possible dose of levonorgestrel or norethisterone. Formulations containing desogestrel or gestodene should only be considered when there are proven clinical benefits, such as in cases of acne or hirsutism. Established users of desogestrel or gestodene formulations who have risk factors such as obesity or a family history of thrombosis should be offered non-steroidal methods of contraception [9].

Screening for thrombophilia

Patients with evidence of thrombophilia or a past history of DVT should not be given oral contraception. Avoid giving the oral contraceptive pill to women with clear risk factors for venous thromboembolism. The background risk of dying from venous thromboembolic disease in the population aged 15–44 is between 0.5 and 4 per million. It usually averages between 1 and 2 per million, which is similar to the estimated figure of 3 per million women years for those using third generation oral contraceptives (Tables 1.4 and 1.5).

To balance the risk involved with DVT there are advantages, explaining the context in which oral contraceptives are taken.

- The overall safety of any combined oral contraceptive when compared to pregnancy
- The non-contraceptive benefits of the combined oral contraceptives
- The wide range of alternatives available, including the progesterone-only pill, injectables, implants, intrauterine contraceptives and barrier method
- The nature and consequences of deep vein thrombosis.

The 4.3 per cent of women with thrombophilia account for one third of deep vein thromboses in oral contraceptive users, so investigating women with a family history of thrombophilia is worthwhile.

Emergency postcoital contraception [10]

The likelihood of pregnancy after a single act of intercourse at days 10–14 is 20 per cent, 30 per cent on the day of maximum risk. At other times during the cycle the risk is 0–10 per cent. The probability of conception is lowest in the days before the expected date of the next menses unless the cycle is unusually long. The most fertile period is between days 7 and 17 of a 28-day cycle with the peak risk at day 13. Therefore if there is any doubt about the possibility of pregnancy, give emergency postcoital contraception, as side effects of postcoital contraception are minimal.

Yuzpe regimen

Until recently, this was the most commonly used regimen. It prevents 75 per cent of pregnancies that would have occurred without treatment.

- Ethinyloestradiol 100 µg plus
- Levonorgestrel 0.5 mg or DL-norgestrel 1.0 mg repeated 12 hours later, e.g. Schering PC4 or Ovran, which contains 250 µg levonorgestrel and 50 µg ethinyloestradiol but is not licensed or packed for postcoital contraception. Two tablets may be taken stat and two tablets 12 hours later.
- Give an extra two tablets in advance in case the treatment is vomited within 3 hours of ingestion.

Alternative regimen

Levonorgestrel 0.75 mg repeated 12 hours later; Postinor 2.

The levonorgestrel regimen is better tolerated than the Yuzpe regimen with greater efficacy in terms of both crude and adjusted pregnancy rates, and pregnancies prevented.

A dose of 750 µg levonorgestrel has few side effects, except acute porphyria, and the only contraindication to taking it is pregnancy.

Treatment should be given as soon as is practicable after unprotected coitus. The success rate is diminished for every 12-hour delay (Table 1.6). The dosage of levonorgestrel should be increased by 50 per cent in those taking enzyme inducers such as St John's Wort. Two tablets should be given stat and one tablet 12 hours later.

Table 1.6 Pregnancy rates with postcoital contraception.

	Levonorgestrel	Yuzpe regimen
Crude pregnancy rate (%)	1.1	3.2
Proportion of pregnancies prevented (%) (compared with the expected number without treatment)	85 (74–93)	57 (39–71)
Nausea (%)	23.1	50.5
Vomiting (%)	5.6	18.8

The crude relative risk of pregnancy for levonorgestrel compared with the Yuzpe regimen was 0.36 (95%, CI 0.18–0.70, $p < 0.01$).

The efficacy of both treatments declined with increasing time since unprotected coitus ($p = 0.01$).

Alternative emergency contraception

Mifepristone (RU486) 600 mg given within 72 hours of unprotected coitus has been associated with no pregnancies. This dose delays significantly the onset of the next menses. It has been shown that a dose as low as 10 mg may be used with the same efficacy [11]. A dose as low as 10 mg does not result in a delay in the onset of the next menses. Mifepristone is associated with significantly less nausea and vomiting compared with the Yuzpe regimen. Administered in the pre-ovulatory phase of the menstrual cycle, it delays or blocks ovulation and hence menses is delayed. Therefore it has the disadvantage of worrying a woman who is already fearful of an unintended pregnancy. In addition, delayed ovulation means a conception risk later in the prolonged cycle if no contraception is used.

The comparison of mifepristone 10 mg in a randomised multicentre trial with levonorgestrel has not been done.

TYPES OF INJECTABLE CONTRACEPTION

- Depot medroxyprogesterone acetate (MPA) 150 mg (Depo-Provera) every 3 months
- Norethindrone enanthate (NET-EN) 200 mg (Noristerat) every 2 months
- Several once-a-month injections of progestin/oestrogen combinations. MPA is a 17-acetoxy-6-methylprogestin that has progestogenic activity in humans. The 17-acetoxyprogestins do not have androgenic activity and are structurally related to progesterone rather than testosterone.

Depot-medroxyprogesterone acetate (DMPA)

Efficacy

The pregnancy rate at 1 year is only 0.1 per cent. At 2 years the cumulative pregnancy rate is 0.4 per cent.

Mechanisms of action

(1) Inhibition of ovulation
(2) Thinning of the endometrium, depleting secretion of glycogen that provides nutrition for a blastocyst entering the endometrial cavity

(3) Thickening of the cervical mucus, increasing its viscosity, thus preventing sperm from reaching the oviduct and fertilising an egg. It is therefore one of the most effective reversible methods of contraception available.

Pharmacokinetics

After deep intramuscular injection into the gluteal or deltoid muscle MPA is measurable within 30 minutes. Blood levels rise to a level >0.5 ng/ml within 24 hours after the injection. DMPA should be given during the first 5 days of the cycle to ensure the woman is not pregnant at the first injection. DMPA does not decrease endogenous oestradiol levels to the postmenopausal range and does not cause symptoms of oestrogen deficiency. DMPA does not prevent return of fertility. It only delays the time at which conception will occur. Because of its long and unpredictable duration of release from the injection site, resumption of fertility may be delayed for 1 year or more after last injection. Therefore information should be given to women considering this method of contraception on the long duration of action. Median time to conception varies between 9 and 12 months after the last injection. It is possible the reason for this is one related to weight. If body weight increases a concomitant increase has been observed in the median time to resumption of conception, possibly due to absorption of MPA into adipose tissue, from which it is not cleared rapidly.

Side effects of DMPA

In the first 3 months after the first injection, approximately 60 per cent of women become amenorrhoeic. Another 30 per cent have irregular bleeding and spotting. After discontinuing DMPA, 50 per cent of women resume regular menstrual cycles within 6 months. Seventy per cent have regular cycles within 1 year.

The effect of DMPA on body weight is unclear. The incidence of depression is <5 per cent. It is not associated with alteration in blood clotting factors or angiotensinogen levels. It does not affect blood pressure. There is a slight deterioration in glucose tolerance with DMPA use. The risk of endometrial cancer is reduced by 8 years in women after discontinuing use. There is no increased incidence of breast cancer.

DMPA

- Reduces the risk of developing iron deficiency anaemia
- Reduces the risk of pelvic inflammatory disease
- May have a beneficial effect upon haematological parameters in women with sickle cell disease
- Reduces seizure frequency in women with epilepsy
- Reduces the incidence of primary dysmenorrhoea, ovulation pain and functional ovarian cysts by inhibiting ovulation
- Reduces the symptoms of endometriosis
- Reduces the incidence of vaginal candidiasis

DMPA does not affect the quality or quantity of breast milk. The product labelling states that the first injection should not be given until at least 6 weeks postpartum.

Norethindrone enanthate

The pregnancy rate for NET-EN is 0.4 per cent if given every 60 days, and 0.6 per cent if given between 60 and 84 days. NET-EN should be given every 60 days for at least the first 6 months and then at least every 12 weeks thereafter. The World Health Organisation (WHO) recommends that it should be administered at intervals no shorter than 46 days and no longer than 74.

Progestin/oestrogen combinations

Progestogen-only injectable contraceptives are often discontinued because of menstrual irregularity. Combined progestogen/oestrogen injectables given monthly, which produce regular withdrawal bleeding, counteract this. They consist of a low dose of long-acting progestin plus a small amount of an oestradiol.

INTRAUTERINE DEVICES (IUDs)

Main benefits

- High level of efficacy
- Lack of associated systemic metabolic effects
- Need for only a single insertion for long-term use

- They are the ideal contraceptive in which the default state is one of contraception, unlike pills and condoms where the default state is conception.

Types of IUDs

- Copper IUDs: Multiload Cu250, Multiload Cu375, TCu 380, Gyne T 380 Slimline, Nova-T
- Levonorgestrel-releasing intrauterine systems (IUS): Mirena

The most effective IUDs are those with a copper surface area of $300\,mm^2$. Copper-containing IUDs cause a foreign body response in the endometrium. The result is a toxic environment to sperm. The copper prevents fertilisation in the vast majority of cases rather than preventing implantation. Copper IUDs do not affect ovarian function.

The levonorgestrel (LNG)-IUS exerts a strong progestational effect on the cervical mucus, which becomes thick and impenetrable to sperm. It renders the endometrium thin and inactive. It probably causes a foreign body reaction similar to copper-containing devices.

Mechanism of action

An IUD generates a foreign body reaction causing a local sterile inflammatory reaction. There is a 1000 per cent increase in the number of leukocytes present in the endometrial cavity. Leukocytes are toxic to all cells including spermatozoa and the blastocyst. Copper increases the extent of the inflammatory reaction. It also impedes sperm transport and viability in the cervical mucus. Because of the spermicidal action of IUDs very few, if any, sperm reach the oviducts, and the ovum usually does not become fertilised. They therefore have a contraceptive effect, not an effect on implantation. IUDs should be inserted during the menses optimally but may be safely inserted at any time during the cycle.

The blood levels of levonorgestrel with the LNG-IUS are less than half the mean blood levels of those using the POP. Therefore ovarian function is altered less.

Failure rates

Failure rates in the first year are <1 per cent with copper-containing IUDs, and 2 per cent with a progesterone-releasing IUS. The annual incidence of accidental pregnancy decreases steadily with the first year of IUD use. The cumulative pregnancy rate after 7 years using a copper-containing IUD is only approximately 1.6 per cent. The IUD is especially suited for older parous women who wish to prevent further pregnancies. The Mirena IUS (see Chapter 7) has the lowest failure rate of IUDs of 0.1 per cent per year (5 per 1000 at 5 years), and in fact performs better than sterilisation. The ectopic pregnancy rate is 0.02 per 100 woman years.

Advantages of the IUD

- Safe – mortality less than 1 in 500000
- Highly effective; effect immediately; more effective than the COC
- The Gyne T 380 has a cumulative failure at 5 years of only 1.4 per 100 woman years
- No link to coitus
- No pills to remember to take effectively
- High continuation rates (in excess of 10 years)
- May be used post-termination of pregnancy but not the LNG-IUS, because it does not have the efficacy of copper that enables instant effectiveness in copper-containing IUDs
- The LNG-IUS is 12 times more effective for preventing an intrauterine pregnancy or ectopic pregnancy compared to the Nova-T IUD.

Adverse effects

- In the first year of use, there is a 1 per cent pregnancy rate, a 10 per cent expulsion rate, and a 15 per cent rate of removal for adverse symptoms, e.g. bleeding and pain.
- Blood loss in each cycle is significantly greater in women using copper IUDs than in non-users. It increases up to 130 per cent. Reduced blood loss occurs with the progesterone-releasing IUD and the levonorgestrel-releasing IUS (Mirena). Twenty per cent have amenorrhoea; 80–90 per cent have a reduction in the amount of bleeding. Irregular spotting does occur.
- Pelvic infection: a WHO study in 1992 identified 22903 insertions (4301 in China). All countries had a six times increase in the risk of PID within 3 weeks after insertion, except in China, where in the 1980s monogamy was the norm. The insertion interferes with the

normal antibacterial barrier of the cervix and therefore swabs should be taken prior to insertion for *Chlamydia* and the patient seen a week after insertion.

- Any IUD that has perforated the uterus, which can occur at the time of insertion, should be removed from the peritoneal cavity, even if it is asymptomatic, because it can result in adhesions with a bowel obstruction. Perforation can occur through the cervix in approximately 1 per 1000 women. There is no increase in congenital abnormalities with babies born with an IUD in situ. If conception occurs in the presence of an IUD the incidence of spontaneous miscarriage is approximately 55 per cent, three times the normal rate. The incidence of spontaneous miscarriage is significantly reduced if the IUD is removed.

Types of device

The TCu 380 and the GyneFix are the most effective copper IUDs available, at least twice as effective in the first year of use and four or five times as effective cumulatively over 5 years as the Nova-T. The failure rate of the TCu 380 was 0.4 per 100 woman years. No pregnancies at all occurred after 5 years of use.

Duration of use

The TCu 380 is fully approved for 10 years' use in the UK and 13 years in the USA. Nova-T devices should be removed on efficacy grounds after 3 years (or a maximum of 5 years).

The Family Planning Association (FPA) stated in the *Lancet* in 1990 that any copper device fitted in women above the age of 40 may be that woman's last device and never needs to be changed, but it may not be so licensed.

Insertion of device

An IUD or LNG-IUS can be inserted at any time during the menstrual cycle (establish that the woman is not pregnant). A copper-containing IUD can be inserted immediately postpartum or prior to discharge at 48 hours, although expulsion rates are higher at this time. It is recommended that the LNG-IUS be inserted at 6 weeks postpartum.

Before IUD insertion:

- note the last menstrual period (LMP), previous medical history and sexually transmitted disease (STD) screening
- inform the patient of efficacy, mechanism of action, possible side effects, change in menses and risks
- pelvic examintion.

Follow-up:

- At 3–6 weeks after insertion when there is the highest risk of infection.

BARRIER METHODS OF CONTRACEPTION

The average sperm survival is 3–4 days. 'Fringe' sperm can last up to 7 days.

Condoms

Condoms are made of vulcanised, latex rubber. Method failure rates are reported as low as 1 pregnancy per 100 couple years. These are based on selected populations where there has been no sexual contact whatever, without the use of a condom, the only failures being caused by condoms bursting due to manufacturing defect. Rates may be as low as 0.4 per 100 woman years or as high as 32 per 100 woman years. The average is 8–10 failures at 1 year. For the careful user it is 3.1–4.8 woman years. In the Oxford/FPA study, a pregnancy rate of only 0.7 per 100 couple years was reported among women older than 35 compared to a rate of 3.6 per 100 couple-years from women aged 25–34. Spermicides are not mandatory.

Chemical interaction needs to be avoided with condoms. In general, water-based lubricants such as KY jelly, ethylene glycol, glycerol and silicones are all that are safe to use with condoms.

Consistent condom use protects against upper genital tract disease in the woman and against gonorrhoea, *Trichomonas* vaginitis, syphilis, *Chlamydia* and other bacteria and protozoa. The rubber of both male and female condoms is effective against human immuno-deficiency virus (HIV), infectious hepatitis B virus, herpes simplex types I and II and the wart viruses.

Diaphragms

Diaphragms have a first year failure rate of 4–8 per 100 'careful users' but 10–18 per 100 'typical users.' They do not interfere with the sexual mechanism and may be inserted prior to coitus.

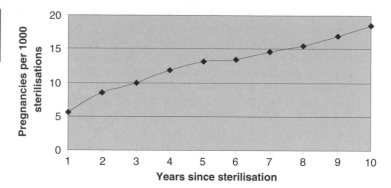

Fig. 1.5 Cumulative pregnancies per 1000 sterilisations (all methods). Source: CREST.

STERILISATION

The CREST study (United States Collaborative Review of Sterilisation) looked at the outcome of female sterilisation in 10 685 women over 14 years [12]. The failure rate of sterilisation was 1.8 per cent. The failure rate went on occurring and late failures occurred presumably due to recanalisation. The Filshie clip is more effective than the clips used in this study, with a failure rate of 3 per 1000 up to 2 years. Therefore the lifetime failure rate on the basis of using the Filshie clip is 1 per 200 women or 5 per 1000 (Fig. 1.5). In the CREST study, one third of all pregnancies were ectopic. Sterilisation therefore is not as good as has been previously quoted (failure rates around 1 per 1000).

VASECTOMY

- Objectively ten times more effective than female sterilisation
- Failure rate of 1 per 1000
- The suspicion of an increased incidence of prostatic carcinoma in men with vasectomies has not been substantiated.

The reliability of vasectomy – long-term follow-up of vasectomised men [13]

Vasectomy can fail at any stage and therefore couples ought to be warned of the risk of failure. In the majority of cases azoospermia is achieved within 4 months of vasectomy. Early failure is recognised when the patient still produces sperm at the first semen analysis. Late failure with the presence of sperm in the ejaculate after the initial negative semen analysis has only been reported rarely.

Recanalisation does occur, leading to pregnancy. The rate is about 1 in 2000 [13,14]. Most episodes of recanalisation are believed to happen soon after vasectomy. Delayed recanalisation after the first year is uncommon and isolated cases have been reported only. Temporary reappearance of the sperm has also been reported, i.e. a positive semen analysis at 12 months after vasectomy clearance, followed by two further negative samples.

The normal criteria for sterility amongst men at the clinic studied by Haldar *et al.* was two consecutive azoospermic semen samples at 16 and 18 weeks post-vasectomy. In the nine failures resulting in pregnancy, the initial two post-vasectomy semen samples were azoospermic, but subsequent samples at the time of pregnancy were positive.

The technique of vasectomy includes intraluminal cautery applied to the ends of the divided vas deferens after removal of a 1–2 cm segment. Of 2250 men, 20 had a positive semen analysis, 15 at the first year, 4 at the second and 1 at the third. Those positive at either the second or third year did not have a positive test the previous year. However, the sperm count was <10000/ml in the majority and the samples were also negative in the majority 1 month later. No pregnancies resulted.

Transient reappearance of sperm with low counts happens in 1 in 165 (0.6 per cent) men after vasectomy clearance. This is ten times greater, approximately, than the reported pregnancy rate after vasectomy.

Other reasons for failure

Some spermatozoa could remain in the terminal vas (ampulla) which are tortuous and formed by many tiny compartments. This makes clearance of sperm unpredictable and often very slow. There are discrepancies in the number of ejaculates necessary for clearance.

Another possible explanation for the lowered rate of positive semen tests with time is that any tiny channels formed between the two ends of the vas, allowing sperm through during the first year, may close over by scarring over time. Reappearance of non-motile sperm does occur after initial azoospermia in 0.8 per cent of men post-vasectomy, but no pregnancies usually result. It is crucial that all patients be informed with vasectomy that, although it is an extremely effective form of contraception, there are biological failures.

STOPPING CONTRACEPTION

Non-hormonal methods of contraception should be continued until a woman has experienced 1 year of amenorrhoea if she is 50 or older, and 2 years of amenorrhoea is she is younger. Use of the COC will mask amenorrhoea, regular withdrawal bleeds will occur and it suppresses gonadotropin secretion. Raised FSH concentrations on two separate occasions in a woman taking the POP usually indicate ovarian failure. The COC must be stopped for about 6 weeks before FSH concentrations will give a reliable estimation of menopausal status, and the measurement probably needs to be repeated. Table 1.7 shows comparative failure rates of all contraceptive methods.

HORMONE REPLACEMENT THERAPY AND CONTRACEPTION

If a woman is prepared to stop hormone replacement therapy (HRT) for 6 weeks, an FSH concentration can be checked after that time and the woman advised accordingly. If she is unwilling to discontinue HRT, contraception can be arbitrarily continued until she reaches the age of 55.

Contraception should be continued in women taking HRT who have not yet reached the menopause, because the natural oestrogens contained in HRT preparations are of lower potency and dose than the synthetic oestrogen within the COC and do not reliably inhibit ovulation. (Most standard HRT preparations contain 1 or 2 mg oestradiol and the contraceptive dose is 4 mg.) A POP can be given in addition to the HRT for adequate contraception in the older woman.

THE PREMENSTRUAL SYNDROME [14]

Symptoms and behaviour may occur intermittently, appear during the late luteal phase of the menstrual cycle, are not easily verifiable by the clinician, are not easily defined by the patient and disappear with menses (Table 1.8).

Table 1.7 First-year user failure rates per 100 women for different methods of contraception. (With permission from Guillebaud (2000) [2].)

Method of contraception[4]	Range in the world literature[1,2]	Oxford/FPA study (*Lancet* report in 1982; all women married and aged above 25)[5]	
		Age 25–34 (≤2 years' use)	Age 35+ (≤2 years' use)[3]
Sterilisation			
Male (after azoospermia)	0–0.05	0.08	0.08
Female	0–0.5	0.45	0.08
Subcutaneous implant			
Implanon	0–0.07		
Injectable (DMPA)	0–1	—	—
Combined pills			
50 µg oestrogen	0.1–3	0.25	0.17
<50 µg oestrogen	0.2–3	0.38	0.23
Progestogen-only pill	0.3–4	2.5	0.5
IUD			
Nova-T	1–2		
Nova-T 380	0.6		
Multiload Cu375	0.2–1		
Gyne T 380	0.2–1		
Levonorgestrel IUS	0.1–0.2		
Diaphragm	4–20	5.5	2.8
Male condom	2–15	6.0	2.9
Female condom	5–15		
Coitus interruptus	6–17	—	—
Spermicides alone	4–25	—	—
Fertility awareness	2–25	—	—
'Persona'	6–?	—	—
No method, young women	80–90	—	—
No method at age 40	40–50	—	—
No method at age 45	10–20	—	—
No method at age 50 (if still having menses)	0–5	—	—

[1] Excludes atypical studies and all extended-use studies. For sterilisation, rates in first column are estimated **lifetime failure rates**.

[2] First figure of range in first column gives a rough measure of 'perfect use' (but is not the same).

[3] Influence of age, all the rates in the fourth column being lower than those in the third column. Lower rates still may be expected above age 45.

[4] Much better results also obtainable in other states of relative infertility, such as lactation.

[5] Oxford/FPA users were established users at recruitment, greatly improving results, especially for barrier methods.

Table 1.8 Common complaints in the premenstrual syndrome.

Emotional symptoms
Depression
Mood swings
Anger
Irritability
Anxiety
Loss of self-control

Physical symptoms
Breast swelling and tenderness
Abdominal bloating
Headaches
Muscle aches and pains
Oedema
Backache
Weight gain
Gastrointestinal disturbance

Generalised symptoms
Decreased interest in usual activities
Fatigue
Difficulty concentrating
Increased appetite
Food cravings
Hypersomnia or insomnia
Change in libido

Diagnosis is by prospective symptom charting and exclusion of other disorders. Treatment strategies are often empirical. Women with identifiable criteria of the premenstrual syndrome may have lower serum concentrations of the progesterone metabolite allopregnanolone in the luteal phase compared to symptom-free women. Some abnormality of the central nervous system has been implicated as the cause of premenstrual syndrome, but it is unexplained why symptoms present in the luteal and not the follicular phase of the cycle.

Management of the premenstrual syndrome

The premenstrual syndrome is managed with psychoactive drugs; alprazolam and selective serotonin reuptake inhibitors (e.g. fluoxe-

Table 1.9 Treatments for the premenstrual syndrome.

Treatments are often empirical and trials are hampered by a large placebo response.
(1) Caffeine restriction (reduces insomnia and irritability)
(2) Salt restriction (minimises premenstrual bloating)
(3) Increasing exercise
(4) Pyridoxine (vitamin B_6) – limit dose to 50 mg per day because of risk of neurotoxicity
(5) Control of the menstrual cycle – COCs
(6) Selective serotonin reuptake inhibitors (SSRIs), e.g. fluoxetine – 20 mg/day in the symptomatic phase
(7) Danazol
(8) Alprazolam – begin in the luteal phase at the onset of premenstrual symptoms with 0.25 mg nocte and increased at 0.125 mg t.d.s. Taper the dose gradually during menses to avoid withdrawal symptoms such as exacerbation of anxiety, shakiness, palpitations, tremor and seizures.
(9) Nortriptyline, 50–175 mg at bedtime.
(10) For mastodynia, tocopherol (vitamin E), 400 units/day; evening primrose oil, one capsule, 500 mg daily up to 1 g t.d.s.

tine or sertraline) are effective. The theory of progesterone deficiency has not been confirmed and progesterone suppositories are an ineffective treatment. A recent theory proposes that women with premenstrual syndrome differ from symptom-free women in the metabolism of progesterone (Table 1.9).

REFERENCES

1 Thorneycroft, I.H., Mishell, D.R., Stone, S.C., Kharma, K.M. & Nakamura, R.M. (1971) The relation of serum 17-hydroxyprogesterone and estradiol-17β levels during the human menstrual cycle. *American Journal of Obstetrics and Gynecology*, **111**, 947–951.

2 Guillebaud, J. (2000) *Contraception Today*, 4th edn. Martin Dunitz, London.

3 WHO Scientific Group on Cardiovascular Disease and Steroid Hormone Contraception (1998) Cardiovascular disease and steroid hormone contraception: report of a WHO Scientific Group. WHO Technical Report Fer. 877. World Health Organisation, Geneva.

4 Collaborative Group on Hormonal Factors in Breast Cancer (1996) Breast cancer and hormonal contraceptives: collaborative reanalysis of individual data on 53 297 women with breast cancer and 100 239 women without breast cancer from 54 epidemiological studies. *The Lancet*, **347**, 1713–1727.

1

5 Schlesselman, J.J. (1995) Net effect of oral contraceptive use on the risk of cancer in women in the United States. *Obstetrics and Gynecology*, **85**, 793–801.

6 Hankinson, S.E., Colditz, G.A., Hunter, D.J. & Rosner, B. (1992) A quantitative assessment of oral contraceptive use and risk of ovarian cancer. *Obstetrics and Gynecology*, **80**, 708–714.

7 Vessey, M.P., Villard-Mackintosh, L., McPherson, K. & Yeates, D. (1989) Mortality among oral contraceptive users: 20-year follow-up of women in a cohort study. *British Medical Journal*, **299**, 1487–1491.

8 Colditz, G.A. for the Nurses' Health Study Research Group (1994) Oral contraceptive use and mortality during 12 years' follow-up: the Nurses' Health Study. *Annals of Internal Medicine*, **120**, 821–825.

9 Mills, A.M., Wilkinson, C.L., Bromham, D.R. *et al.* (1996) Guidelines for prescribing combined oral contraceptives. *British Medical Journal*, **312**, 121–122.

10 Taskforce on Post-Ovulatory Methods of Fertility Regulation (1998) Randomised controlled trial of levonorgestrel versus the Yuzpe regimen of combined oral contraceptives for emergency contraception. *The Lancet*, **352**, 428–433.

11 Taskforce on Post-Ovulatory Methods of Fertility Regulation (1999) Comparison of three single doses of mifepristone as emergency contraception: a randomised trial. *The Lancet*, **353**, 697–702.

12 Peterson, H.B., Xia, Z., Hughes, J.M., Wilcox, I.S., Ratliff Tylor, L. & Trussell, J. (1996) The risk of pregnancy after tubal sterilisation: findings from the US collaborative review of sterilisation. *American Journal of Obstetrics and Gynecology*, **174**, 1161–1170.

13 Haldar, N., Cranston, D., Turner, E., Mackenzie, I. & Guillebaud, J. (1999) How reliable is a vasectomy? Long-term follow-up of vasectomised men. *The Lancet*, **356**, 43–44.

14 Philp, T., Guillebaud, J. & Budd, D. (1984) Late failure of vasectomy after two documented analyses showing azoospermic semen. *British Medical Journal*, **289**, 77–79.

15 Dimmock, P.W., Wyatt, K.M., Jones, P.W. & O'Brien, P.M.S. (2000) Efficacy of selective serotonin reuptake inhibitors in premenstrual syndrome: a systematic review. *The Lancet*, **356**, 1131–1136.

2 Early Pregnancy

DIAGNOSING PREGNANCY

Pregnancy is diagnosed on clinical grounds by a missed period and symptoms and signs including:

- Nausea
- Breast tenderness
- Urinary frequency
- Clinically an enlarged uterus.

Other relevant features of a history in evaluating the state/viability of a pregnancy include:

- Fertility history
- Known tubal disease
- History of previous ectopic pregnancy
- Miscarriage and previous pregnancy outcomes.

The expected date of delivery is calculated (Naegele's formula) as last menstrual period (LMP) plus 7 days and 9 calendar months.

Pregnancy tests

Home kits give a faster and less expensive indication of pregnancy compared to radioimmunoassay.

Types of pregnancy test

(1) Slide or tube latex-particle agglutination inhibition tests are performed within 2–3 minutes. They require 300–500 mIU human chorionic gonadotrophin (hCG)/ml of urine for a positive result. These levels are achieved about 4 weeks after the last menstrual period. The test is performed by taking a urine specimen and mixing it with a solution of hCG antibody which will bind any hCG present in the test specimen. A suspension of hCG-coated latex heads or erythrocytes is then added. If hCG is present in the test specimen, the binding of the hCG-coated latex particles or erythrocytes to the antibody will be blocked and the agglutination reaction inhibited. No agglutination indicates a positive pregnancy test. Agglutination (i.e. the presence of a fine floccular precipitant) indicates a negative pregnancy test.

(2) The enzyme-liked immunosorbent assay (ELISA) method is performed in 4–5 minutes. It can detect 50 mIU hCG/ml of urine as early as 10–12 days after ovulation.

(3) Quantification of hCG by radioimmunoassay. These assays are performed in 70–180 minutes and can detect as little as 1 mIU hCG as early as 7 days after ovulation.

Ultrasound imaging of early pregnancy

The pregnancy is imaged to identify a viable intrauterine fetus, confirm the gestational age and exclude any other abnormality or normal variant, e.g. multiple pregnancy.

• The first sign of pregnancy is thickening of the endometrium but this may not be recognized for what it is.

• With vaginal scanning, a 1 mm gestational sac may be imaged at 4 weeks and 2 days from the LMP of a regular cycle. Early gestational structures can usually be seen about 1 week earlier by transvaginal (TV) rather than transabdominal (TA) ultrasound.

• An intrauterine pregnancy is visible on vaginal ultrasound scan at a β-hCG level of 1000 IU/l, and at 5000 IU/l for transabdominal ultrasound scanning.

• Sac size at 6 weeks transabdominal is about 25 mm with an embryo with a heartbeat. Transvaginally, sac size is 15 mm with an embryo with a heartbeat, corresponding to an earlier gestation.

• With an embryo of 3 mm TA or TV, a heartbeat should be visualised with most machines, which is a gestation of about 6 weeks. However, if a heartbeat is not seen up to a crown rump length (CRL) of 5 mm, rescanning 1 week later is indicated. It does not necessarily indicate fetal demise.

• In normal pregnancy the sac diameter increases by 1 mm/day. Growth of less than 1 mm/day is a poor prognostic sign. The sac diameter should be greater than 30 mm at 6–7 weeks' gestation.

• The yolk sac is the first structure that can be accurately identified within the gestational sac (5 weeks and 5 days) – a little earlier than the embryo, and initially it is much larger than the embryo.

• Because the yolk sac is part of the embryo when seen, it means it is a gestational sac and not a fluid collection and therefore in most cases there is not an extrauterine pregnancy. The incidence of heterotopic pregnancy is 1 per 30 000, but the risk is increased with assisted reproductive techniques (ART).

- A diagnosis of an anembryonic pregnancy (blighted ovum) is suggested when a gestational sac is larger than 20 mm in diameter with no yolk sac, or greater than 25 mm without a fetus or the yolk sac is large (greater than 10 mm in diameter).
- Fetal crown rump length should be measured.
- Fetal cardiac activity can be first identified at 41–43 days of gestation using a 2.5 MHz transabdominal sector transducer.
- Over 90 per cent of embryos with cardiac activity identified on ultrasound develop normally. The risk of miscarriage is reduced from about 40–50 per cent to between 1 and 3 per cent, depending on the gestational age when the fetal heart is first imaged and the age of the woman. If the heart rate is less than 85 beats per minute, miscarriage is likely [1].

BLEEDING IN EARLY PREGNANCY (THREATENED MISCARRIAGE OR MISSED MISCARRIAGE)

- A diagnosis of missed miscarriage should not be made if no fetal pole is seen and the gestation sac diameter is less than 20 mm.
- If the CRL is ≤6 mm, the pregnancy should be rescanned in 7–10 days. A missed miscarriage can be confirmed by correlating β-hCG levels with the ultrasound findings.
- If CRL is >6 mm with no cardiac activity, the pregnancy is non-viable.
- Any intrauterine haematoma should be noted.
- Retained products of conception are shown as tissue of mixed echogenicity with no gestation sac. If the volume is <30 mm (maximum diameter) with mild blood loss, and no evidence of infection, expectant management is all right. Evacuation of the uterus is indicated for women with a large volume of products of conception and/or heavy blood loss.
- The adnexa should be imaged and peritoneal fluid looked for.
- If the uterus is empty with a positive pregnancy test, the pregnancy is very early, a complete miscarriage or an ectopic pregnancy.

FIRST TRIMESTER MISCARRIAGE

Definition

The World Health Organisation (WHO) definition of miscarriage is 'the expulsion or extraction from its mother of an embryo or fetus weighing 500 g or less' (approximate gestational age of 20–22 weeks, which is considered pre-viable).

Incidence of miscarriage

- Spontaneous miscarriage occurs in 15–20 per cent of all clinically diagnosed pregnancies. However, the actual loss may be as high as 60 per cent of 'chemical pregnancies' diagnosed before the first missed period by estimation of the β-hCG level.
- Even after three or more consecutive losses, the chance of a successful pregnancy in the subsequent pregnancy is still at best 75 per cent and at worst about 50 per cent.

Threatened miscarriage

History is typically vaginal spotting or mild vaginal bleeding but with minimum pelvic or lower back pain without loss of any tissue vaginally. Threatened miscarriage complicates 15 per cent of pregnancies, and 20 per cent of these will progress to a miscarriage. Threatened miscarriage tends to be associated with a high likelihood of adverse subsequent perinatal outcome with complications including prematurity, small for gestational age, breech presentation, perinatal asphyxia, and increased risk of perinatal death. An ultrasound scan should be done weekly (see Chapter 6) until bleeding has settled.

Inevitable miscarriage

The internal cervical os is dilated, usually preceded by lower abdominal pain and vaginal bleeding.

Septic miscarriage

Septic miscarriage presents with the patient febrile, with significant tenderness over the uterus and lower abdomen. The uterus should be evacuated as soon as the patient is stable. Swabs are taken to identify bacteria for sensitivity to antibiotics. Antibiotics should be commenced. Anaerobic organisms are common (anaerobic streptococci, bacteroides and clostridia). A broad-spectrum antibiotic such as co-amoxiclav 1.2 mg i.v. 8-hourly is an ideal single agent for anaerobic and aerobic organisms as it is a potent β-lactamase inhibitor. Alterna-

Table 2.1 Features of septic shock syndrome.

Sepsis
Tachypnea (>20 breaths/min)
Tachycardia (>90 beats/min)
Hypotension
Hypothermia (<35°C) or hyperthermia (>38.3°C)
Evidence of inadequate organ perfusion
Hypoxaemia
Elevated plasma lactate
Oliguria (<0.5 ml/kg body weight for at least 1 hour in patients with a catheter)
Positive blood cultures

tive antibiotics include crystalline penicillin G (10 million units i.v. 4-hourly), ampicillin (2 g 4-hourly), and ofloxacin (400 mg once-daily).

Treatment of anaerobic organisms

Septic shock (Table 2.1) is caused by Gram-negative organisms in up to 80 per cent of cases and by Gram-positive organisms in up to 20 per cent of cases. It should be treated with metronidazole (500 mg i.v. 8-hourly), clindamycin (300–600 mg i.v. 6-hourly) or chloramphenicol (1 g in 100 ml saline 6-hourly).

Early septic shock is responsive to conventional therapy (i.v. fluids and antibiotics). Refractory septic shock is treated with vasopressors such as dopamine (>6 mg/kg/hour).

Complete miscarriage

The fetus, placenta and membranes are passed intact with minimal bleeding or pain. On pelvic examination the uterus is well contracted and the cervix is closed. Retained products of conception are diagnosed by ultrasound scan (Chapter 6).

Incomplete miscarriage

Incomplete miscarriage presents with a history of increased vaginal bleeding with crampy lower abdominal pain and the passage of some products of conception. On vaginal examination, tissue may be seen coming through the dilated cervical os. It should be removed with sponge forceps to decrease the uterine bleeding and prevent cervical (vasovagal) shock. If there is profuse vaginal bleeding, 20 units oxy-tocin in 1000 ml normal saline, 5% dextrose or Plasma-Lyte should be given to enhance uterine contractility. It should be run at 10–12 milliunits/min. Evacuation should be carried out as soon as the patient is stable, to reduce blood loss.

Missed miscarriage

Missed miscarriage is the failure to expel the products of conception after death of the embryo. It is clinically recognised by the uterus not being as large as expected for gestation. The symptoms of pregnancy may have disappeared. Ultrasound scanning identifies no fetal heart-beat. Often there is morphological abnormality of the gestation sac.

Management of first trimester miscarriage (Fig. 2.1) [2]

1 Expectant

A randomised controlled trial at a gestation of less than 13 weeks has shown that surgical curettage may not be necessary for the resolution of miscarriage [3]. Up to 80 per cent of women may be managed by expectant management. Expectant management results in no subsequent impairment in cumulative conception rates or pregnancy outcome [4,5].

2 Medical evacuation

Evacuation is performed with mifepristone and misoprostol.

3 Surgery

Surgical evacuation of the uterus may be preferred for those bleed-ing heavily with pain, or to avoid inconvenience of not knowing when a miscarriage will take place.

Products of conception

It is usual practice to send products of conception for histology.

Histological analysis of products of conception (histology, karyotype, culture)

The incidence of miscarriage overall is approximately 11.3 per cent [6], but for women aged 35–40 it is double at 21 per cent and for

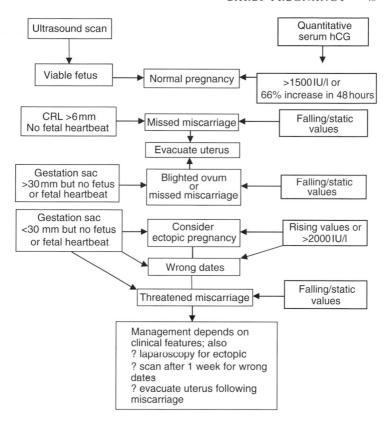

Fig. 2.1 Amenorrhoea, positive pregnancy test and vaginal bleeding. Summary of management options. (With permission from Rosevear (1999) [2].)

women over 40 it is double this at 41 per cent. There is a 70 per cent rate of successful outcome of subsequent pregnancies after many treatment regimens, attributable to chance than to specific therapy.

Causes of miscarriage

A diagnosis can be established in up to 50 per cent of cases (Table 2.2) [7].

Table 2.2 Causes of recurrent miscarriage in 195 couples. (Stray-Pederson & Stray-Pederson (1984) [7].)

Causative factors	First trimester		Second trimester		Primary miscarriage		Secondary miscarriage		Total	
	No.	%	No.	%	No.	%	No.	%	No.	%
Uterine defects	15	12.1	15	12.1	27	20.0	3	5.5	30	15
Cervical incompetence	4	3.2	21	29.6	17	12.6	8	13.3	25	12
Endocrine	9	7.3	1	1.4	9	6.7	1	1.7	10	5
Endometrial infection	20	16.1	9	12.7	21	15.6	8	13.3	29	14
Chromosomal	5	4.0	0	0	4	3.0	1	1.7	5	2
Systemic disorder	0	0	2	2.8	2	1.5	0	0	2	1
Oligospermia	7	5.6	1	1.4	8	5.9	0	0	8	4
Excessive smoking	1	0.8	0	0	1	0.7	0	0	1	0
Total known	61	49.2	49	69.0	89	65.9	21	35.0	110	56
Total unknown	63	50.8	22	31.0	46	34.1	39	65.0	85	43

Chromosomal abnormalities

Forty to sixty per cent of first trimester abortuses have chromosomal anomalies. Five per cent of abnormal karyotypes are abnormalities in the structure of individual chromosomes such as translocation. The majority are numerical abnormalities as a result of errors occurring during gametogenesis (chromosomal non-disjunction during meiosis), during fertilisation (triploidy as a result of disgyny or dispermy) or during the first division of a fertilised ovum (tetraploidy or mosaicism). Autosomal trisomy is the most common with chromosomes 13, 16, 18, 21 and 22 (50–60 per cent incidence).

Polyploidy is a deviation from the normal diploid number of chromosomes ($2n = 46$) in a cell by a multiple of the haploid number ($n = 23$). Polyploidy occurs in 10 per cent of abortuses. Triploidy and tetraploidy occur, triploidy most commonly. It originates by dispermy or by the failure of the first or second meiotic division of oocytes or spermatocytes, or less commonly through participation of the second polar body in fertilisation, or by defective segregation of one haploid set of chromosomes during the first zygotic division. Tetraploids originate from the suppression of the first cleavage division (cytokinesis) of a diploid zygote after the duplication of chromosomes. It is associated with hydropic degeneration that may occur as an incomplete hydatidiform mole. The karyotype 45 XO occurs in 7 per cent. Most fetuses with this karyotype are miscarried. In the few who survive (1 in 300) the karyotype is clinically recognisable as Turner Syndrome [8].

The prevalence of major chromosomal abnormalities in either parent is 3 per cent in those with two or more pregnancy losses. This is five to six times higher than in the general population. About half of all chromosomal abnormalities are balanced reciprocal translocations; 25 per cent are Robertsonian translocations; 12 per cent are sex chromosome mosaicism in the female. The rest are inversions and other sporadic abnormalities. Therefore karyotype of both partners with two or more spontaneous miscarriages should be performed. If a translocation is found in one parent, about 80 per cent of their subsequent pregnancies will miscarry. If miscarriage does not occur in a subsequent pregnancy, fetal cytogenetic studies are indicated because there is about a 3–5 per cent incidence of unbalanced fetal karyotype in these pregnancies. Among couples with a history of both miscarriage and fetal anomalies, the frequency of a chromosomal abnormality in one parent is 23 per cent.

Anomalies of uterine development

Uterine abnormalities occur from 1 in 200 to 1 in 600 women. In women with anomalies of uterine fusion, 20–25 per cent have problems with reproduction. Surgical correction of bicornuate and septate uteri is possible by using transfundal metroplasty techniques or by transcervical hysteroscopic incision of the uterine septum. Hysteroscopic incision of a septate uterus can reduce the pregnancy loss from as high as 95 per cent to 10 per cent [9].

Other causes/associations with miscarriage

Infections:

- Toxoplasmosis
- *Ureaplasma urealyticum* (T-mycoplasma)
- *Chlamydia*
- Cytomegalovirus
- Herpes simplex.

Other:

- Severe congenital heart disease
- Renal disease with hypertension
- Maternal and paternal age.

Antiphospholipid syndrome

A recent consensus statement for the preliminary classification criteria for definite antiphospholipid syndrome has been formulated [10] (Table 2.3).

Lupus anticoagulant activity is measured by one of the phospholipid-dependent coagulation tests:

- The activated partial thromboplastin time (APTT)
- The kaolin clotting time
- Dilute Russell's viper venom time.

Presence of lupus anticoagulant is determined using dilute Russell's viper venom time (DRVVT).

Anticardiolipin antibody can be determined by specific solid phase or enzyme-linked immunoassays. Lupus anticoagulant is found in about 10 per cent of women with recurrent spontaneous miscarriage of undetermined aetiology. Prevalence of either lupus anticoagulant or anticardiolipin antibodies in a normal obstetric population is only about 1 per cent for each antibody. If one of these antibodies is present in women with recurrent miscarriage and no treatment

Table 2.3 Preliminary criteria for the classification of the antiphospholipid syndrome. (With permission from Wilson *et al.* (1999) [10].)

Clinical criteria:

(1) Vascular thrombosis

One or more clinical episodes of arterial, venous, or small vessel thrombosis, in any tissue or organ, confirmed by imaging or Doppler studies or histopathology that does not identify significant inflammation in the vessel wall

(2) Pregnancy morbidity

(a) One or more unexplained deaths of a morphologically normal fetus at or beyond the 10th week of gestation, with normal fetal morphology documented by ultrasound or by direct examination of the fetus; or

(b) One or more premature births of a morphologically normal neonate at or before the 34th week of gestation because of severe pre-eclampsia or eclampsia, or severe placental insufficiency; or

(c) Three or more unexplained consecutive spontaneous miscarriages before the 10th week of gestation, with maternal anatomic or hormonal abnormalities and paternal and maternal chromosomal causes excluded

Laboratory criteria:

(1) Anticardiolipin antibody of IgG and/or IgM isotype in blood, present in medium or high titre, on two or more occasions, at least 6 weeks apart, measured by a standardised ELISA for β_2-glycoprotein I-dependent anticardiolipin antibodies

(2) Lupus anticoagulant present in plasma, on two or more occasions at least 6 weeks apart, detected according to the guidelines of the International Society on Thrombosis and Haemostasis in the following steps:

(a) Prolonged phospholipid-dependent coagulation demonstrated on a screening test, e.g. activated partial thromboplastin time, kaolin clotting time, dilute Russell's viper venom time, dilute prothrombin time, Textarin time

(b) Failure to correct the prolonged coagulation time on the screening test by mixing with normal platelet-poor plasma

(c) Three or more unexplained consecutive miscarriages before the 10th week of gestation, with maternal anatomic or hormonal abnormalities and paternal and maternal chromosomal causes excluded

(d) Exclusion of other coagulopathies, e.g. factor VIII inhibitor or heparin, as appropriate

Definite antiphospholipid antibody syndrome is considered to be present if at least one of the clinical criteria and one of the laboratory criteria are met

---

given, spontaneous miscarriage occurs in 90 per cent of the next pregnancies. In women with recurrent miscarriage without these antibodies present, miscarriage occurs in approximately 34 per cent of subsequent pregnancies.

Furthermore, fetal heart activity is detected in up to 90 per cent of these pregnancies. Thus, first trimester loss is embryonic, not anembryonic in those with antiphospholipid antibodies.

A recent randomised study in those with a history of three or more fetal losses and persistently positive for antiphospholipid antibodies (excluding those with systemic lupus erythematosus (SLE) or a history of thrombosis) found that low-dose aspirin (75 mg daily) gave a subsequent live birth rate of 80 per cent, compared to placebo who had an 85 per cent live birth rate, who otherwise received supportive care (see Table 2.4) [11].

Recurrent miscarriage

- Three consecutive pregnancy losses before the 20th week of gestation.
- Recurrent miscarriage is infrequent, affecting 1 in 200 couples or 1 in 500 pregnancies.
- Only 30 per cent of all possible fertilisations result in a viable fetus.
- There is a lack of randomised treatment trials of sufficient power to demonstrate a significant effect of treatment. Therefore the use of a variety of treatments is often empirical.
- There is a high placebo response with treatment of miscarriage with 'TLC' (tender loving care) [7].

Treatment

- There is no general agreement about therapy for women with recurrent miscarriage in the presence of lupus anticoagulant or anti-cardiolipin antibodies, because in randomised control trials the birth rate is of the order of 75 per cent in the treatment regimen for women with a history of recurrent miscarriage in the presence of either anti-cardiolipin or antiphospholipid antibodies [11,12]. The avoidance of stress and supportive care give very good results in randomised trials. Table 2.4 outlines 'rules' to achieve stress avoidance, not just coping skills, as based on empirical experience by observation of circumstances that may have contributed to recurrent pregnancy loss.

Table 2.4 Empirical 'rules' – TLC or stress-reducing guidelines for management of recurrent pregnancy loss.

Listen lying down to relaxation tapes on a Walkman $\frac{1}{2}$–1 hour per day
Stop work for 9 weeks (sick leave)
Once fetal heart is seen, practise creative visualisation
60 per cent threaten miscarriage – treat any bleeding with bed rest for 1 week
No sexual intercourse until 13 weeks, or until 2 weeks after gestation of previous loss
No moving house. If house is on the market, take it off
No exercise except walking 10 minutes per day and swimming
No gym, no tennis
No driving until 13 weeks
No house guests
No dinner parties
No weddings
No funerals except immediate family
No natural herbs
5 mg folic acid until 15 weeks
No hot baths, spa pools
Avoid chemicals and sprays
No housework, gardening, sweeping floors, vacuuming
No other children – to be minded for 3 days per week
No travel
Out for lunch 11.30a.m., home by 2.30p.m.
Out for dinner 6.30p.m., home by 9.00p.m. only, Sunday–Wednesday
Only go to the cinema during the day
Avoid crowds

- Women with a history of recurrent miscarriage have a high perinatal mortality rate. They are particularly at risk of severe sepsis and life-threatening haemorrhage and should be cared for by a perinatal team.
- A recent study [13] has shown that in a recurrent miscarriage clinic, excluding those with known associations with recurrent miscarriage (antiphospholipid syndrome, oligomenorrhoea, midtrimester loss, abnormal parental karyotype and other rare abnormalities), there was a 70 per cent conception rate and 75 per cent live birth rate. Of 55 miscarriages, 3 per cent occurred following detection of fetal cardiac activity (Table 2.5). In women with a history of idiopathic recurrent miscarriage, the most perilous time is between 6 and 8 weeks' gestation. Between these gestations, 78 per cent of the pregnancy losses occurred, with 89 per cent occur-

Table 2.5 Important gestational milestones for success and loss prediction. (Brigham *et al.* (1999) [13].)

Gestational age (weeks)	Success rate (%)	Miscarriage rate (%)
6	78	22
8	98	2
10	99.4	0.6

ring without the detection of fetal cardiac activity (this discriminates a pregnancy as 'embryo loss', rather than fetal loss). Therefore, identification of the fetal heartbeat by 8 weeks gives a chance of successful outcome in a subsequent pregnancy of 98 per cent, increasing to 99.4 per cent if a fetal heartbeat is seen at 10 weeks.

▪ Where there is a history of thrombosis or SLE, treatment consists of 80 mg aspirin daily throughout the pregnancy and heparin (10 000 units subcutaneously) as soon as fetal heart activity is demonstrated by ultrasound, with or without steroids. Aspirin (70–80 mg) inhibits platelet aggregation. Heparin prevents thrombosis. Heparin requires parenteral administration and may cause osteoporosis and thrombocytopenia. Prednisone is associated with glucose intolerance, skin and bone changes and preterm rupture of the membranes.

▪ Human leukocyte antigen (HLA) testing or any alternative immune tests are reported. However, these studies remain controversial.

▪ Maternal age has a profound effect on pregnancy outcome. A 20-year-old woman with two miscarriages has a 92 per cent (CI 86–98) chance of success in a subsequent pregnancy compared to a 45-year-old woman, where the chance of success is 60 per cent (CI 41–79) with two previous losses (Tables 2.6, 2.7, 2.8) [6,14,15].

Investigations for miscarriage are summarised in Table 2.9 and for recurrent miscarriage in Fig. 2.1. The psychological effects of miscarriage can be traumatic [16].

SECOND TRIMESTER MISCARRIAGE

Cervical incompetence

▪ The risk of an incompetent cervix relates to history, in particular trauma, to the cervix. The relative risk increases with the number of prior induced terminations of pregnancy.

Table 2.6 Overall risk of miscarriage, according to maternal age. (Knudsen *et al.* (1991) [6].)

Maternal age	Number of pregnancies	% spontaneous abortions (confidence interval)
–19	1105	10.8 (9.0–12.7)
20–29	13173	9.7 (9.2–12.7)
30–34	3900	11.5 (10.6–12.6)
35–39	1299	21.4 (19.2–23.7)
40+	260	42.2 (35.1–47.4)
Overall	19737	11.3 (10.9–11.8)

Table 2.7 Miscarriages according to success of previous pregnancy or not (*n* = 630). (Regan *et al.* (1989) [15].)

Incidence of clinically recognised spontaneous miscarriages (half before 8 weeks' gestation)	12%
Primagravida	5%
Gravida	14%
Women whose last pregnancy was successful	5%
Women who had miscarried their last pregnancy	20%
All prior pregnancies resulting in miscarriage	24%

Table 2.8 Risk of subsequent pregnancy ending in a spontaneous miscarriage. (Knudsen *et al.* (1991) [6].)

Number of previous miscarriages	Number of pregnancies studied	Miscarriage risk (%)
1	21054	15
2	2231	25
3	353	45
4	94	54

Thus the chance of having a subsequent miscarriage after three prior miscarriages is about 50 per cent.

- It is asymptomatic dilatation of the internal cervical os. Spontaneous rupture of the membranes occurs, leading to fetal loss.
- Dilatation of the cervix occurs without bleeding or contractions in the second trimester with a viable fetus.

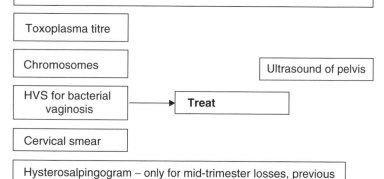

Karyotype of husband/partner

**Antinuclear antibodies (ANA)
Anti-double-stranded DNA**

Extractable nuclear antigen
(ENA) screen
Anti-Sm
Anti-RNP
Anti-Ro (SSA)
Anti-La (SSB)

Lupus anticoagulant
Anticardiolipin antibodies

Kaolin clotting time (50–100)
Prothrombin ratio (0.8–1.2)
APTT (25–40)
Dilute Russell's viper venom (<46 seconds)

APC resistance – If low, do a full factor V Leiden mutation and physician review

Toxoplasma titre

Chromosomes

Ultrasound of pelvis

HVS for bacterial vaginosis → **Treat**

Cervical smear

Hysterosalpingogram – only for mid-trimester losses, previous retained placentas or previous breech presentation

Fig. 2.2 Investigations for recurrent miscarriage.

Table 2.9 Investigations for recurrent miscarriage.

History – gynaecological, obstetric and medical
Time taken to conceive
Gestation of previous miscarriages
Details of previous investigations and treatments
Chromosome karyotyping of both partners
Mid-follicular phase gonadotrophin concentrations (follicle-stimulating hormone, FSH; luteinising hormone, LH)
Pelvic ultrasound scan for morphology of the uterus and ovaries
Calculation of body mass index
Antiphospholipid antibodies (APA) which includes lupus anticoagulant (LA) and anticardiolipin antibody (ACA)
Microbiological culture of the lower genital tract

Monitoring in the pregnancy
See as early as possible in the pregnancy
Serial ultrasound scans
Serum β-hCG levels
Emotional support with liberal admission policy
24-hour-a-day telephone support
Perinatal obstetric care after the first trimester

- Typical ultrasonographic appearances are 'beaking' or 'funneling' of the cervix and loss of length (see Chapter 6).
- On ultrasound scanning an internal os of 23 mm or greater in diameter is suggestive of cervical incompetence, while that of less than 19 mm excludes the diagnosis.
- Insertion of a cervical suture correcting competence has resulted in up to a 90 per cent success rate, together with multiple sutures to achieve pregnancy viability. Transabdominal cervicoisthmic cerclage may be indicated in the management of previous recurrent second trimester miscarriage and preterm delivery, where fetal survival may be as high as 85 per cent.
- Vaginal and intracervical swabs should be taken to exclude β-haemolytic streptococci, in particular.
- Cervical cerclage should be performed in a subsequent pregnancy of 14 weeks' gestation. A 5 mm double-needled Shirodkar suture is placed in a purse string manner through the cervical stroma just distal to the level of the internal cervical os. This is then cut and removed at 38–39 weeks' gestation.

Guidelines for rhesus (D) immunoprophylaxis with miscarriage

(1) Haemolytic disease of the newborn has largely been prevented since 1969 by the use of Rh immunoprophylaxis.

(2) Potentially sensitising events include:
- (a) miscarriage
- (b) invasive prenatal diagnosis
  - (i) amniocentesis
  - (ii) chorionic villus sampling
  - (iii) fetal blood sampling
  - (iv) intrauterine procedures
- (c) antepartum haemorrhage
- (d) closed abdominal injury
- (e) ectopic pregnancy
- (f) intrauterine death.

(3) Prophylaxis to prevent the development of anti-Rh(D) should be considered for all rhesus-negative women without antibodies with miscarriage both threatened and otherwise.

Anti-D products available in the UK

Bio Products Laboratory (BPL) Intramuscular:
(1) 250 IU (50 µg)
(2) 500 IU (100 µg)
(3) 2500 IU (500 µg)

Plasma Fractionation Laboratory (PFL) Intramuscular:
(1) 250 IU (50 µg)
(2) 500 IU (100 µg)
(3) 5000 IU (1000 µg)

Dosage: 100–125 IU (20–25 µg) of anti-D immunoglobulin (Ig) suppresses sensitisation by 1–1.25 ml of RhD-positive fetal red blood cells. Intramuscular anti-D is best given into the deltoid muscle as injections into the gluteal region often only reach the subcutaneous tissues and absorption may be delayed.

For successful immunoprophylaxis, anti-D Ig should be given as soon as possible after the sensitising event but always before 72 hours. If for some reason it is not given within 72 hours, it may still offer some protection if given within 9–10 days.

Women who have a weak expression of the Rh blood group D^u do not form anti-D and therefore do not require prophylaxis.

Prophylaxis following miscarriage (Reproduced with permission from [17])

Anti-D immunoglobulin must be given:

- To all RhD-negative women having a therapeutic termination of pregnancy, whether by surgical or medical methods, regardless of gestational age, unless they are known from previous blood tests to already have immune anti-D.
- To all non-immunised RhD-negative women who have an ectopic pregnancy.
- To all non-immunised RhD-negative women who have a spontaneous complete or incomplete miscarriage after 12 weeks' gestation.
- When the miscarriage is earlier than 12 weeks in RhD-negative women, published data on which to base recommendations for using anti-D immunoglobulin in their management are scant. There is evidence that significant fetal maternal haemorrhage (FMH) only occurs after curettage to remove products of conception but does not occur after complete spontaneous miscarriage. Anti-D immunoglobulin should therefore be given when there has been an intervention to evacuate the uterus. The risk of sensitisation by spontaneous miscarriage before 12 weeks is negligible when there has been no instrumentation to evacuate the products of conception. Anti-D immunoglobulin is not required in this situation.
- Opinion is divided about the need to administer anti-D where there is uterine bleeding in the first trimester in a pregnancy which is viable and continues. There are rare examples of sensitisation. Therefore routine immunisation is not recommended but it may be prudent to administer anti-D where bleeding is heavy or repeated, or where there is associated abdominal pain, particularly if these events occur as gestation approaches 12 weeks. When bleeding continues intermittently after 12 weeks' gestation, anti-D immunoglobulin should be given at approximately 6-week intervals.

Dose of anti-D

A dose of 250 IU (50 μg) is recommended for prophylaxis following sensitising events up to 20 weeks' gestation. For all events after 20 weeks, 500 IU (100 μg) anti-D immunoglobulin should be given followed by a test to identify FMH greater than 4 ml red blood cells.

Additional anti-D immunoglobulin should be given as determined by the level of spill. The standard postnatal dose given in the UK is 500 IU (100 μg) which suppresses sensitisation by 4–5 ml of RhD-positive red blood cells. A Kleihauer test identifies if the FMH is greater than 4 ml, thus requiring more anti-D immunoglobulin.

Occasionally, where a macerated stillbirth has occurred, following an intrauterine death, the RhD type cannot be determined. Anti-D immunoglobulin should be given to the mother and a Kleihauer test performed to exclude a large spontaneous FMH.

ECTOPIC PREGNANCY [18]

- Ectopic pregnancy is part of the differential diagnosis of bleeding in early pregnancy (Tables 2.10 and 2.11).
- It is a pregnancy implanted outside the decidualised endometrium mostly in the fallopian tube (98 per cent; ampulla, 81 per cent; isthmus, 12 per cent; fimbrial end, 5 per cent; interstitial segment, 2 per cent). Other sites include the ovary, cervix, peritoneal cavity (abdominal pregnancy, 1 per cent).
- The incidence is approximately 20 per 1000 pregnancies.
- Reversal of sterilisation – rate of ectopic pregnancy is about 4 per cent (it is increased if the tubes have not been damaged by infection).
- Incidence of ectopic pregnancy after *in vitro* fertilisation and embryo transfer (IVF-ET) is 4–7 per cent of clinical pregnancies. It is more common with transplantation of cryo-preserved embryos from unstimulated cycles than with fresh embryos.

Table 2.10 Risk factors for ectopic pregnancy.

Past history of ectopic pregnancy
History of infertility
Use of ovulation induction agents
History of tubal reconstruction (14% of women)
Endometriosis
History of termination of pregnancy
Use of an intrauterine contraceptive device
History of sexually transmitted disease – *Chlamydia* (identified by
    antichlamydial IgG antibodies), trachomatous or *Neisseria gonorrhoeae*
History of salpingitis (40%)

Table 2.11 Clinical features of an ectopic pregnancy.

History
Irregular menstrual cycles
Irregular bleeding
Amenorrhoea

Symptoms
Irregular vaginal bleeding
Unilateral pain
Generalised pain
Fainting and signs of abdominal tenderness
Unilateral or generalised plus/minus guarding and peritonism
Possibly pallour, shock, sweating, tachycardia, decreased blood pressure
On vaginal examination irregular bleeding, closed os, signs of pregnancy, small
   uterus for gestational age, adnexal mass with or without tenderness, cervical
   excitation

Ectopic pregnancy and a quantitative hCG

- A β-hCG level >1500 IU/l (first international reference) and no gestational sac visualised in the endometrial cavity on vaginal ultrasound suggest ectopic pregnancy.
- In normal pregnancy, β-hCG should increase by 66 per cent in 48 hours.
- β-hCG level should increase by 1000 IU/l in 2 days.
- A serum progesterone level <30 IU/l suggests an abnormally developing pregnancy. Progesterone levels <10 IU/l are associated with either an ectopic or non-viable intrauterine pregnancy, compared with 50 IU/l indicating a viable intrauterine pregnancy.

Management of ectopic pregnancy (Fig. 2.3)

- With increasing diagnosis at earlier gestation, it is possible to observe the ectopic pregnancy when indicated, and await natural resolution [19] (Table 2.12).
- The success rate of expectant management is up to 70 per cent.
- Follow-up requires measurement of β-hCG levels twice weekly for the first 2 weeks, and thereafter weekly until it disappears.
- Surgery is indicated if at any time there are peritoneal signs or haemodynamic instability. Resolution may take up to 50 days.

2

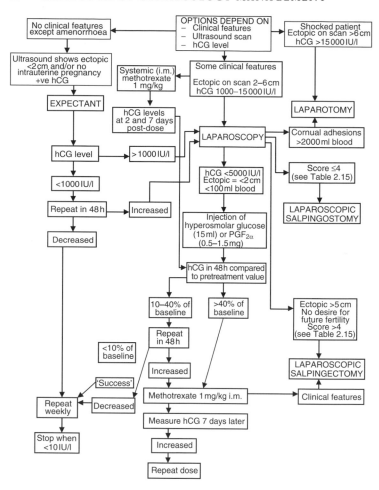

Fig. 2.3 Ectopic pregnancy: summary of management options.

Medical management

The ectopic pregnancy may be injected under ultrasound guidance with methotrexate, prostaglandins (PGF$_{2\alpha}$) or hyperosmolar glucose.

Methotrexate is a cytotoxic agent which may be used either systemically, by intramuscular injection or by localised injection into

Table 2.12 A scoring system for non-surgical treatment of ectopic pregnancy. (Fernandez *et al.* (1994) [19].)

	Score		
	1	2	3
Gestational age, weeks, amenorrhoea	>8	7–8	6
hCG level (IU/l)	>1000	1000–5000	>5000
Progesterone level	<5	5–10	>10
Abdominal pain, absent, induced, spontaneous, haematosalpinx (cm)	<1	1–3	>3
Haematoperitoneum	0	1–100	>100

the ectopic pregnancy. Methotrexate is an antimetabolite that interferes with the synthesis of deoxyribonucleic acid (DNA) by inhibiting the action of dihydrofolate reductase in the conversion of dihydrofolic acid into tetrahydrofolic acid. It interrupts the synthesis of the purine nucleotide thymidylate and the amino acids serine and methionine. The intramuscular dose is $50\,mg/m^2$ or $1\,mg/kg$ body weight.

Methotrexate stops DNA synthesis and to some extent ribonucleic acid (RNA) synthesis. The trophoblast, therefore, with its rapid cellular turnover, is very susceptible.

With methotrexate only 5 per cent of women experience minor side effects. These include stomatitis and elevated serum glutamic-oxalo-acetic transaminase levels. Intramuscular methotrexate preserves the potential for reproductive function. The rates of recurrent ectopic pregnancy in subsequent intrauterine pregnancy are very similar to those seen after laparoscopic salpingotomy. Methotrexate is widely used for the treatment of gestational trophoblastic disease in much higher doses. Follow-up of women who have received such treatment in subsequent pregnancies has identified no increase in stillbirths, premature deliveries, ectopic pregnancies or repeat molar pregnancies, or first and second trimester spontaneous miscarriages. There was no increase in major or minor congenital anomalies.

Recognising treatment complications

With methotrexate patients can have an exacerbation of low abdominal pain in up to 60 per cent. This may confuse the pain of impending tubal rupture. Pain is typically bloating or full feeling. If it is not relieved by anti-inflammatory medication, check the haemo-globin level to make certain there is no intra-abdominal blood loss.

Surgical treatment of ectopic pregnancy [20]

Surgical treatment is the principal mode of treatment for ectopic pregnancy. Increasingly salpingotomy via a laproscopic approach is both effective and advantageous.

Advantages of surgical treatment
- Confirmation of the diagnosis of tubal pregnancy
- Assessment of the status of the affected and contralateral tubes and the pelvis in general
- Effective and prompt treatment irrespective of the size of gestation, tubal rupture and presence of haemoperitoneum. Treatment may be either conservative (salpingotomy) or radical (salpingectomy), depending on the history of the patient, the pelvic findings and the patient's wishes for future fertility.

Laparoscopic surgery

Surgical treatment for unruptured ectopic pregnancies is essentially either linear salpingotomy or salpingectomy at laparoscopy. The advantages of laparoscopy are less blood loss, a lower requirement for analgesia and a shorter stay in hospital with subsequent cost savings. There is no difference in reproductive outcome with salpingostomy by laparoscopy or laparotomy.

The complication rate from laparoscopic salpingectomy is 0.6 per cent. Approximately 5 per cent require a second laparoscopy or laparotomy for persistent trophoblastic disease. Intramuscular methotrexate (1 mg/kg) is given when asymptomatic with β-hCG levels rising as previously outlined.

Laparoscopic linear salpingotomy (conservation of the tubes)

A three-puncture laparoscopy technique is used with two operative port sites, placed one to the left and one to the right one third of the distance to the umbilicus. Any haematoperitoneum is aspirated.

Marcaine with adrenaline diluted in 20 ml of Plasma-Lyte is injected into the mesosalpinx through a 20-gauge spinal needle. Blanching of the fallopian tube and transient ischaemia occurs. A

10–15 mm incision is made into the antemesenteric border of the haematosalpinx with the needle electrode (15 W coagulation and 30 W cutting, force II diathermy). A suction/irrigation apparatus is used for evacuating the clot and trophoblast. Alternatively, if the clot and trophoblast are too organised, making suction difficult, 10 mm spoon-shaped grasping forceps (Semm spoon forceps) may be introduced through a 10 mm port to remove the trophoblast. Alternatively a combined instrument (the triton-needlepoint diathermy and suction/irrigation) is efficient for opening the tube and removing the ectopic. The salpingotomy site is left open for healing. This decreases the incidence of tubal damage and allows better healing of the circumferential mucosal fold. Bleeding points are diathermied.

Laparoscopic salpingectomy

Salpingectomy is performed laparoscopically either by using a suture loop or by coagulation with bipolar diathermy forceps (3 mm) before cutting the tube. The excised tube together with the ectopic pregnancy is removed through a 10 mm port. Laparotomy is indicated in approximately 10 per cent of cases of ectopic pregnancy.

If the patient is shocked and haemodynamically unstable, or the serum β-hCG is >15 000 IU/l or there are extensive intra-abdominal adhesions or conservative surgery has failed, a mini laparotomy incision is made. The salpingectomy is performed by clamping the mesosalpinx and dividing the tube at the cornual end. It is transected and sutured with vicryl. The abdomen is closed after irrigation.

Overall rates for subsequent intrauterine pregnancy following linear salpingostomy are about 50 per cent (Table 2.13). Approximately 12 per cent will have a further ectopic and 5 per cent require treatment for persisting trophoblastic tissue. After total or partial

Table 2.13 Intrauterine pregnancy rates and recurrent ectopic pregnancy rates with past history of ectopic pregnancy. (Yao & Tulandi (1997) [18].)

	n	Intrauterine pregnancy rate	Recurrent ectopic pregnancy rate
Future pregnancy	1514	61.4	15.4
Partial or total salpingectomy	3584	38.1	9.8

salpingectomy, the intrauterine pregnancy rate was 38.1 per cent in 3584 patients desiring fertility, with a recurrent ectopic rate of 9.8 per cent. Among 176 women attempting to conceive with one tube, the intrauterine pregnancy rate was 54.5 per cent with a recurrent ectopic rate of 20.5 per cent. Previous infertility is by far the most important factor for subsequent pregnancy outcome. Successful conception is four times more likely without such a history. Subsequent intrauterine pregnancy rates are lowered and there is an increase in the recurrent ectopic rate with:

- ipsilateral periadnexal adhesions
- a history of infertility
- damage to the contralateral tube.

Most spontaneous pregnancies occur within 18 months of surgical treatment of an ectopic pregnancy. Even with a history of two repeat ectopic pregnancies, approximately 66 per cent will have a further ectopic. However, between 10 and 20 per cent will have an intrauterine pregnancy.

Results of fertility after conservative laparoscopic treatment of ectopic pregnancy in 223 patients are shown in Table 2.14 [21]. Twelve per cent had a recurrent ectopic pregnancy, nearly 85 per cent recurred in the ipsilateral tube; 33 per cent failed to conceive. Parity did not make a difference to recurrence risk. If infertility has not been a prior problem, the rate of intrauterine pregnancy following an ectopic is 85 per cent, with 7.5 per cent recurrent, and 7.5 per cent infertile. Future fertility is unrelated to the characteristics of the ectopic pregnancy, i.e. the size of the haematosalpinx, the volume of haemoperitoneum and tubal rupture had no significant

Table 2.14 General fertility results per cases and per patients. (Pouly *et al.* (1991) [21].)

	Ectopic pregnancy			Total per case	Total per patient
	1st	2nd	3rd		
No.	223	24	11	258	223
Ectopic pregnancy	27 (12%)	11 (46%)	1 (9%)	39 (15%)	
Intrauterine pregnancy	143 (64%)	5 (21%)	1 (9%)	149 (58%)	149 (67%)
Infertility	53 (24%)	8 (33%)	9 (82%)	70 (27%)	74 (33%)

influence on the rates of intrauterine pregnancy, ectopic pregnancy recurrence or infertility. Similarly, the location of ectopic pregnancy in a tube was of no predictive value in terms of future intrauterine pregnancy, ectopic pregnancy, recurrence or infertility.

Future fertility is dramatically affected by the incidence of ipsilateral periadnexal adhesions. With no adhesions present, 67.5 per cent had an intrauterine pregnancy, compared with 45.7 per cent with ipsilateral adhesions. The prognosis is worse for those where the function of the contralateral tube is compromised. In 21.1 per cent the contralateral tube was non-functional. For these patients the rates found for intrauterine pregnancy, recurrent ectopic and infertility were 21.3, 21.3, and 57.4 per cent respectively.

If there was a patent contralateral tube, 75.5 per cent achieved an intrauterine pregnancy, 9.7 per cent had an ectopic recurrence and 14.8 per cent were infertile. If the contralateral tube was patent but with periadnexal adhesions, the rate of intrauterine pregnancy was 41.9 per cent, the rate of infertility 38.7 per cent. If there were no adhesions and a patent contralateral tube, the intrauterine pregnancy rate was 82.8 per cent with 9.6 per cent infertility.

Previous history

If there was no history of prior abdominal surgery, IUD use or prior history of ectopic pregnancy, infertility or salpingitis, subsequent intrauterine pregnancy was 88.7 per cent with 3.8 per cent infertile versus 56 per cent intrauterine pregnancy and 30 per cent infertility in those with that history. There is no difference in rates of recurrence, 7.5 per cent without a history, compared to 13.5 per cent with.

Fifty per cent intrauterine pregnancy rates occur in the first year, and 70 per cent within 2 years, of the management of the ectopic pregnancy. Conservative surgical treatment may be contraindicated when the probability of an intrauterine pregnancy is lower than that of a recurrent ectopic pregnancy. A therapeutic scoring system for ectopic pregnancy is given in Table 2.15 for risk factors [20].

TERMINATION OF PREGNANCY (TOP) [22]

The indications for terminating pregnancy are based on legal constraints of various countries which medical personnel certifying and carrying out terminations of pregnancy must comply with. Termination of pregnancy rates per thousand estimated mean number of

Table 2.15 Risk factors and therapeutic score of the ectopic pregnancy. (Chapron *et al.* (1993) [20].)

	Score
One previous ectopic pregnancy	2
Each additional ectopic pregnancy	1
Previous laparoscopic adhesiolysis	1
Previous tubal microsurgery	2
Solitary tube	2
Previous salpingitis	1
Homolateral adhesions	1
Contralateral adhesions	1

Score

0–3	Laparoscopic conservative treatment
4	Laparoscopic salpingectomy
5 or more	Laparoscopic salpingectomy and contralateral sterilisation and IVF for future fertility

Table 2.16 Regimens for cervical priming.

Gemeprost	1 mg vaginally 3 hours prior to surgery
Misoprostol	400 µg (2 × 200 µg tablets) vaginally 3 hours prior to surgery
Mifepristone	200 mg or as in data sheet

women aged 15–44 years vary in countries of low fertility from approximately 14.77 (England and Wales), 10.4 (Finland), 12.4 (France), 7.9 (Germany), 11.2 (Scotland), 22.9 (United States), 18.2 (New Zealand) (1995–1999 figures).

Guidlines for termination (Tables 2.16–2.20)

- Medical termination of pregnancy has up to a 90 per cent success rate up to 83 days of gestation [23–25].
- The dose of oral mifepristone (RU486) can be reduced from formerly 600 mg to 200 mg without any effect on the efficacy [26].
- Misoprostol (800 µg 36–48 hours later, administered vaginally) is cheaper and does not require special storage facilities compared to gemeprost as the type of prostaglandin to use in conjunction with

Table 2.17 Regimens for early medical termination of pregnancy.

Mifepristone 200 mg in combination with a prostaglandin
Misoprostol (a prostaglandin E_1 analogue, given vaginally, is a cost-effective
   alternative for all abortion procedures for which the E_1 analogue gemeprost is
   given)
Alternative regimens for early medical TOP: mifepristone 600 mg orally followed
   36–48 hours later by gemeprost 1 mg vaginally.
Mifepristone 200 mg orally followed 36–48 hours later by misoprostol 800 µg (4
   × 200 µg tablets) vaginally
Mifepristone 200 mg orally followed 36 hours later by gemeprost 0.5 mg
   vaginally
Conventional suction TOP is an appropriate method of termination of pregnancy
   at gestations of 7–15 weeks. Cervical preparation is beneficial prior to suction
   termination and should be routine if the woman is aged under 18 years or the
   gestation >10 weeks.

Table 2.18 Methods of termination of pregnancy at more than 15 weeks' gestation.

Mifepristone 600 mg orally followed 36–48 hours later by gemeprost 1 mg
   vaginally every 3 hours to a maximum of five pessaries
Mifepristone 200 mg orally followed 36–48 hours later by misoprostol 800 µg
   vaginally then misoprostol 400 µg orally to a maximum of four doses
Mifepristone 200 mg orally followed 36 hours later by gemeprost 1 mg vaginally
   every 6 hours

mifepristone. Vaginal administration of misoprostol is associated with fewer side effects and improved efficacy [27].

- At gestations up to 7 weeks, misoprostol appears to be as effective as gemeprost, but efficacy is reduced at 7–9 weeks' gestation.
- Termination usually occurs within 8 hours.
- If a response has not occurred within 24 hours of misoprostol administration surgical termination may be offered. Alternatively, a repeat ultrasound scan could be done at 1 week. If there is doubt about the completeness of medical termination then a follow-up ultrasound scan vaginally should be done 10 days later.
- As misoprostol is unlicensed for use in early TOP, qualified doctors are permitted by the EC Pharmaceutical Directive 89/349/EEC to use licensed medications for indications or in doses or routes of

Table 2.19 Examples of prostaglandin administration protocols for evacuation of missed miscarriage and late fetal death *in utero*. [Mackenzie (1999) [29].)

Drug administration protocol	Vomiting (%)	Diarrhoea (%)	Expulsion time (hours) (mean or median)
Vaginal PGE_1 (misoprostol) 50–100 µg/day	0	0	11.6
Vaginal PGE_2 20 mg every 3–6 hours	87	70	14.6
Vaginal PGE_2 25 mg single instillation + i.v. oxytocin after 15–20 hours	31	8	14.4
Vaginal 16,16-dimethyl-PGE_1, 1 mg every 3 hours × 3 + i.v. oxytocin after 15–20 hours	15	10	14.2
Extra-amniotic PGE_2 1–4 µg/min infusion	29	0	10.0±
Intramuscular 16-phenoxy-PGE_2 500 µg every 4–6 hours	48	48	12.4
Intramuscular 15-methyl-$PGF_{2\alpha}$ 125–500 µg every 2 hours	52	59	8.6
Intravenous 16-phenoxy-PGE_2 1 µg/min infusion	19	2	12.0
Intravenous 16-phenoxy-PGE_2 3 µg/min infusion	38	14	12.0

Intra-amniotic PGE_2 5–10 mg + i.v. oxytocin at 6 hours
Intra-amniotic $PGF_{2\alpha}$ 25 mg + 25 mg every 6 hours
Intra-amniotic 15-methyl-$PGF_{2\alpha}$ 2.5 mg single injection

administration outside the recommendation given in the licence. Informed consent should be obtained.

Antibiotics

Doxycycline for 7 days or azithromycin 1 g, which is more cost effective and ensures compliance. This covers bacterial vaginosis and chlamydial infection as opposed to screening and treatment of positive cases [28].

Other medications required

- Anti-D at the time of termination.

Table 2.20 Complications of TOP.

Complication	Incidence
Haemorrhage	1.5 per 1000 1.2 per 1000 at <13 weeks 8.5 per 1000 at >30 weeks
Uterine perforation	1.4 per 1000 (rate is lower the earlier the gestation)
Cervical trauma	<1% (rate is lower the earlier the gestation)

Failed termination of pregnancy requiring a further procedure
    Surgical
    Medical
	
	2.3 per 1000
	6 per 1000

Infection – pelvic inflammatory disease	Up to 10% of cases. Risk is reduced with prophylactic antibiotics or when lower genital tract infection has been excluded by bacteriological screening
Future reproductive outcome	No proven association between induced abortion and subsequent infertility or preterm delivery
Psychological sequelae	Minimal

- Human immunodeficiency virus (HIV) seropositivity rate in women attending for TOP in inner-city London in an anonymous survey in 1994 was 1 in 160.
- Future contraceptive plans need to be established.
- Up to 70 per cent require no analgesia. Co-proxamol may be needed in up to 25 per cent. Less than 5 per cent require intramuscular opioid analgesia. Increasing analgesic requirements are associated with increasing gestational age.

Side effects of TOP

- In developed countries the safety of both medical and surgical TOP is well established – mortality <1 in 100 000 with surgical TOP.
- Ongoing pregnancy rate is approximately 3 per 1000.
- Incomplete TOP rate is 2 per cent.

- Vomiting occurs in 25 per cent and diarrhoea in 13 per cent undergoing medical TOP.
- Mean blood loss is <100 ml. A clinically significant blood loss occurs in 1 per cent.
- Transfusion rate is 1 in 2000.

After termination of pregnancy [22]:

- Anti-D immunoglobulin should be given to all non-sensitised RhD-negative women following termination of pregnancy whether surgical or medical methods are used, regardless of gestational age (see above for anti-D regimens).
- A follow-up visit should occur at 2 weeks and adequate contraception supplied. An intrauterine device (IUD) may be inserted at the time of termination of pregnancy.

Mid-trimester termination of pregnancy

Extra-amniotic infusion [29]

Under aseptic condition the self-retained 14- or 16-gauge Foley's catheter is introduced through the cervical canal. The balloon is distended with 20–50 ml of sterile isotonic saline. The catheter is connected to an infusion pump. Prostaglandin E_2 (PGE$_2$) solution is infused into the extra-amniotic space at 20–150 µg/hour with 10 µg/hour incremental increases at 15-minute intervals as necessary using a solution concentration of 1.5–5 µg/ml. The infusion is maintained until the catheter is naturally expelled into the vagina when labour has caused cervical dilatation. Oxytocin augmentation is started 3 hours or more after discontinuing the prostaglandin infusion. It is preferable not to rupture the membranes because of the risk of ascending infection.

Alternatively, a single bolus injection of prostaglandin may be given using a disposable polyethylene catheter introduced into the extra-amniotic space. PGE$_2$ (240–500 µg in 7–10 ml of viscous gel) is injected and the catheter withdrawn. Oxytocin is commenced as previously once labour has commenced.

The optimal treatment protocol for a mid-trimester termination of pregnancy has not been established. Examples may be seen in Tables 2.18 and 2.19. Clotting status should be made if fetal death has occurred 3 weeks previously. Adequate analgesia should be provided. Ergometrine or intramuscular prostaglandin analogues should be given to enhance uterine contractility following delivery to reduce the chances of excessive haemorrhage.

Intra-amniotic protocols have been used for terminations beyond 15 weeks' gestation. Many protocols have been developed over the past 20 years and involve either single instillation of prostaglandins at amniocentesis or repeated injections through an indwelling trans-abdominal intra-amniotic catheter inserted through a Tuohy needle at the time of amniocentesis. An additional 200 ml of hypotonic saline solution is inserted to ensure fetal demise before delivery.

Embolisation procedures

Alternatively, 10 ml of air into the umbilical cord under ultrasound for pregnancies smaller than 24 weeks' gestation. Embolisation procedures are better done with prostaglandins given vaginally, since the myometrium is increasingly sensitive as the gestation advances. Vaginal pessaries of prostaglandins offer a relatively non-invasive method which can be enhanced by subsequent intravenous infusion of oxytocin. The oral administration of the anti-progestational agent epostane, a 3β-hydroxy steroid dehydrogenase inhibitor, or mifepristone (RU486), the progesterone-receptive blocker, 200 mg 24–72 hours prior to prostaglandin treatment, reduces the induction to TOP interval by up to 60 per cent, thus lowering the dose of prostaglandins needed with a decreased incidence of gastrointestinal side effects and the need for analgesia.

The placenta should deliver within 2 hours of TOP. The longer the delay before surgical removal the greater the rate of excessive bleeding.

Ergometrine (0.5 mg intramuscularly) should be given at the time of termination of pregnancy, to reduce excessive blood loss (>500 ml).

GESTATIONAL TROPHOBLASTIC DISEASE (FIG. 2.4) [30]

Gestational trophoblastic disease (GTD) is identified as an abnormal proliferation histologically of trophoblastic tissue (Table 2.21). Trophoblastic disease manifests itself clinically as irregular vaginal bleeding and typical ultrasound features of a classic 'snowstorm' appearance with an absence of fetal parts and heartbeat.

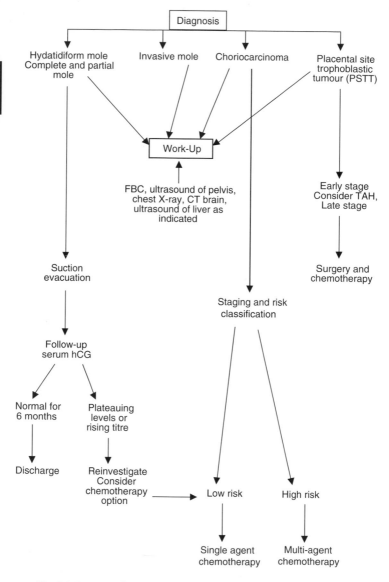

Fig. 2.4 Gestational trophoblastic disease – clinical practical guidelines summary. (With permission from Benedet *et al.* (2000). *International Journal of Gynecology and Obstetrics*, **70**, 209–262.)

Table 2.21 World Health Organisation (WHO) classification of trophoblastic disease. (With permission from Benedet *et al.* (2000) [30].)

1 Hydatidiform mole
   Complete
   Partial
2 Invasive hydatidiform mole
3 Choriocarcinoma
4 Placental site trophoblastic tumour
5 Trophoblastic tumour, miscellaneous
   Exaggerated placental site
   Placental site nodule or plaque
6 Unclassified trophoblastic lesions

Table 2.22 Staging of gestational trophoblastic diseases. (With permission from Benedet *et al.* (2000) [30].)

FIGO stages[1]		TNM categories
	Primary tumour cannot be assessed	TX
	No evidence of primary tumour	T0
I	Tumour confined to uterus	T1
II	Tumour extends to other genital structures: vagina, ovary, broad ligament, fallopian tube by metastasis or direct extension	T2
III	Metastasis to the lung(s)	M1a
IV	Other distant metastasis with or without lung involvement	M1b

[1] Stages I–IV are subdivided into A–C according to the number of risk factors: A, without risk factors; B, with one risk factor; C, with two risk factors.

Occasionally grape-like hydropic villi may be passed vaginally. See Table 2.22 for staging.

Hydatidiform mole

- May be complete and incomplete or partial.
- Complete moles are diploid lesions with 46XX karyotype being the most common.

- Incomplete moles have chromosomes that are paternally derived.
- Characterised by hydropic swelling of the chorionic villi with diffuse trophoblastic proliferation.
- Absent embryonic or fetal tissue.
- 10–30 per cent of evacuated complete moles may be followed by persistent gestational trophoblastic disease requiring therapy.
- The risk of requiring chemotherapy is 1 in 10

Partial moles

- Karyotype is triploid (69 chromosomes).
- Two paternal sets and a maternal chromosome complement.
- Varying size chorionic villi with focal hydropic changes and trophoblastic hyperplasia.
- Fetal or embryonic tissues are usually identified. They have lower frequency of progressing to choriocarcinoma.
- The risk of requiring chemotherapy after partial hydatidiform mole is about 1 in 200.
- A complete or partial hydatidiform mole may undergo malignant transformation. Even after surgical evacuation it may persist and remain confined to the uterine cavity or penetrate into the myometrium. Embolisation to the lungs or vagina may occur or it may transform to choriocarcinoma.

Follow-up (Fig. 2.5)

- If the serum hCG falls to <5 IU/l by 56 days post-evacuation, the follow-up period may be reduced to 6 months.
- If the hCG has not fallen to <5 IU/l, follow-up should continue for 2 years.
- The risk of requiring chemotherapy after partial hydatidiform mole is about 1 in 200, compared with a risk of about 1 in 10 after a complete hydatidiform mole.
- Patients treated for a persisting trophoblastic lesion within 6 months of evacuation of a mole usually respond completely to a low-toxicity methotrexate/folinic acid regimen.
- Twenty-five per cent require additional cytotoxics.
- The overall cure rate in the post-hydatidiform mole group is more than 99 per cent.
- Etoposide, methotrexate, actinomycin D/cyclophosphamide with vincristine regimen is used to treat patients with persisting disease, which achieves eradication in 85 per cent of choriocarcinomas [31].

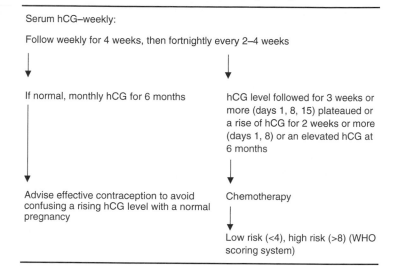

Serum hCG–weekly:

Follow weekly for 4 weeks, then fortnightly every 2–4 weeks

If normal, monthly hCG for 6 months

hCG level followed for 3 weeks or more (days 1, 8, 15) plateaued or a rise of hCG for 2 weeks or more (days 1, 8) or an elevated hCG at 6 months

Advise effective contraception to avoid confusing a rising hCG level with a normal pregnancy

Chemotherapy

Low risk (<4), high risk (>8) (WHO scoring system)

Fig. 2.5 Follow-up after surgical evacuation of gestational trophoblastic tumour. (With permission from Benedet (2000).)

- The placental site of trophoblastic tumours should be identified because of the need for possible early hysterectomy.
- Drug resistance requires additional therapeutic agents and often surgery.
- Central nervous system metastases also require treatment, and may be eradicated in up to 70 per cent of cases.
- Fertility is not significantly impaired by chemotherapy.
- There is no increased risk of secondary tumours but therapy-induced leukaemias have occurred.
- The incidence of choriocarcinoma following hydatidiform mole is about 1 in 30; 1 in 50 000 occurs after a term pregnancy.

Treatment of a molar pregnancy

Suction evacuation of the uterine cavity is the treatment of choice. There are significant risks of perforation and haemorrhage. All tissue should be sent for histological examination.

Table 2.23 Gestational trophoblastic disease prognostic score. (With permission from Benedet *et al.* (2000) [30].)

	0	1	2	4
Age (years)	<39	>39		
Antecedent pregnancy	Mole	Miscarriage/TOP	Term pregnancy	
Interval (months)	4	4–6	7–12	>12
Pretreatment hCG (log)	<3	<4	<5	<5
ABO group (female × male)		O × A A × O	B AB	
Largest tumour (cm)		3–5	5	
Site of metastasis		Spleen, kidney	GI tract, liver	Brain
Number of metastases identified		1–4	4–8	>8
Previous chemotherapy failed			Single drug	Two or more

Chemotherapy

Chemotherapy protocols are initiated to minimise the risk of progressive disease by timely intervention without subjecting more patients than necessary to cytotoxic agents. Approximately 8 per cent of patients with hydatidiform mole using these protocols require chemotherapy.

The risk of relapse at 6 months if the β-hCG is <5 IU/l is less than 1 in 2000. This means that for approximately 65 per cent of patients whose β-hCG results fall into this normal range by the 56th day post-evacuation, they do not need to wait before trying for a further pregnancy.

The risk of a second hydatidiform mole is 1 in 76 and that of a third 1 in 6.

A scoring system for risk and prognostic factors in trophoblastic neoplasia can be seen in Table 2.23 [32].

Choriocarcinoma

- Malignant tumour of the trophoblast.
- Generally follows an identifiable gestational event such as a molar pregnancy, abortion, ectopic or term pregnancy.
- Approximately 50 per cent of cases of choriocarcinoma are preceded by a hydatidiform mole.

- Twenty-five per cent occur after a miscarriage.
- Twenty-two per cent occur after a normal pregnancy.
- Three per cent occur after an ectopic pregnancy.
- Haemoptysis may occur due to blood-borne metastases.
- Thyrotoxicosis may occur because of the thyrotrophic effect of β-hCG.

2

Good prognostic factors for choriocarcinoma
- Urinary hCG <100 000 IU/l for 24 hours.
- Serum hCG <40 000 IU/l.

Symptoms
- Pregnant for <4 months.
- Absence of brain or liver metastases.
- No prior chemotherapy where the pregnancy was not a term delivery.

Treatment for low and high risk prognostic score of GTD

Low risk GTD (WHO score 4 or less)
- Commence treatment as soon as possible.
- A low risk of GTD can be managed with single-agent chemotherapy using methotrexate with folinic acid.
- Other drugs include etoposide.
- If single-agent chemotherapy is used and is not working, a more aggressive treatment is warranted to prevent the emergence of drug resistance.

Intermediate risk GTD (WHO score 5–7)
- Commence on regimen that includes combination chemotherapy – methotrexate and actinomycin D, as well as an alkylating agent.
- If a complete response is not achieved on this regimen the patient should be commenced on etoposide, methotrexate and actinomycin D, alternating with cyclophosphamide and vincristine (EMA-CO).

High risk GTD (WHO score 8 or more)
- These patients require significant chemotherapy because they include those with brain metastases, liver and gastrointestinal tract metastases and they are at significant risk from massive bleeding.

- A combination of chemotherapy, either EMA-CO or methuotrexate and folinic acid chemotherapy is indicated.

Surgical treatment

- Surgery is indicated if profuse vaginal or intraperitoneal haemorrhage occurs and cannot be managed conservatively.
- Hysterectomy may be indicated for intramyometrial invasion.

How long should patients be followed up after evacuation of hydatidiform mole?

- Patients whose β-hCG became normal, i.e. <5 IU/l by the 56th day post-evacuation (8 weeks) have little or no risk of late recurrence.
- More than half of patients will have a fall of β-hCG to normal by the 56th day post-evacuation and they may be followed up for a period of 6 months only, after which a further pregnancy is not contraindicated.
- The risk of subsequent relapse in this group is of the order of <1 in 2000.
- The risk of a second hydatidiform mole is 1 in 76 and a third is 1 in 6.

Oral contraception following trophoblastic
disease (E.S. Newlands, personal communication)

- All forms of exogenous hormones should be avoided until the hCG is clearly normal. This is because taking exogenous hormones when the hCG is raised means that the proportion of patients needing chemotherapy goes up from 7–8 per cent to 30 per cent (a significant increase over a very large database of over 20 000 patients).
- Once the hCG is clearly normal, there is no contraindication to patients going onto oral contraceptives or, later in life, going onto hormone replacement therapy (HRT).
- There is controversy between the data from the UK, which are from a larger database with a more conservative policy of treating patients with chemotherapy, and data from the USA. The main difference between the data from the two sides of the Atlantic is that policy in the USA is for all patients to be given chemotherapy if the hCG is not normal by 8 weeks following evacuation of their molar

pregnancy. In the USA a higher proportion of patients are treated than in the more conservative approach adopted in the UK.

REFERENCES

1 Hill, L.M., Guzick, D. & Fries, J. (1990) Fetal loss rate after ultrasonically documented cardiac activity between 6 and 24 weeks menstrual age. *Journal of Clinical Ultrasound*, **19**, 221–223.

2 Rosevear, S. (1999) Bleeding in early pregnancy. In: *High Risk Pregnancy, Management Options*, (eds D.K. James, P.J. Steer, C.P. Weiner & B. Gonik), 2nd edn, pp. 61–89. Harcourt Brace, London.

3 Nielsen, S. & Hahlin, M. (1995) Expectant management of first-trimester spontaneous abortion. *The Lancet*, **345**, 84–86.

4 Blohm, F., Hahlin, M., Nielsen, S. & Milsom, I. (1997) Fertility after a randomised trial of spontaneous abortion managed by surgical evacuation or expectant treatment. *The Lancet*, **349**, 995.

5 Nielsen, S., Hartkainen-Sorri A.-L., Oja, H. & von Wendt, L. (1999) Randomised trial comparing expectant with medical management for first trimester miscarriages. *British Journal of Obstetrics and Gynaecology*, **106**, 804–807.

6 Knudsen, U.B., Hansen, V., Juul, S. & Secher, N.J. (1991) Prognosis of a new pregnancy following previous spontaneous abortions. *European Journal of Obstetrics and Gynaecology*, **39**, 31–36.

7 Stray-Pedersen, B. & Stray-Pedersen, S. (1984) Etiologic factors and subsequent reproductive performance in 195 couples with a prior history of habitual abortion. *American Journal of Obstetrics and Gynecology*, **148**, 140–146.

8 Tharapel, A.T., Tharapel, S.A. & Bannerman, R.M. (1985) Recurrent pregnancy losses and parental chromosome abnormalities: a review. *British Journal of Obstetrics and Gynaecology*, **92**, 899–914.

9 Heinonen, P.K., Saarikoski, S. & Pystynen, P. (1982) Reproductive performance of women with uterine anomalies. *Acta Obstetrica Gynecologica Scandinavica*, **61**, 157–162.

10 Wilson, W.A., Gharavi, T.K., Lockshin, M.D. *et al.* (1999) International consensus statement on preliminary classification criteria for definite antiphospholipid syndrome. *Arthritis and Rheumatism*, **42**, 1309–1311.

11 Pattison, N.S., Chamley, L.W., Birdsall, M., Zanderigo, A.M., Liddell, H.S. & McDougall, J. (2000) Does aspirin have a role in improving pregnancy outcome for women with antiphospholipid syndrome? A randomised controlled trial. *American Journal of Obstetrics and Gynecology*, **183**, 1008–1012.

12 Clifford, K., Rai, R. & Regan, L. (1997) Future pregnancy outcome in unexplained recurrent first trimester miscarriage. *Human Reproduction*, **12**, 387–389.

13 Brigham, S.A., Conlon, C. & Farquharson, R.G. (1999) A longitudinal study of pregnancy outcome following idiopathic recurrent miscarriage. *Human Reproduction*, **14**, 2868–2871.

14 Clifford, K., Rai, R., Watson, H. & Regan, L. (1994) An informative protocol for the investigation of recurrent miscarriage: preliminary experience of 500 consecutive cases. *Human Reproduction*, **9**, 1328–1332.

15 Regan, L., Braude, P.R. & Trenbath, P.L. (1989) Influence of past reproductive performance on risk of spontaneous abortion. *British Medical Journal*, **299**, 541–545.

16 Lee, C. & Slade, P. (1996) Miscarriage as a traumatic event: a review of the literature and implications for intervention. *Journal of Psychosomatic Research*, **40**, 232–245.

17 Joint Working Group of the British Blood Transfusion Society and the Royal College of Obstetricians and Gynaecologists (1999) Recommendations for the use of anti-D immunoglobulin for rhesus prophylaxis. *Transfusion Medicine*, **9**, 93–97.

18 Yao, M. & Tulandi, T. (1997) Current status of surgical and non-surgical management of ectopic pregnancy. *Fertility and Sterility*, **67**, 421–433.

19 Fernandez, H., Laidier, C., Thouvenez, V. & Frydman, R. (1994) The use of a pre-therapeutic, predictive score to determine inclusion criteria for the non-surgical treatment of ectopic pregnancy. *Human Reproduction*, **6**, 995–998.

20 Chapron, C., Pouly, J.L., Wattiez, A. *et al.* (1993) Laparoscopic management of tubal ectopic pregnancy. *European Journal of Obstetrics, Gynecology and Reproductive Biology*, **49**, 73–79.

21 Pouly, J.L., Chapron, C. & Manhes, H. (1991) Multifactorial analysis of fertility after conservative laparoscopic treatment of ectopic pregnancy in a series of 223 patients. *Fertility and Sterility*, **56**, 453–460.

22 Royal College of Obstetricians and Gynaecologists (1997) Induced abortion clinical 'Greentop' guidelines. No.11, July 1997. RCOG, London.

23 Spitz, I.M., Bardin, C.W., Benton, L. & Robbins, A. (1998) Early pregnancy termination with mifepristone and misoprostol in the United States. *New England Journal of Medicine*, **338**, 1241–1247.

24 UK Multicentre Study: final results (1997) The efficacy and tolerance of mifepristone and prostaglandin in termination of pregnancy of less than 63 days' gestation. *Contraception*, **55**, 1–5.

25 Henshaw, R.C., Naji, S.A., Russell, I.T. & Templeton, A.A. (1994) A comparison of medical abortion (using mifepristone and gemeprost) with surgical vacuum aspiration: efficacy and early medical sequelae. *Human Reproduction*, **9**, 2167–2172.

26 World Health Organisation Task Force on Post-ovulatory Methods of Fertility Regulation (1993) Termination of pregnancy with reduced doses of mifepristone. *British Medical Journal*, **307**, 532–537.

27 Jannet, D., Aflak, N., Abankwa, A., Corbonne, B., Marpeau, L. & Milliez,

J. (1996) Termination of second and third trimester pregnancies with mifepristone and misoprostol. *European Journal of Obstetrics, Gynecology and Reproductive Biology*, **70**, 159–163.

28 Sawaya, G., Grady, D., Kerlikowske, K. & Grimes, D. (1996) Antibiotics at the time of induced abortion: the case for universal prophylaxis based on a meta-analysis. *Obstetrics and Gynecology*, **87**, 884–890.

29 MacKenzie, I.Z. (1999) Labour induction including pregnancy termination for fetal anomaly. In: *High Risk Pregnancy, Management Options* (eds D.K. James, P.J. Steer, C.P. Weiner & B. Gonik), 2nd edn, pp. 1079–1101. Harcourt Brace, London.

30 Benedet, J.L., Bender, H., Jones III, H., Ngan, H.Y.S. & Pecorelli, S. (FIGO Committee on Gynecologic Oncology) (2000) FIGO staging classifications and clinical practice guidelines in the management of gynecological cancers. *International Journal of Gynecology and Obstetrics*, **70**, 209–262.

31 Newlands, E.S., Bagshaw, K.D., Bergent, R.H.J., Rustin, G.J.S. & Holden, L. (1991) Results with the EMA/CO (etoposide, methotrexate, actinomycin D, cyclophosphamide, vincristine) regimen in high risk gestational trophoblastic tumours (1979–1989). *British Journal of Obstetrics and Gynaecology*, **98**, 550–557.

32 Bagshaw, K.D. (1976) Risk and prognostic factors in trophoblastic neoplasia. *Cancer*, **38**, 1373–1385.

3 Cervical Screening and Premalignant Disease of the Cervix

The cervical smear is a screening test of asymptomatic women with the object of detecting treatable preinvasive squamous abnormalities of the cervix. Screening with the cervical smear can prevent up to 93 per cent of cases of invasive carcinoma of the cervix.

PREVENTION

Primary prevention of cervical cancer

- Delay of age of sexual intercourse.
- Use of barrier methods of contraception in addition for control of viral load (protects the vulnerable squamocolumnar junction especially in the young).
- Bilateral monogamy.

Secondary prevention of cervical cancer

- Education for cervical screening to target under-screened populations.
- Improvement of sensitivity and specificity of screening for the precursors of cervical cancer.

SCREENING FOR CERVICAL CANCER

- Regular screening should commence at age 20 years in women who have had sexual intercourse.
- A further smear is taken 1 year after the first smear and then at 3-yearly screening intervals, or if the gap from her last smear has been more than 5 years.
- Screening may cease at the age of 70 years in a woman with a history of normal cervical smears.

• No further smear needs to be done in women who have had a hysterectomy for benign conditions with a history of normal smears and where the cervix, completely removed, histologically is normal.

• Women who have had a total abdominal hysterectomy (TAH) with histological evidence of a high grade lesion, should have annual vault smears until the age of 70 years. If the lesions has been low grade, 3-yearly screening is adequate.

• Immunosuppressed women should have yearly smears.

• If a cervical smear is negative in the presence of symptoms and signs suggestive of cervical cancer, further gynaecological investigation should be carried out.

3

Reporting of cervical cytology

Reports should indicate:
• The adequacy of the specimen
• A general categorisation as to whether the smear is within normal limits or not
• A descriptive diagnosis.

An abnormal smear refers to all smears showing epithelial cell abnormalities that may need further management, including atypical squamous cells of undetermined significance (ASCUS) and atypical glandular cells of undetermined significance (AGUS), but not including benign cellular changes, i.e. infection and reactive epithelial cell changes.

The Bethesda system for reporting cervical/vaginal cytological diagnoses (1991) [1]

Adequacy of the specimen
• Satisfactory for evaluation
• Satisfactory for evaluation but limited by . . . (specify reason)
• Unsatisfactory for evaluation . . . (specify reason)

General categorisation
• Within normal limits
• Benign cellular changes: see descriptive diagnosis
• Epithelial cell abnormality: see descriptive diagnosis.

Descriptive diagnosis

Benign cellular changes
Infection:
- *Trichomonas vaginalis*
- Fungal organisms morphologically consistent with *Candida*
- Predominance of coccobacilli consistent with shift in vaginal flora
- Bacteria morphologically consistent with *Actinomyces*
- Cellular changes associated with herpes simplex virus
- Other.

Reactive epithelial changes:
Reactive cellular changes associated with:
- Inflammation (includes typical repair)
- Atrophy with inflammation ('atrophic vaginitis')
- Irradiation
- Intrauterine contraceptive device
- Other.

Epithelial cell abnormalities
Squamous cell:
- Atypical squamous cells of undetermined significance (ASCUS)
Qualify: favour reactive or favour premalignant/malignant process
- Low grade squamous intraepithelial lesion (LSIL): encompassing cervical intraepithelial neoplasia (CIN) 1 and/or human papillomavirus (HPV)
- High grade squamous intraepithelial lesion (HSIL): encompassing moderate and severe dysplasia, CIN 2 and CIN 3/carcinoma in situ (CIS)
- Squamous cell carcinoma.

Glandular cell:
- Endometrial cells in a postmenopausal woman who is not on hormone replacement therapy
- Atypical glandular cells of undetermined significance (AGUS)
Qualify: favour reactive or favour premalignant/malignant process
- Endocervical adenocarcinoma in situ (AIS)
- Endocervical adenocarcinoma
- Endometrial adenocarcinoma
- Extrauterine adenocarcinoma
- Adenocarcinoma, not otherwise specified.

Other malignant neoplasms: Specify.

Interpretation of the adequacy of the smear

(1) Satisfactory but limited smear

The smear may be adequate for an evaluation, but the report is limited for a variety of reasons. These include: abundant neutrophils or blood obscuring 50–75 per cent of the squamous cells present, poor fixation, scanty squamous cells or the presence of cytolysis. Although the quality of the smear is limited, enough clearly visible squamous cells are present for a report to be satisfactory. The absence of an endocervical cell component is also included in this category, but evidence suggests that there is no increase in the incidence of abnormality in this group of women, so the usual 3-yearly screening interval can prevail.

Follow-up for satisfactory but limited smears should be as if the smear result is normal. If there has been an abnormal smear within the previous 5 years (ASCUS, AGUS or CIN), the next smear should be taken at 6 months. If the smear result is abnormal, follow-up depends on the abnormality detected.

Follow-up for women who repeatedly have smears that are satisfactory but limited by information is controversial. Smears should be taken annually. Investigation should try to identify a cause for the findings, including microbiological culture.

(2) Cytolytic smear

This results from a proliferation of lactobacilli normally found in the vaginal flora. These bacteria cause a breakdown in the squamous cell cytoplasm, making detection of abnormalities difficult. Cytolysis commonly occurs in the latter part of the menstrual cycle. A further smear taken around mid-cycle will usually resolve the problem. An endocervical component includes endocervical columnar glandular cells and/or metaplastic squamous cells, and indicates that the transformation zone has been sampled, which is the area most at risk of metaplastic and malignant change. It is an indicator of good smear-taking technique. An endocervical component may never be obtained in some women, particularly those postmenopausal or women who have had previous surgery to the cervix. There is no clear evidence that women whose smears lack an endocervical component are at greater risk of concurrent or subsequent abnormalities than women whose smears contain an endocervical component [2].

(3) Unsatisfactory smear

- Insufficient squamous epithelial cells
- Poor fixation
- Marked cytolysis
- Abundant neutrophils or blood obscuring more than 75 per cent of the squamous cells present.

Smears repeated at short time intervals are less likely to detect significant lesions.

Follow-up of unsatisfactory smears should be repeated at 1–3 months, ideally around mid-cycle. Referral for colposcopy should be considered after three consecutive unsatisfactory smears.

DIAGNOSES

Reactive epithelial changes (inflammation/repair)

Inflammation of the cervix is common and some neutrophils are present in most cervical smears. When they are abundant the squamous cell component may be obscured, resulting in satisfactory but limited smears or unsatisfactory smears. Inflammatory smears may be associated with a specific infectious agent, e.g. *Candida*. The organisms may be apparent in the smear, but in many women specific microbiological culture will be required to identify them.

The presence of inflammatory cells may or may not be associated with reactive epithelial cell changes. These reactive cells can usually be distinguished from dysplastic cells. If there is any doubt the smear will be reported as showing atypia of undetermined significance, with a comment as to whether a reactive or neoplastic process is favoured. The term 'inflammatory smear' should be avoided because of the confusion as to whether the term refers to smears with abundant and obscuring neutrophils, or to smears showing reactive epithelial cell changes.

Follow-up

If the smear shows reactive epithelial cell changes the next smear should be obtained at the normal screening interval. Repeated satisfactory smears with reactive epithelial changes are not an indication to repeat the smear early or to refer for colposcopy.

Some infections occasionally induce epithelial cell changes which can be difficult to distinguish from dysplasia. In these cases the laboratory may report the smear as showing atypical cells of undetermined significance and recommend another smear after treatment of the infection.

Atypical cells of undetermined significance

Atypical squamous cells of undetermined significance

This defines a variety of squamous cellular changes which cannot be specifically classified. They are usually more than a benign reactive process, but are insufficient for a diagnosis of HPV or squamous intraepithelial lesion (SIL). For women with a persisting ASCUS lesion, a significant number show SIL on colposcopic biopsy which is usually low grade but may be high grade. In a small number of smears, there are specific cell changes that are suspicious of high grade SIL, while not diagnostic (ASCUS – possible HSIL). These smears should be specifically identified in the cytology report with a recommendation for referral for colposcopy.

Atypical glandular cells of undetermined significance

These are glandular cells which demonstrate changes exceeding those normally expected in a benign reactive process, but which are insufficient for a diagnosis of AIS. The atypical cells are usually identified as endocervical or endometrial in origin. Smears showing 'equivocal AIS' should be reported as AGUS with features suggestive of AIS. The concept of a precursor lesion to AIS, i.e. endocervical glandular dysplasia, is controversial. In follow-up studies of women who have 'atypical endocervical cell reports', squamous lesions are the most common abnormalities detected on biopsy.

Endocervical adenocarcinoma (in situ or invasive) is found in a minority of cases.

Figure 3.1 shows recommendations for follow-up.

Cervical dysplasia

Low grade squamous intraepithelial lesion

This category includes CIN 1 (mild dysplasia) and/or a definite diagnosis of HPV – the cytological distinction between HPV alone and HPV with CIN 1 can be difficult.

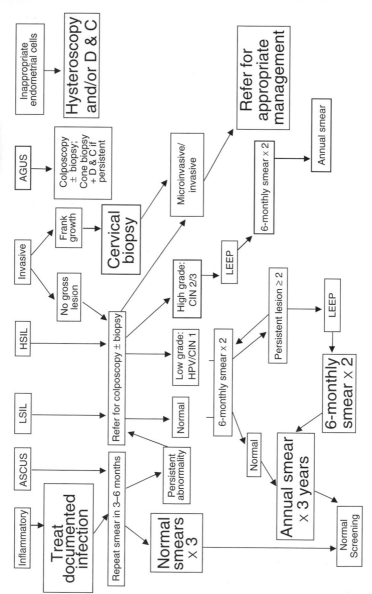

Fig. 3.1 Management of the abnormal cervical smear. LEEP, loop electrosurgical excision procedure [3].

Discriminating the cytological abnormality may be subjective and this is most marked with low grade abnormalities [4].

A proportion of smears reported as LSIL will have histologically proven high grade abnormalities.

There is a high spontaneous regression rate of LSILs. Therefore, a low grade abnormality should have a further smear taken at 6 months. If that smear is abnormal then referral for colposcopy is recommended. More than half of LSILs are reported to regress spontaneously. Follow-up is by 6-monthly smears and annual colposcopy if they remain abnormal. Treatment is indicated if there is persistence or progression.

After treatment for LSIL, annual smears for life after a diagnosis are not necessary. A 3-yearly screening interval is satisfactory provided there have been three normal smears after the diagnosis and/or treatment of the low grade abnormality [5].

Once 3-yearly screening is established, if there are further abnormal smears they are managed as a new episode of abnormality. Colposcopy is recommended the first time a follow-up smear shows LSIL if there has been no treatment for a previous LSIL.

High grade squamous intraepithelial lesion

This category includes CIN 2 and CIN 3 (moderate dysplasia, severe dysplasia/carcinoma in situ).

All women whose smears indicate HSIL should be referred for colposcopy. If the colposcopic examination of the cervix shows no sign of any abnormality, the whole genital tract should be reviewed with careful clinical inspection and colposcopy of the entire lower genital tract to identify the site of origin of the dysplastic cells.

Long-term follow-up after histologically confirmed diagnosis of HSIL and treatment is annual smears until the age of 70. If any further abnormal smears occur the woman should be referred again for colposcopy.

Any woman with a history of high grade vulval or vaginal intraepithelial neoplasia (VIN, VAIN) should have annual cervical or vaginal vault smears until the age of 70.

High grade glandular lesions, adenocarcinoma in situ (AIS)

These lesions require a cone biopsy for diagnosis to exclude carcinoma.

Carcinoma

Women whose smears show squamous carcinoma, adenocarcinoma or any other malignant neoplasm should be referred immediately to an experienced colposcopist for tissue diagnosis and treatment. Long-term follow-up for women treated for invasive carcinoma should be on the recommendations of a gynaecological oncologist.

Treatment methods for histologically confirmed high grade lesions [6,7]

(1) Ablative therapy. This method requires thorough colposcopic examination and biopsy so that any suspicion of invasion is completely excluded. Ablative therapy does not enable a sample of tissue to be reviewed histologically. Ablative therapy may be by electro-coagulation, needle diathermy, cryocautery (has the lowest rate of postoperative bleeding) or laser.

(2) Excision biopsy. The efficacy of all three methods is similar. In general these techniques are preferable because tissue is available for histological examination. This is especially important because up to 2–3 per cent of specimens ablated may be unexpectedly an AIS or microinvasive carcinoma.

   (a) Loop excision (large loop excision of the transformation zone, LLETZ).

   (b) Laser conisation.

   (c) Cold knife cone biopsy – this is indicated where the whole lesion cannot be visualised or if there is a suspicion of invasive disease. If the canal is involved, a LLETZ procedure can raise doubt as to whether excision is complete if there is abnormality extending to the zone of thermal artefact on the edge of the specimen.

(3) Hysterectomy. This is a possibility for women with both a cervical abnormality and other gynaecological pathology. It may be the best management for persistent or recurrent disease in women who have completed childbearing. Ideally the hysterectomy should be done vaginally.

Risk factors for persistent disease

- Lesions affecting more than two thirds of the surface of the cervix (19 times the risk). The following gave twice the risk:

- Age over 30 years
- Positivity for HPV 16 or 18
- Previous treatment of CIN.

Follow-up after treatment

A cervical smear and colposcopy should be done 4–6 months after treatment.

Colposcopy enables the early diagnosis of treatment of failures in the presence of false-negative smears.

Women who have had a total hysterectomy and who at any time in the past have had histological evidence of a high grade lesion should be followed with annual vaginal vault smears until aged 70 years. Those who have had histological evidence of CIN 1 should have 3-yearly vaginal vault cytology until the age of 70.

Women who have had a total hysterectomy for a benign condition with no histological evidence of cervical dysplasia or malignancy, either previously or in the hysterectomy specimen, do not require vaginal vault cytology.

HPV DNA typing may be useful to identify which group of women with dysplastic disease, particularly with HSIL or ASCUS, are at higher risk of an invasive lesion on the basis of the HPV viral type. Studies applying the technology to population screening are awaited. HPV develops in approximately two thirds of all people who have sexual contact with an infected partner, usually within 3 months. There are over 70 different types of HPV. Forty affect the urogenital area. HPV types 6 and 11 are low risk types. HPV types 16, 18, 31 and 45 are high risk types and account for more than 80 per cent of all invasive cervical cancers. Up to 50 per cent of all sexually active women have DNA evidence of HPV infection. Infection lasts on average 8 months with 70 per cent disappearing at 1 year. It is not clear why some individuals have lesions which clear spontaneously while others persist with progression to invasive cancer [8,9].

Complications of treatment of high grade lesions

- Post-operative bleeding and infection
- Persistent or recurrent disease.

Treatment of CIN can impair fertility by:

- Cervical stenosis

- Decreased volume of cervical mucus
- Cervical incompetence
- Tubal scarring induced by post-treatment infection.

Cold knife cone biopsy can increase the risk of second trimester miscarriage, breech presentation and low birth weight babies, because a greater amount of tissue is removed. The amount of tissue removed by laser, cryotherapy and LLETZ is small, so that these techniques usually have no adverse effect on pregnancy. Risks are increased if biopsies are very large or second and third procedures have been done for recurrent or persistent dysplasia [10].

Carcinoma of the cervix develops if dysplasia is left untreated. Figure 3.2 shows the probability of patients remaining free of invasive carcinoma comparing group 1 (n = 817 women) with normal

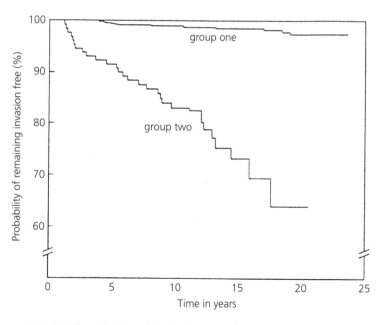

Fig. 3.2 The probability of the development of invasive carcinoma in two groups of women. Group 1 had normal follow-up cytology after a diagnosis of carcinoma in situ, and group 2 had abnormal cytology after a diagnosis of CIS. (With permission from McIndoe *et al.* (1984) [11].)

cytology follow-up after a diagnosis of carcinoma in situ of the cervix and a second group of 131 women who continued to have abnormal cytology [10]. Of the original 948 women, 41 (4.3 per cent) women with CIS developed invasive carcinoma of the cervix when followed from 5 to 28 years, but only 12 (1.5 per cent) of the 817 women with normal cytology follow-up after diagnosis and treatment subsequently developed invasive carcinomas.

In group 1 (normal cytology to follow-up), 12 (1.5 per cent) developed invasive carcinoma, and in group 2, 29 (22 per cent) developed invasive carcinoma of the cervix or vaginal vault.

From these data it may be concluded that follow-up gives an incidence rate of 0.89 for normal cytology and 16.64 per 10 000 women months respectively for abnormal cytology for invasive carcinoma. The relative risk is therefore 18.78 with abnormal follow-up cytology compared to normal. This provides conclusive evidence for the necessity for treatment of cervical dysplasia to avoid the natural progression to carcinoma of the cervix.

Recurrence of CIS occurred in 6 of the 817 women (0.7 per cent). Of the 139 group 1 patients with incomplete excision of the original lesion, only 5 (3.5 per cent) later developed invasive carcinoma.

Patients with normal follow-up cytology after treatment of CIS of the cervix are 3.2 times more likely to develop invasive cervical or vaginal vault carcinoma, compared with those women who have never had CIS of the cervix.

In the second group of patients with continuing abnormal cytology follow-up after an initial diagnosis, invasive carcinoma developed in 29 of 131 (22 per cent) of patients followed from 5 to 19 years. These women with continuing abnormal cytology are 24.8 times more likely to develop invasive carcinoma than women of the same age with normal cytology after diagnosis.

Regression of CIS only occurred in 5 per cent naturally. Figure 3.2 indicates that women with cytological evidence of continuing neoplasia after an initial diagnosis of CIS of the cervix have an 18 per cent chance of developing invasive carcinoma of the cervix or vaginal vault at 10 years and a 36 per cent chance at 20 years [11].

The data in Table 3.1 show that excision or ablation of high grade dysplasia reduces the risk of invasive cancer of the cervix by 95 per cent for the following 8 years after treatment [12]. However, even with careful long-term follow-up the risk of invasive cervical cancer among these women is about five times greater than that amongst

Table 3.1 The rate of invasive disease and duration of the risk of developing invasive cervical cancer after ablative or excisional techniques for CIN. (Soutter *et al.* (1997) [12].)

Women years of follow-up	44 699
Observation for 8 years	2116
Women with invasive cancer	33
Microinvasion	14
Cumulative rate of invasion 8 years after treatment	5.8 per 1000 women
Rate of invasive cancer during this period	85 (95% CI 60–119) per 100 000 women years

the general population of women throughout that period. This is why careful annual follow-up is essential after excision or ablative techniques (i.e. not hysterectomy) for high grade lesions.

Loop diathermy may result in an inappropriately short biopsy being taken in older women who may have more severe disease higher up in the endocervical canal. Cold knife cone biopsy, with histologically identifiable margins clear of the high grade lesions, may be a better form of treatment for older women.

Cervical glandular neoplasia

Glandular neoplastic lesions of the cervix include cervical intra-epithelial glandular neoplasia (CIGN) and invasive adenocarcinoma of the cervix. Mostly they are diagnosed on smear. Colposcopy is always indicated. If the smear shows malignant glandular cells, a cone biopsy and endometrial sampling is always indicated. With a low grade lesion there is always a risk of undetected lesion in the endocervical canal. Conisation is an acceptable form of treatment providing the resection margins are clear. If excision margins are involved, a repeat cone is indicated or if fertility is not desired, a hysterectomy. After hysterectomy, follow-up with vault smears should be done.

REFERENCES

1 Anonymous (1993) The Bethesda system for reporting cervical/vaginal cytologic diagnoses: revised after the 2nd National Cancer Institute Workshop, April 29–30, 1991. *Acta Cytologica*, **37**(2), 115–124.

2 Mitchell, H. & Medley, G. (1993) Cytological reporting of cervical abnormalities according to endocervical status. *British Journal of Cancer*, **67**, 585–588.

3 Benedet, J.L., Bender, H., Jones III, H., Ngan, H.Y.S. & Pecorelli, S. (FIGO Committee on Gynecologic Oncology) (2000) FIGO staging classifications and clinical practice guidelines in the management of gynecological cancers. *International Journal of Gynecology and Obstetrics*, **70**, 209–262.

4 Ismail, S.M., Colclough, A.B., Dinnen, J.S. *et al.* (1989) Observer variation in histopathological diagnosis and grading of cervical intraepithelial neoplasia. *British Medical Journal*, **298**, 707–710.

5 Macgregor, J.E., Campbell, M.K., Mann, E.M.F. & Swanson, K.Y. (1994) Screening for cervical intraepithelial neoplasia in North East Scotland shows fall in incidence and mortality from invasive cancer with concomitant rise in preinvasive disease. *British Medical Journal*, **308**, 1407–1411.

6 Mitchell, M.F., Tortelero-Luna, G., Cook, H., Whittaker, L., Rhodes-Morris, H. & Silva, E. (1990) A randomised clinical trial of cryotherapy, loop electrosurgical excision for treatment of squamous intraepithelial lesions of the cervix. *Obstetrics and Gynecology*, **92**, 737–744.

7 Flannelly, G., Langhan, H., Jandial, L., Mann, E., Campbell, M. & Kitchener, H. (1997) A study of treatment failures following large loop excision of the transformation zone for the treatment of cervical intraepithelial neoplasia. *British Journal of Obstetrics and Gynaecology*, **104**, 718–722.

8 Ylitalo, N., Sorensen, P., Josefsson, A.M. *et al.* (2000) Consistent high viral load of human papillomavirus 16 and risk of cervical carcinoma in situ: a nested case-control study. *The Lancet*, **355**, 2194–2198.

9 Manos, M.M., Kinney, W.K., Hurley, L.B. *et al.* (1999) Identifying women with cervical neoplasia using human papillomavirus DNA testing for equivocal Papanicolaou results. *Journal of the American Medical Association*, **281**, 1605–1610.

10 Montz, F.J. (1996) Impact of therapy for cervical intraepithelial neoplasia on fertility. *American Journal of Obstetrics and Gynecology*, **175**, 1129–1136.

11 McIndoe, W.A., McLean, M.R., Jones, R.W. & Mullins, P.R. (1984) The invasive potential of carcinoma in situ of the cervix. *Obstetrics and Gynecology*, **64**, 451–458.

12 Soutter, W.P., deBarros Lopes, A., Fletcher, A. *et al.* (1997) Invasive cervical cancer after conservative therapy for cervical intraepithelial neoplasia. *The Lancet*, **349**, 978–980.

4 Gynaecological Endocrinology

POLYCYSTIC OVARY SYNDROME

Polycystic ovary syndrome (PCOS) is a heterogeneous disorder with variable clinical and endocrine features. There is no universally agreed definition or criteria. The diagnosis of PCOS is made when, in addition to the ultrasound finding of polycystic ovaries, there are associated symptoms (menstrual irregularity, hyperandrogenisation, obesity) or endocrine abnormalities (raised serum luteinising hormone (LH) and testosterone concentrations) [1].

Symptoms [2,3]

- Obesity – up to 40 per cent
- Acne, hirsutism and alopecia – 70 per cent
- Irregular periods and oligomenorrhoea (cycle interval longer than 35 days but less than 6 months)/amenorrhoea (no menstruation for more than 6 months) – up to 70 per cent
- Subfertility – inhibition of production of insulin-like growth factor 1 (IGF1) binding protein results in an increased concentration of circulating free IGF1, further enhancing ovarian androgen production. IGF potentiates the action of follicle-stimulating hormone (FSH) in granulosa cells. It may initiate or perpetuate the ovulatory dysfunction in PCOS.
- Alopecia
- Acanthosis nigrans.

Features of the endocrine and metabolic disturbance in PCOS

- Hyperinsulinaemia. Obese women (body mass index, BMI >30 kg/m^2) with PCOS hypersecrete insulin which stimulates ovarian secretion of androgens and is associated with hirsutism, menstrual disturbance and infertility [4]. Measure fasting insulin levels. Raised serum concentrations of insulin are commoner in women with PCOS compared with weight-matched controls. Hyperinsulinaemia is the key to the pathogenesis of this syndrome because insulin stimulates androgen secretion by the ovarian theca and seems to affect the normal development of ovarian follicles, through the adverse effects of androgens on follicular growth. It also may suppress apoptosis, enabling survival of follicles that would have otherwise disappeared.

- Genetic studies have revealed abnormalities both in the steroidogenic pathway for androgen biosynthesis and in the regulation of expression of the insulin gene. The locus that regulates insulin gene expression is an insulin gene minisatellite, known as the insulin variable number of tandem repeats (INS VNTR) on chromosome 11p15.5. It is associated with hyperinsulinaemia, higher birth weight and susceptibility to non-insulin-dependent diabetes mellitus.

- Insulin excess augments the pituitary LH response to gonadotrophin-releasing hormone (GnRH) and amplifies androgen bioactivity by decreasing the hepatic production of sex hormone-binding globulin (SHBG).

- Elevated mid-follicular phase LH (day 8 ± 1 IU/l/day) (LH > 10 IU/l in >40 per cent) may occur.

- Elevated testosterone >3.0 nmol/l (mean and 95th percentiles 2.6 (1.1–4.8) nmol/l). If levels are >4.8 nmol/l, exclude androgen-secreting tumours of the ovary or adrenal gland, Cushing's syndrome and congenital adrenal hyperplasia. Give dexamethasone 1 mg at 23.00 hours followed by measurement of plasma cortisol at 09.00 hours. Normal values of cortisol are 180–800 nmol/l. Suppression of plasma cortisol below 150 nmol/l excludes a diagnosis of Cushing's syndrome.

- Oestrogen levels in PCOS are usually normal (>100 pmol/l).

- Elevated prolactin.

- BMI >30 kg/m^2 correlates with increased hirsutism, serum testosterone concentration, cycle disturbance and sub-fertility. These women should lose weight and the symptoms will improve.

- Assess glucose tolerance (the incidence of diabetes in obese women with PCOS is 11 per cent).

- Eating disorders may be due to a link with leptin, which affects the hypothalamic pulsatility of GnRH.

Ultrasound findings in PCOS

- Enlarged ovaries (volume of >9 ml) with ≥10 cysts 2–8 mm in diameter, in one plane usually peripherally situated with an echo-dense thickened central stroma.

- Ovarian volume ($\frac{4}{3}\Pi$ ($\frac{1}{2}$ diameter)^3) where the diameter is the mean of the height, width and depth of the ovary in the absence of a dominant follicle.
- Transvaginal ultrasonography is indicated because transabdominal ultrasound may miss up to 30 per cent of cases of PCOS.
- Polycystic ovaries are an inherited phenotype found in about 20 per cent of healthy women. They are present in over 90 per cent of women with hirsutism and in 75 per cent of women with anovulatory infertility.
- An endometrial thickness of >5 mm indicates adequate oestrogenisation. If it is >15 mm, a withdrawal bleed should be induced and if the endometrium fails to shed, an endometrial sample taken to exclude endometrial hyperplasia.

Basis for treatment strategies of PCOS

BMI should be normalised. An increased rate of hirsutism, cycle disturbance and infertility is correlated with a raised BMI. The incidence of diabetes in obese women with PCOS is 11 per cent. Weight loss improves the symptoms of PCOS and improves the patient's endocrine profile [5], particularly by reducing hyperinsulinaemia and hyperandrogenism. Weight loss should be encouraged prior to ovulation induction treatment (see Chapter 5 for ovulation induction in PCOS where cycles are anovulatory).

Women with PCOS are not oestrogen deficient. Treatment depends on symptoms being complained about. Those with amenorrhoea are not at risk of osteoporosis, but are at risk of endometrial hyperplasia or adenocarcinoma. Cycle control and regular withdrawal bleeding may be managed with the oral contraceptive pill but a raised BMI has always been a contraindication because of the risk of venous thromboembolism. The combined oral contraceptive (COC) pill suppresses serum testosterone concentrations and improves hirsutism and acne. Ethinyloestradiol combined with cyproterone acetate is most suitable.

HIRSUTISM

Treatment – general

- Weight reduction can lead to re-establishment of regular menstrual cycles.

- Bleaching with hydrogen peroxide removes hair pigments.
- Temporary methods of removing hair include plucking, shaving, waxing and depilatory creams. Plucking encourages hair growth and may cause folliculitis. Electrolysis is the only established physical method that offers the potential for permanent hair removal. It is time-consuming, painful and expensive; regrowth occurs.
- Pharmacological treatment slows the growth of new hair but does not lead to loss of established hair.
- The degree of hirsutism may be quantified [6], but usually a semi-quantitative subjective report from the patient as to rate of growth and need for cosmesis is satisfactory to gauge the response to therapy.

Pharmacological treatment of hirsutism

1 Suppression of androgen secretion [7]

The combined oral contraceptive pill

- The COC is the drug of first choice for most women, as it has been shown to be effective in the treatment of hirsutism.
- It suppresses LH secretion and hence LH-mediated androgen secretion by the ovary.
- The oestrogen component increases the concentration of SHBG by slowing its clearance rate and so decreases the amount of free testosterone available.
- The progesterone component of the contraceptive pill gives cycle control and prevents endometrial hyperplasia.

Side effects of the COC include weight gain, nausea, emotional lability, breast tenderness. Contraindications include a past history of venous thrombosis, and obesity (BMI ≥30) because it is a risk factor for a thrombotic event. Relative contraindications include hypertension and a family history of both breast cancer and thromboembolic phenomena.

Cyproterone acetate

- Cyproterone acetate is a competitive inhibitor of dihydrotestosterone, binding to its receptor.
- It is a potent progestogen with weak corticosteroid-like effects.
- It suppresses gonadotrophin secretion and decreases ovarian androgen production.

- Because it is highly lipophilic its progestational activity is prolonged. Therefore it is given in doses of 25–100 mg on days 5–15 of the menstrual cycle combined with 20–35 µg ethinyloestradiol on days 5–25, i.e. a 'reversed sequential regimen'.
- Alternatively a COC may be used. Dianette/Diane is useful in women with mild symptoms of hirsutism. It contains 35 µg ethinyloestradiol and 2 mg cyproterone acetate.

Side effects: Cyproterone acetate is generally well tolerated. Side effects include weight gain, oedema, headache, fatigue, mood changes, reduced libido and breast tenderness. Isolated cases have been reported of hepatocellular carcinoma in patients using high doses (>200 mg per day). Conception is not recommended for 3 months after ceasing the drug because of its lipophilic nature.

GnRH analogues
- These are expensive as a first-line therapy in the treatment of hirsutism.
- They suppress ovarian hormone secretion to a greater degree than the COC alone and therefore are expected to be more effective. However, the oestrogen in the COC increases the concentration of SHBG and thus decreases the concentration of unbound testosterone.
- A GnRH analogue combined with a low-dose COC or with a postmenopausal oestrogen regimen has been shown to be more effective than either alone, although these results are not absolutely conclusive. They cannot be used long term because of the risk of osteoporosis.

2 Peripheral blockade of androgen action, androgen receptor antagonists

Two classes of drugs are used in clinical practice. The receptor competitor inhibits binding of testosterone and dihydrotestosterone (DHT) to the androgen receptor. 5α-reductase inhibitors reduce the conversion of testosterone to the more potent androgen DHT. COCs should be used with these two classes of drugs since the antiandrogen medication may adversely affect the genital development of the male fetus.

Spironolactone
- Spironolactone is an aldosterone antagonist and a potassium-sparing diuretic.

- It also has potent peripheral antiandrogen activity.
- It inhibits cytochrome P450 link enzymes involved in both ovarian and adrenal steroidogenesis. In addition to decreasing testosterone production it increases the metabolic clearance of testosterone.
- The clinical efficacy of spironolactone is dose dependent. The dosage is 50–200 mg daily with treatment being commenced at 25–50 mg.

Side effects: Polymenorrhoea due to the mild progestational activity of the drug occurs in up to 80 per cent of cases and can be avoided by giving the COC concomitantly. Gastrointestinal disturbances such as nausea, vomiting, diarrhoea and discomfort occur in about 20 per cent of women taking 200 mg per day. Neurological sequelae – headache, confusion, dizziness, breast tenderness – are not uncommon in up to 40 per cent. The diuretic action of spironolactone is rarely clinically significant. Hyperkalaemia is rarely a problem but spironolactone should be avoided in women with renal impairment and those using potassium-sparing diuretics, angiotensin-converting enzyme inhibitors or angiotensin II receptor blockers. Blood pressure and serum potassium concentration should be checked at the start of medication and regularly, particularly with high doses. Adequate contraception is obligatory.

Flutamide
- Flutamide inhibits the androgen receptor.
- A dosage of 250–375 mg/day is usual but there are reports of efficacy with a dosage as low as 62.5 mg/day. Monitoring of liver function tests is essential. Hepatoxicity, particularly with doses of 500–750 mg/day has been reported.

Finasteride
- Inhibits 5α-reductase activity which reduces the conversion of testosterone to the more potent androgen DHT.
- It primarily inhibits type II 5α-reductase activity. As hirsutism is a combination of type I and II effects, this agent is only partially effective.
- In a dose of 5 mg/day it significantly improves hirsutism without significant side effects.

Treatment of hirsutism requires time. Anagen on the face lasts 2–3 months, and changes in hair growth are only evident after 4–6 months of treatment.

Metformin [8]

- Metformin inhibits the production of hepatic glucose and enhances the sensitivity of peripheral tissue to insulin, thereby decreasing insulin secretion.
- It reduces hyperandrogenism and abnormalities of gonadotrophin secretion in women with PCOS.
- It can restore menstrual cycles, ovulation and fertility.
- Metformin (1.5–2.5 g/day, given in divided doses) elevates SHBG.

Glucocorticoid therapy

- Suppression of adrenal androgens decreases serum androgen concentrations by suppressing adrenocorticotrophic hormone (ACTH)-mediated adrenal secretion. Since many women with hirsutism from PCOS have a degree of adrenal hyperandrogenism, this may seem appropriate. However, giving an optimal dose to suppress adrenal androgen production without causing symptoms of glucocorticoid excess, such as weight gain and depression, together with the increase in insulin resistance that glucocorticoids cause make this treatment unwarranted. Even with an adrenal enzyme defect such as late onset 21-hydroxylase deficiency, peripheral blockade with antiandrogen medication is probably more beneficial unless fertility is required.

Long-term associated medical conditions with PCOS

- Hypertension
- Cardiovascular disease
- Diabetes mellitus
- Dyslipidaemia – increased low density lipoproteins (LDL), decreased high density lipoproteins (HDL) and increased triglycerides
- Endometrial carcinoma.

Screen longitudinally for diabetes, dyslipidaemia and hypertension.

OVULATION INDUCTION IN ANOVULATORY WOMEN WITH PCOS [9]

Indications

Women with anovulatory infertility and oligomenorrhoea (menses occurring at intervals of more than 35 days) need ovulation induction. Clomiphene is the drug of first choice. The dose is commenced at 25–50 mg from days 2 to 6 of the cycle and an oestradiol level measured to check for a response. When it is 500 pmol/l, an ultrasound scan should be done to look for follicular size. If there is no response to clomiphene, ovarian diathermy may be done in the first instance because this has excellent pregnancy rates, subsequently, without the risk of multiple pregnancy that occurs with the use of gonadotrophins for ovulation induction [10,11]. Occasionally a patient with PCOS has an all or nothing response to gonadotrophin stimulation. The only way to control for this is to do in vitro fertilisation (IVF) (see Chapter 5).

AMENORRHOEA (see Fig. 5.6)

4

Physiological causes of amenorrhoea are pregnancy, lactational and menopausal. Iatrogenic causes are due to exogenous hormones. Amenorrhoea may be due to anatomical causes (defects or absence of the uterus or vagina) or endocrine causes (lack of stimulation of the uterus by ovarian hormones).

Primary amenorrhoea

Normal puberty
- Cryptomenorrhoea is diagnosed by a history of monthly cyclic pain with the physical findings of a blue bulge of the imperforate hymen with or without a palpable uterus. Incision of the hymen releases fluid of chocolate consistency with normal reproductive potential.
- Vaginal atresia requires more extensive plastic surgery and use of vaginal dilators.

Abnormal puberty
- Gonadal dysgenesis: the uterus may be atretic or tiny. Gonadotrophin concentrations are typically high. Check karyotype for Y chromosome.
- Turner's syndrome (45XO): phenonotypic features include short stature, webbing of the neck, cubitus valgus, and widely spaced nipples. Congenital heart disease and hypothyroidism may occur. Some evidence of oestrogenic activity suggests a slower rate of oocyte atresia or mosaicism of karyotype.

- Kallman's syndrome: anosmia, due to the failure of secretion of normal amounts of GnRH into the hypothalamic–hypophyseal portal blood.
- Mass lesion of the pituitary such as a craniopharyngioma or granuloma.
- Androgen resistance syndrome (testicular feminisation): the gonads in such patients ought to be removed because of the high risk of malignancy.

Secondary amenorrhoea

- Psychological stress, travel, weight related: functional defects in hypothalamic function are due to a reduction in the activity of the GnRH neurones in the hypothalamus, leading to a corresponding reduction in secretion of FSH and LH. In normal women during the follicular phase of the cycle, LH is secreted from the pituitary in pulses approximately once an hour in response to hourly bursts of activity of GnRH neurones. If LH pulses occur less frequently than 2-hourly, normal follicular development and ovulation do not occur.
- Polycystic ovarian syndrome: exclude the possibility of Cushing's disease. Congenital adrenal hyperplasia (or partial) is identified by measuring 17α-hydroxyprogesterone in the follicular phase. These patients often present with pubic hair, before breast development and menarche, indicating a high testosterone level. Dexamethasone (0.25 mg at night) suppresses the testosterone.
- Hyperprolactinaemia.
- Resistant ovary syndrome: the ovaries contain many primordial follicles which are apparently resistant to the action of gonadotrophins.

PREMATURE OVARIAN FAILURE [12]

- Premature ovarian failure (POF) results because of a decreased number of follicles being formed during development or an increased rate of follicle loss (atresia) during reproductive life.
- It results in amenorrhoea, hypo-oestrogenism and elevated gonadotrophins (FSH >40 IU/l) before 40 years.
- It is a common disorder affecting approximately 1 in 100 women over 40 years of age:

15–29 years, 10 per 100000
30–39 years, 76 per 100000
40–44 years, 881 per 100000.

- Most cases are idiopathic. A cause is identified in 30 per cent.
- It is important to consider POF as a diagnosis because there are no signs or symptoms of impending ovarian failure.
- The incidence of POF with primary amenorrhoea is 10–28 per cent, and with secondary amenorrhoea it is 4–18 per cent.
- Ten per cent of women with mumps have a diffuse oophoritis that can result in ovarian atrophy and fibrosis with loss of follicular structures.
- Irradiation with a dose >6 Gy usually results in permanent ovarian failure.
- The gonads of prepubertal girls are particularly resistant to irradiation. Lateral transposition of the ovary prior to irradiation maintains normal ovarian function.
- Cyclophosphamide is gonadotoxic, leading to early depletion of follicles. Gonadotrophin-releasing hormone agonist (GnRHa) may protect the ovary from cyclophosphamide-induced damage as indicated in a prospective randomised controlled trial.

POF and fertility

- POF may be intermittent, and particularly early on, the occasional ovulation may occur.
- Not all cases are permanent or irreversible. The COC pill should be offered to women with POF who do not wish for pregnancy, since the lifetime chance of conception in women with karyotypically normal spontaneous POF is approximately 10–15 per cent.
- No treatment is proven to improve spontaneous chances of fertility.
- Assisted reproductive techniques (donor oocyte) are the only definitive management for POF.
- Psychological support is very important when the diagnosis was unexpected with an incompleted family.
- Women with POF need hormone replacement therapy (HRT) for the oestrogen deficiency, to protect against osteoporosis and cardiovascular disease.
- Consideration should be given to androgen replacement in women who have persistent symptoms of poor libido and decreased energy.

Further investigations in POF

- It frequently is familial with a dominant maternal and/or paternal transmission with incomplete penetrance. The long arm (Xq) of the X chromosome may be affected. Turner's syndrome (karyotype 45XO) results in rapid depletion of ovarian follicles before puberty. Studies have indicated the gene (*POF1*), localised to either Xq21.3-q27 or Xq62.1-q27, is responsible for ovarian failure [13]. Women carrying one X chromosome with a fragile X premutation are at increased risk of premature menopause (ten times). Screening of women with POF for fragile X premutations will identify 3 per cent of women with the sporadic form of POF and 13 per cent with familial POF (the expected prevalence is 1 in 590).
- Exclude other causes of autoimmune disease such as Addison's disease, myasthenia gravis, diabetes mellitus and hypothyroidism.

ANOREXIA NERVOSA

This is a complex psychosomatic eating disorder primarily affecting adolescent girls and young women. Its incidence in Western cultures is 0.5 per cent amongst young women. Up to 95 per cent of women with anorexia nervosa are typically white and middle to upper-middle socioeconomic status. Anorexia nervosa is distinguished by a refusal to maintain the minimal normal body weight for age and height (i.e. loss of weight of >15 per cent weight for height), an intense fear of gaining weight or becoming fat, while being under-weight, a disturbance in the way in which one's weight or shape is perceived, and amenorrhoea for at least three consecutive menstrual cycles in postmenarchal women.

There are two types of anorexic women:

(1) The restricting type that are quite controlled of their behaviour. They fast and undergo excessive exercise. There is a preoccupation with food and its avoidance becomes an obsession to the exclusion of other activities.

(2) The bulimic anorexic. These women tend to be more distressed, depressed, overtly angry and impulsive. Binge eating and purging are regular behaviours as well as self-induced vomiting. They may misuse laxatives, diuretics, diet pills, enemas or even thyroid medication.

Endocrine mechanisms of amenorrhoea

Amenorrhoea in anorexia nervosa is a result of hypothalamic dysfunction. Gonadotrophin concentrations are low, together with low oestrogen levels caused by inhibition of GnRH pulsatility, a blunted response of LH to GnRH and diminished pulsatile release of LH, loss of feedback effect of oestrogen and multifollicular changes in the ovary, resulting in failure of follicle selection and dominance.

Oestrogen metabolism – the effects of anorexia

- Aromatisation of androgens to oestrogens occurs in adipose tissue. Because of the loss of body fat there is a severe lack of adipose tissue, leading to a decrease in aromatisation.
- There is a shift in oestrogen metabolism from the active form of oestradiol towards catecholoestrogen, which has no direct oestrogenic activity. Catecholoestrogen competes with catecholamine for the enzyme chol-O-methyltransferase. This competition may cause an increase in dopamine secretion. Dopamine is a known inhibitor of GnRH pulsatility, which ultimately will have a negative effect on oestrogen production.
- Hypo-oestrogenism results in a decrease in size and volume of breasts, uterus and ovaries.
- Osteoporosis leads to a low bone mass with an increase in the occurrence of fractures with minimal stress. It may not be fully reversible. Adolescence is the critical time for bone mineral accretion as more than half of the bone calcium in an individual is normally laid down during these years. Once 90 per cent of the predicted weight for height is achieved, most anorexic patients will resume menses within 6 months to 1 year.

Recovery

Seventy per cent have a good to moderate improvement; 20–30 per cent remain chronically ill with no improvement. The mortality rate is 5–10 per cent, mainly due to suicide.

HYPERPROLACTINAEMIA [14]

Prolactin is secreted by lactotrophs from the posterolateral aspects of the adenohypophysis. It responds to inhibiting and releasing

Table 4.1 Serum prolactin levels and likely pathological conditions.

Serum prolactin level (mIU/l)	Condition
<3000	Large non-functioning tumour
>8000	Prolactin-secreting macroadenoma
1500–4000	Prolactin-secreting microadenoma
<2500	PCOS, hypothyroidism, drugs, e.g. dopaminergic antagonist phenothiazines, domperidone and metoclopramide

factors. The most important factor is dopamine (prolactin inhibitor factor, PIF) which exerts its effect on dopamine receptors in the hypophysis.

There are a group of patients with no demonstrable structural lesion – known as 'functional hyperprolactinaemia'. Hyperprolactinaemia otherwise may be caused by an increased secretion of prolactin from a prolactin-secreting pituitary adenoma, or from a non-functioning 'disconnection' tumour in the region of the hypothalamus or pituitary, which disrupts the inhibitory influence of dopamine on prolactin secretion (Table 4.1). Hyperprolactinaemia may cause anovulation and infertility.

Prolactin levels should be measured between 9.00 a.m. and 12.00 noon as peak levels occur between 3.00 and 5.00 a.m. Prolactin levels are increased during pregnancy due to the increased oestrogen secretion. High concentrations of oestrogen induce hyperplasia and hypertrophy of the lactotrophs, which in turn stimulate the secretion of prolactin. Prolactin concentrations are also increased by stress and exercise. Stress can inhibit the release of hypothalamic prolactin inhibitory factor which increases prolactin secretion and galactorrhoea.

Symptoms and signs of hyperprolactinaemia

- Galactorrhoea is non-puerperal watery or milky breast secretion that contains neither pus nor blood. It may occur in up to one third of women with hyperprolactinaemia. Its presence is not correlated with prolactin levels or a tumour.
- Menstrual irregularities.

- Hypo-oestrogenisation – vaginal dryness, dyspareunia, reduced libido. If prolonged, osteoporosis occurs.
- Visual field defects occur in 5 per cent.
- Hyperprolactinaemia causes primary or secondary amenorrhoea by inhibiting the release of LH and FSH. High levels of prolactin may also affect the frequency or amplitude of GnRH pulses through changes in dopamine release.

Disorders affecting prolactin concentration

Pituitary causes

The most common pituitary tumour is an adenoma. Most prolactin-secreting adenomas are microadenomas, i.e. adenomas of <1 cm diameter confined to the sella turcica. Prolactin-secreting macro-adenomas are adenomas of more than 1 cm in diameter that extend beyond the sella; they are very uncommon.

Hyperprolactinaemia with or without a microadenoma usually has a benign clinical course without treatment. Spontaneous remission may occur. Any lesion of the hypothalamus or pituitary stalk that interferes with delivery of PIF (dopamine) will cause hyperprolactinaemia.

Brain, pituitary, hypothalamic mass lesions

- Tumour
- Metastases
- Germinoma encephalitis
- Cranial radiation
- Craniopharyngioma
- Glioma
- Meningiomas
- Gonadotroph.

Metabolic

- Hypothyroidism
- Renal failure.

Functional infiltrators

- Histiocytosis, sarcoid tuberculosis, granuloma
- Pituitary – macro- or microprolactinoma
- Hyperplasia

- Empty sella syndrome. This is usually caused by a congenital abnormality of the sellar diaphragm, in which the arachnoid membrane herniates into the sella turcica. It may also be secondary to trauma, surgery or tumours and may cause gonadotroph compression
- Acromegaly.

Vascular
- Pituitary stalk section
- Sheehan's syndrome
- Cushing's disease.

Metastases
- Malignant tumours with ectopic production of prolactin.

Drugs (Table 4.2)
- Hormonal
- Anxiolytic
- Antihypertensive
- Serotonergic (i.e. amphetamines and hallucinogens)
- Histamine (H_2) receptor antagonist (i.e. cimetidine).

Hypothyroidism

Some 3–5 per cent of women with galactorrhoea and hyperprolactinaemia have primary hypothyroidism. Hypothyroidism is characterised by a low serum level of thyroxine (T_4) and decreased negative feedback on the hypothalamic–pituitary axis. The resulting increased secretion of thyrotrophin-releasing hormone (TRH) stimulates thyrotrophs and lactotrophs, thereby increasing the levels of both thyroid-stimulating hormone (TSH, thyrotrophin) and prolactin. The negative feedback of T_4 and triiodothyronine (T_3) is mostly directed towards the pituitary, rather than the hypothalamus. TRH levels may therefore be elevated minimally. The decreased T_4 and T_3 may induce changes in the sensitivity of the pituitary cells, prompting an exaggerated response to normal or slightly elevated levels of TRH. With the diminished need to feed back, patients with primary hypothyroidism have an alteration in the positive feedback loop between T_4 and dopamine. The decreased dopamine secretion will also lead to elevated levels of serum TSH and prolactin. To

Table 4.2 Pharmacological agents affecting prolactin concentration.

Stimulators	Inhibitors
Anaesthetics	L-dopa
Psychoactive drugs	Dopamine
Phenothiazines	Bromocriptine
Tricyclics	Pergolide
Antidepressants	Cabergoline
Opiates	
Amphetamines	
Haloperidol	
Antipsychotics – chlorpromazine	
Hormones	
Oestrogen	
Oral contraceptives	
Steroids	
Thyroid-releasing hormones	
Antihypertensives	
Methyldopa	
Reserpine	
Verapamil	
Dopamine receptor antagonists	
Metoclopramide	
Antiemetics	
Cimetidine	

4

identify primary hypothyroidism in women with galactorrhoea, serum prolactin and TSH should be measured. If serum TSH is elevated a diagnosis of primary hypothyroidism (usually Hashimoto's thyroiditis) is made.

Therapy

Hypothyroidism is treated with thyroxine replacement (0.05 mg for 2 weeks with the dose increasing by 0.05 mg every 2 weeks until a maintenance dose of 0.15 mg/day is reached). This dose lowers the elevated serum TSH and prolactin levels to within the normal range.

Effect of pregnancy or exogenous oestrogen on prolactinomas in hyperprolactinaemia

Hyperoestrogenism may cause significant growth of the macroadenoma. Pre-pregnancy dopaminergic suppression, radiation or surgery and close supervision during pregnancy is essential. Inter-disciplinary care is recommended. Breastfeeding does not stimulate tumour growth. Pregnancy may increase the chance of spontaneous regression of hyperprolactinaemia.

Acromegaly

Women with acromegaly have galactorrhoea and elevated serum prolactin, due to increased secretion.

Sheehan's syndrome

This is the only known condition with lower than normal levels of serum prolactin due to destruction of lactotrophs.

Renal disease

Hyperprolactinaemia results from delayed clearance.

Diagnosis

Because prolactin levels may only be modestly high in patients with non-functioning pituitary adenomas, baseline magnetic resonance imaging (MRI) is useful in those with no extrapituitary–hypothalamic cause (drugs, renal disease, etc.) with levels >1000 mIU/l.

A serum sample taken after 60 minutes of rest and an MRI or computerised tomography (CT) scan of the pituitary should be performed in women with normal TSH and prolactin levels exceeding 1000 mIU/l or those with symptoms of headaches and visual field changes. MRI is more sensitive than CT and avoids the use of radiation. It permits fine delineation of the gland, especially the lateral margins. MRI is superior in identifying the optic chiasma, optic nerves, cavernous sinuses and carotid arteries. A CT scan provides information on the bony structures of sella turcica and soft tissue lesions extending into the extracellular space. Traditionally a skull X-ray has identified typical radiological changes of an asymmetrically enlarged pituitary fossa, a double contour to the floor and erosion of the clinoid processes, but these are late-stage changes.

Treatment of prolactin-secreting pituitary macroadenomas

Aims

- Elimination of galactorrhoea
- Normalisation of oestrogen secretion
- Induction of ovulation and fertility if desired.

Management – observation

Where women with galactorrhoea have regular ovulatory cycles and normal or slightly elevated serum prolactin levels (<1000 mIU/l), treatment is not absolutely necessary while the galactorrhoea is not troublesome and regular or irregular menstruation is present. If anovulation with unopposed oestrogen secretion occurs, cyclic progestogen or oral contraceptives should be given to induce regular uterine bleeding. Long-term treatment with a dopaminergic agent is not necessary, as women with normal oestrogen levels and idiopathic hyperprolactinaemia have no additional risks. Women with radiological evidence of microadenomas may be observed by yearly measurements of serum prolactin, because microadenomas grow very slowly.

Hyperprolactinaemia with low oestradiol levels

For those who do not wish to conceive, oestrogen replacement therapy prevents osteoporosis. Appropriate regimens include postmenopausal HRT regimens or the COC. Oestrogen replacement therapy does not usually increase the size of pituitary microadenomas.

Dopaminergic agents

Elevated prolactin levels interfere with the normal cyclic discharge of GnRH from the hypothalamus. They may also reduce gonadotrophin release from intact gonadotrophin-releasing cells, resulting in amenorrhoea and low production of oestrogen. Hyperprolactinaemia suppresses LH pulsatile secretion by decreasing the pulse amplitude and the pulse frequency. Dopaminergic agents exert a direct effect on the pituitary gland to lower serum prolactin levels, thus removing the block to gonadotrophin release. Through receptors in the hypothalamus, they possibly stimulate release of prolactin-inhibiting factor. In more than 80 per cent of women with amenorrhoea due to hyperprolactinaemia, dopaminergic agents lower prolactin levels, suppress lactation and induce ovulatory menstrual cycles. The size of both microadenomas and macroadenomas is reduced and visual field defects are reversed.

Hyperprolactinaemia, galactorrhoea and amenorrhoea will recur in 70 per cent of women if therapy is discontinued. Ten per cent of women with microadenomas have complete regression of their lesions after 1 year of use of dopaminergic agents and an increasing proportion over time. Therapy should be discontinued for 6 weeks every year to determine whether prolactin levels have come back to normal and regular menstruation has occurred.

Women not oestrogen deficient, but who wish to become pregnant, may have hyperprolactinaemia treated with clomiphene. If ovulation does not occur then bromocriptine should be given with or without clomiphene. Women with low levels of oestrogen will not ovulate with clomiphene alone and require dopaminergic agents. Almost all women with hyperprolactinaemia can achieve ovulation following administration of dopaminergic agents. Ovulation and normal menstrual cycles and pregnancy may occur without serum prolactin levels being in the normal range.

Dopaminergic agents can be discontinued as soon as pregnancy is confirmed, unless there is a macroadenoma. If a macroadenoma is present, treatment may be maintained throughout pregnancy or re-instituted if tumour enlargement occurs. Microadenomas do not grow substantially in pregnancy, however a visual field examination should be done at 20, 28 and 38 weeks of pregnancy. If an extra-sellar extension is suspected because of an abnormal visual field, or if headaches develop or worsen, an MRI or limited CT scan is indicated. If suprasellar extension occurs, treatment with dopaminergic agents should be instituted or increased, and maintained for the rest of the pregnancy. In patients with a macroadenoma, MRI or CT scanning should be done. If an enlarged macroadenoma does not shrink with dopaminergic agents, adenomectomy can be performed during pregnancy as no increase in surgical morbidity has been reported.

Dopaminergic agents cause regression of most pituitary macroadenomas, usually within 3 months but sometimes up to 6 months. Patients with a pituitary macroadenoma should have a repeat MRI or CT scan 6 months after initiation of dopaminergic therapy. For as long as the adenoma continues to shrink, drug therapy should be continued and then maintained long term to maintain tumour suppression. Visual function may improve within days of initiating therapy.

Bromocriptine

- It has dopaminergic activity that suppresses prolactin secretion. It lowers prolactin levels, restores gonadal function, stops galactorrhoea and shrinks the prolactinoma if present.
- Bromocriptine is a derivative of lysergic acid substituted with bromine that binds to dopamine receptors and inhibits pituitary prolactin secretion. The half-life of bromocriptine is 3–7 hours (relatively short) and so oral administration should be given every 8–12 hours (two to three times daily). Bromocriptine treats symptomatic galactorrhoea and induces ovulation.
- Bromocriptine is given as a starting dose of 1.25 mg (half a 2.5 mg tablet) given at bedtime for 5 days; 1.25 mg in the morning is added in. It should then be increased slowly every 5 days to reduce the likelihood of side effects up to a dose range of 2.5–7. 5 mg daily in divided doses with food. The minimum effective dose should be used. Dosage should be maintained at the lowest amount needed to keep serum prolactin levels in the normal range.
- Prolactin concentrations fall within a few days and tumour volume reduces within 6 weeks. Prolactin measurements should return to normal and then require only infrequent monitoring.

Common side effects with bromocriptine
Side effects include nausea, nasal stuffiness and postural hypotension, which is dose-related. Nausea is a mild and mostly transient problem, occurring in only 50 per cent of patients. That is the reason for starting slowly by one half to one tablet per day, given with a meal in the evening or by the vaginal route of administration, depo injection or a slow-release oral preparation.

Five per cent of patients are intolerant of the side effects that include nausea, vomiting and abdominal cramps due to a local effect on the gastric mucosa. Other unusual side effects are vertigo, postural hypotension, headaches and drowsiness due to smooth muscle relaxation in the splanchnic beds and inhibition of sympathetic activity.

Unusual long-term side effects include Raynaud's syndrome, constipation and psychiatric changes, especially aggression. Side effects can be reduced when the medication is taken at bedtime or with food. Regular menses should be resumed after 6 weeks in those without evidence of a microadenoma and within 9 weeks in those with an adenoma. Galactorrhoea should resolve by 6 weeks in women without an adenoma.

For severe side effects of bromocriptine, it may be administered vaginally (2.5 mg/day) as serum levels remain elevated longer with this route than with oral administration.

Cabergoline and quinagolide

Cabergoline and quinagolide are δ_2 receptor agonists with longer biological half-lifes than bromocriptine. The dose of cabergoline is 0.5–1 mg twice a week, and quinagolide, 0.075–0.15 mg once daily. Dopaminergic drugs should be stopped if pregnancy occurs, although in patients with a prolactinoma the drugs may need to be restarted if the tumour enlarges in pregnancy. Prepregnancy endocrine consultation is recommended for those women with prolactinomas.

Cabergoline is better tolerated than bromocriptine as well as being a potent and long-lasting inhibitor of prolactin secretion. Cabergoline appears to be more advantageous than bromocriptine in the treatment of women with hyperprolactinaemia in that it is more effective (i.e. higher number of ovulatory cycles and pregnancies), better tolerated and only needs to be taken once or twice weekly.

However, unlike bromocriptine, the teratogenetic effects of cabergoline have not been extensively investigated in humans. Therefore it ought not to be used as a first-line treatment of hyperprolactinaemia for infertility, although normal pregnancies have been reported using this drug.

Quinagolide is more potent and better tolerated than bromocriptine.

Lysuride

The starting dose is 0.1 mg/day, after 2 weeks increasing slowly to 0.1–0.2 mg three times daily. If side effects occur with either bromocriptine or lysuride the new specific δ_2 receptor agonists, specific for prolactin suppression and with fewer effects on emesis and vascular reactivity, are suitable.

Serotonin antagonists

Serotonin stimulates prolactin release.

Bromocriptine and pregnancy

Women with a microprolactinoma who wish to conceive can be reassured that they may stop bromocriptine when pregnancy is diagnosed. They require no further monitoring as the likelihood of significant tumour expansion is very small (<2 per cent).

Women with a macroprolactinoma have a 25 per cent risk of the tumour expanding and therefore ought to be treated. This risk is probably also present if the tumour has been treated but has not shrunk, as assessed by CT or MRI scan. Therefore treatment of macroprolactinomas is a dopaminergic agent combined with barrier methods of contraception. In women with suprasellar extension, a follow-up CT or MRI scan should be done after 3 months of treatment to identify tumour regression before a pregnancy is commenced. Dopaminergic agents are safe to use in pregnancy but may be discontinued. If symptoms suggestive of tumour re-expansion occur, an MRI should be done, and if there is continuing suprasellar expansion, bromocriptine is necessary. In these women, expert assessment of the visual fields should be done in pregnancy. There is no increase in fetal defects using it throughout pregnancy.

4

Surgery

Surgery in the form of a trans-sphenoidal adenomectomy is done for cases of drug resistance (failure to shrink a macroadenoma) or intolerable drug side effects. Non-functioning tumours should be removed surgically, and are usually detected by imaging and a serum prolactin concentration of <3000 mIU/l. When the prolactin level is >3000 mIU/l, a trial of bromocriptine is warranted, and if the prolactin level falls, it can be assumed the tumour is a prolactin-secreting macroadenoma. Surgery is also required for a suprasellar extension of the tumour that has not regressed during treatment with bromocriptine and if pregnancy is desired.

The trans-sphenoidal route (by sublabial incision) for the microsurgical exploration of the sella turcica enables removal of the pituitary adenoma and usually preserves function of the pituitary. Long-term cure rates vary between 10 and 30 per cent. Considering that drug therapy with dopaminergic agents has low rates of side effects and a potential for reducing adenoma size, surgical excision of macroadenomas should be performed only with a complete or partial failure of medical therapy or if poor compliance occurs. Medical therapy should be continued even when surgery takes place as rapid regrowth of the adenoma can occur.

Radiation (45 Gy of cobalt) may arrest the progressive growth of a pituitary adenoma and may be an alternative to surgery, where tumour regression is not occurring on a dopaminergic agent.

REFERENCES

1 Hopkinson, Z.E.C., Sattar, N., Fleming, R. & Greer, I.A. (1998) Polycystic ovarian syndrome: the metabolic syndrome comes to gynaecology. *British Medical Journal*, **317**, 329–332.

2 Balen, A.H., Conway, G.S., Kaltsas, G. *et al.* (1995) Polycystic ovary syndrome: the spectrum of the disorder in 1741 patients. *Human Reproduction*, **10**, 2107–2111.

3 Franks, S. (1995) Polycystic ovary syndrome. *New England Journal of Medicine*, **333**, 853–861.

4 Dunaif, A. (1995) Hyperandrogenic anovulation (PCOS): a unique disorder of insulin action associated with an increased risk of non-insulin-dependent diabetes mellitus. *American Journal of Medicine*, **98**, 335–395.

5 Jacobs, H.S. & Conway, G.S. (1999) Leptin, polycystic ovaries and polycystic ovary syndrome. *Human Reproduction*, **5**, 166–171.

6 Ferriman, D. & Gallway, J.D. (1961) Clinical assessment of body hair growth in women. *Journal of Clinical Metabolism*, **21**, 1440–1447.

7 Conn, J.J. & Jacobs, H.S. (1998) Managing hirsutism in gynaecological practice. *British Journal of Obstetrics and Gynaecology*, **105**, 687–696.

8 Velazquez, E.M., Mendoza, S., Hamer, T., Sosa, F. & Glueck, C.J. (1994) Metformin therapy in polycystic ovaries reduces hyperinsulinaemia, insulin resistance, hyperandrogenaemia and systolic blood pressure, while facilitating normal menses and pregnancy. *Metabolism*, **43**, 647–654.

9 Balen, A. (1997) Anovulatory infertility and ovulation induction. *Human Reproduction*, **12**, 83–87.

10 Abdel Gadir, A., Al Naser, H., Mowafi, R. & Shaw, R. (1992) The response of patients with polycystic ovarian disease to human menopausal gonadotropin therapy after ovarian electrocautery or luteinising hormone-releasing hormone agonist. *Fertility and Sterility*, **57**, 309–313.

11 Donesky, B.W. & Adashi, E.Y. (1995) Surgically induced ovulation in the polycystic ovary syndrome: wedge resection revisited in the age of laparoscopy. *Fertility and Sterility*, **63**, 439–463.

12 Laml, T., Schulz-Lobmeyr, I., Obruca, A., Huber, J.C. & Hartmann, B.W. (2000) Premature ovarian failure: etiology and prospects. *Gynecological Endocrinology*, **14**, 292–302.

13 Krauss, C.M., Turksoy, R.N., Atkins, L., McLaughlin, C., Brown, L.G. & Page, D.C. (1987) Familial premature ovarian failure due to an interstitial deletion of the long arm of the X chromosome. *New England Journal of Medicine*, **317**(3), 125–131.

14 Yazigri, R.A., Quintero, C.H. & Salameh, W.A. (1997) Prolactin disorders. *Fertility and Sterility*, **67**, 215–225.

4

5 Infertility and Assisted Reproductive Techniques

FECUNDITY

Infertility is the inability of a couple to conceive after 1 year of sexual intercourse without using any type of contraception. Fecundity indicates the rate of conception occurring in a population in a given time period, usually 1 month. In clinical practice infertility is usually defined as a failure to become pregnant during a 12-month period of regular unprotected intercourse. Each couple has a more or less constant monthly probability of conceiving, but between couples the probabilities vary widely, from 0 per cent (3–5 per cent of couples) to an upper limit of about 60 per cent. Up to 25 per cent of all women attempting to conceive had an episode of subfertility defined as 1 year failure to conceive with regular unprotected intercourse or the occurrence of more than two spontaneous miscarriages or stillbirths at some time in their reproductive life [1]. Three per cent of all women aged 25–44 were found to be involuntarily childless and 6 per cent of parous women were not able to have as many children as they wished [2].

As the duration of inability to achieve a pregnancy increases, the probability of success during the subsequent year sharply decreases. However, if the period of infertility is short (12 months) there is a 50 per cent chance of conception in the subsequent year. Therefore, depending on the cause of infertility, it may be useful to wait rather than pursue assisted reproductive techniques (ART) early in the period of infertility (Fig. 5.1) [3].

Infertility and age (Table 5.1) [4]

Infertility risk correlates with age as follows:
- 30–34, 1 in 7
- 35–40, 1 in 5
- 40–44, 1 in 4.

For couples who stop using contraception in order to conceive, only 50 per cent conceive in 3 months, 75 per cent in 6 months and 90 per cent by 1 year.

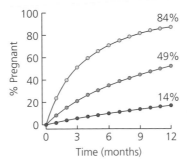

Probability of conceiving for periods up to 12 months

–○– Directly after stopping birth control

–●– If no pregnancy has been achieved within a year

–●– If no pregnancy has been achieved within 3 years

Fig. 5.1 Probability of conceiving for periods up to 12 months. (With permission from Te Velde *et al.* (2000) [3].)

Table 5.1 Infertility and age. [3]

Age	Risk of never having a child (%)
20–24	6
25–29	9
30–34	15
35–40	30
40–44	64

After 2 years of trying to conceive, about 5 per cent of original couples will not have conceived. To determine that any treatment of infertility is superior to no treatment, statistical analysis of the effect of treatment on the incidence of pregnancy over time needs to be calculated [5].

The human ovum is capable of being fertilised for only about 24 hours after ovulation. Spermatozoa retain their fertilising ability for about 48 hours after intercourse. Ovulation usually occurs 12–16 days (14 ± 2 days) before the onset of the subsequent menses. The egg is fertilised within a few hours after it reaches the ampulla of the oviduct. It is best that sperm are present when the egg arrives so that fertilisation can occur. Intercourse should occur before ovulation for maximal likelihood of pregnancy. Pregnancy therefore can arise from day 8 (likelihood of pregnancy is 8 per cent) until day 14, the day of ovulation (likelihood is 36 per cent). Pregnancy does not occur after ovulation or more than 6 days before ovulation based on studies done on a single act of sexual intercourse and pregnancy rates. Because ovulation is sometimes inaccurately determined, the advice is that intercourse should not be timed, but should occur regularly throughout the cycle. Sperm transport to the oviduct from the cervix normally occurs from 5 minutes to 5 days after intercourse. Ovulation occurs 1–3 days after the basal body temperature nadir and 1 day after the luteinising hormone (LH) peak. There is only a 20 per cent chance of conceiving in each ovulatory cycle even with optimally timed intercourse [6].

Conception

The greatest possibility of conception is in the 2 days before ovulation and the day of ovulation itself. Semen quality measured in terms of motility and morphology declines with more than 10 days' abstinence. Regular intercourse – two to three times a week – should ensure that it falls within the fertile period.

Change in cervical mucus is a good indicator of the fertile period. After menstruation there are a variable number of days where there is no vaginal loss of mucus. The change in cervical mucus correlates well with the fertile period. The onset of the fertile mucus is characterised by the appearance of increasing quantities of 'cloudy' or sticky secretion. The sensation is one of dampness. In the immediate pre-ovulatory period the mucus is clear, slippery, lubricative and stringy like raw egg white. The last day of the presence of this mucus is the 'peak symptom' indicating the maximal day of fertility (1 day before the LH surge). After ovulation, the mucus becomes thick, tacky, opaque and diminished in volume. Basal body temperature charts are poor predictors of the day of ovulation and are not indicated in clinical practice. LH detection kits may be better at detecting the onset of the LH surge, but there is no evidence that using the detection of the LH surge improves the conception rate.

A mid-luteal serum progesterone estimation is proof of ovulation at a value of 30 nmol/l. Up to 9 per cent of regular menstrual cycles (defined by the World Health Organisation (WHO) as a cycle length of 25–35 days) are thought to be anovulatory. If the woman has a long or unpredictable cycle the sample may need to be performed later in the cycle than day 21 (e.g. day 28 for a regular 35-day cycle), or be repeated weekly until the next menstrual cycle starts.

Prognosis

Prognosis in infertility treatment (likelihood of pregnancy) generally is inversely related to the time spent trying to conceive (Figs 5.2 and 5.3) [7]. For unexplained infertility, IVF is indicated after 3 years of trying (Fig. 5.4).

5

Lifestyle modification with infertility

- Both partners should stop smoking. Smoking is detrimental to fertility [8]. Infertile women should be advised to stop smoking to enhance their fecundity and reduce the risk of miscarriage and growth retardation in the fetus. Fertilisation rates in smokers are one

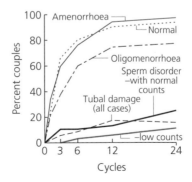

Fig. 5.2 Cumulative pregnancy rates of some of the most common causes of infertility in a complete population of infertile couples treated by conventional methods, compared with normal. (Courtesy of M.G.R. Hull.)

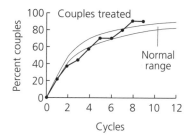

Fig. 5.3 Cumulative pregnancy rates with subfertility treated by IVF. (Courtesy of M.G.R. Hull.)

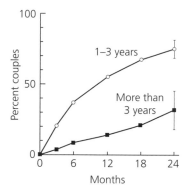

Fig. 5.4 Cumulative fertility in couples with unexplained infertility of less than 3 years and greater than 3 years. (Courtesy of M.G.R. Hull.)

third that of normal couples with ART. Smoking affects sperm quality adversely [9].

• Alcohol intake should be limited to one to two units once or twice a week. Women trying to become pregnant or at any stage of pregnancy should drink no more than one or two units twice a week [10].

• Body mass index (BMI = weight (kg)/height (m)^2) ideally should be in the normal range [11]. The internationally accepted range for BMI is: underweight <18.5, normal 18.5–24.9, overweight 25.0–29.0, obesity 30.0–39.9, extreme obesity ≥40. Underweight women (BMI

$<20\,kg/m^2$ or $<47\,kg$) are frequently hypo-oestrogenic and anovulatory. Similarly overweight women are often anovulatory particularly with polycystic ovary syndrome (PCOS). BMI should be not greater than 30. Fat needs to comprise at least 22 per cent of body weight. Short-term weight reduction, even for a period of 6 months, is often effective in restoring ovulation. Calorie restriction of itself may be more important than the actual weight loss.

- Male partners should be advised to limit their drinking. Men with poor quality sperm should be advised to wear loose-fitting underwear and trousers and avoid occupational or social situations that might cause testicular hyperthermia. Hyperthermia does have a detrimental effect on sperm quality. This may be important in terms of fertility outcome if the man already has suboptimal semen parameters [12]. Advising loose-fitting underwear and trousers is a simple, effective intervention.

- Advise 0.4 mg folic acid as a supplement to take when trying to conceive and during the first 12 weeks of pregnancy in order to prevent neural tube defects. The dose should be increased to 4 mg daily in women who have previously had a baby with a neural tube defect, or those taking medication, or with epilepsy and in recurrent miscarriage.

- Advice should be given concerning risk in any subsequent pregnancy both of the technique and the pregnancy in a relative way (Table 5.2).

Investigations of infertility [13–15]

Investigations conducted into infertility are detailed in Tables 5.3–5.7 and Figs 5.5 and 5.6.

Female partner

- Rubella status: If it is negative, rubella vaccination should be offered and the woman advised not to become pregnant within 1 month of immunisation.

- Thyroid function tests should be done in infertile women with irregular menstrual cycles and in women with signs or symptoms of thyroid disease.

- Prolactin levels should only be done in those women with amenorrhoea, oligomenorrhoea or clinical symptoms of hyperprolactinaemia such as galactorrhoea.

Table 5.2 Risks for counselling for infertility treatment.

Risks related to pregnancy outcome

Event	Material risk
Miscarriage	1 in 7
Premature birth	1 in 15
Birth defect in the baby	1 in 20
Death of the baby	1 in 100
Cerebral palsy in the baby	1 in 400
Death of the mother	1 in 14 000

Material risks related to a woman's age

Age (years)	Chance of death in 1 year when otherwise fit and healthy
40	1 in 1000
50	1 in 500
60	1 in 170
Women aged 50 years, no family history, chance of developing breast carcinoma in the next 12 months	1 in 500
Ovarian carcinoma	1 in 90

'Life risks'

Activity	Chance of death in 1 year
Driving a car	1 in 6000
Motorcycling	1 in 1000
Continuing pregnancy	1 in 14 000
Laparoscopy	1 in 67 000
Termination of pregnancy	1 in 500 000
Jumbo jet flight	1 in 2 000 000

- Evidence of ovulation: measure follicle-stimulating hormone (FSH) and LH levels on days 3–5 of the cycle together with oestradiol levels; if these are high they produce a negative feedback effect on FSH levels. High FSH levels are inversely proportional to the ability

Table 5.3 Factors which influence infertility.

Duration of infertility
Age of the woman

BMI in the female partner
History of male urethritis
Percentage of motile spermatozoa
Quality of motility
Motile sperm concentration
Total motile sperm
Sperm morphology

Sociodemographic factors
Male profession
Alcohol consumption
Sauna bathing
Physical exercise
Mumps
Orchitis
History of prostatitis
Smoking
Coital frequency
Conception rate decreases by 15% per 1 year's duration of infertility and by up
  to 3% per year of the female partner's increasing age

5

Table 5.4 Causes of infertility.

Anovulation	10–15%
Pelvic factors – adhesions from endometriosis or infection or tubal occlusion	30–40%
Abnormalities in male reproductive system – oligozoospermia, high viscosity of semen, low sperm motility, or low volume of semen (male factor)	30–40%
Abnormal sperm–cervical mucus penetration (cervical factor)	5%
Unexplained infertility	10–25%

to get pregnant. This is particularly significant in the older woman where higher FSH levels suggest a poorer response of the ovary to ovulation induction agents.

- A serum progesterone of >20 IU/l on day 21 is indicative of ovulation.

Table 5.5 Initial investigations for infertility.

FSH should be less than 3–5 IU/l in the early follicular phase of the cycle. If elevated it is a useful indicator that the woman's ovarian age is more advanced than her chronological age. Check on oestradiol at the same time because a level >250 pmol/l will cause a decrease in the FSH by negative feedback

Fasting blood glucose – serum progesterone in the mid-luteal phase (5–7 days after the basal body temperature shift)

Chlamydia – IgG antibodies to *Chlamydia trachomatis* – if positive, indicates possible tubal adhesions

Thyroid function tests

Pelvic ultrasound

Prolactin if amenorrhoeic

Semen analysis

Hysterosalpingography in the follicular phase of the cycle

Table 5.6 Ovulation disorders.

---

(1) Intrinsic ovarian failure: genetic, autoimmune, others, e.g. cytotoxic chemotherapy
(2) Secondary ovarian dysfunction
    (a) disorders of gonadotrophin regulation
       (i) specific hyperprolactinaemia, Kallmann's syndrome (WHO group I)
       (ii) functional (WHO group I): weight loss, exercise, drugs, idiopathic
    (b) gonadotrophin deficiency (WHO group I): pituitary tumour, pituitary necrosis or thrombosis
    (c) disorders of gonadotrophin action (WHO group II): polycystic ovary syndrome

---

- Test tubal patency: a hysterosalpingogram may be used as a screening test for tubal patency in a low risk couple. When an evaluation of the pelvis is indicated a diagnostic laparoscopy with dye insufflation should be done. Screen women for *Chlamydia trachomatis* and give antibiotic prophylaxis if positive. If detected, partners should be treated (see Chapter 10). Fallopian tube obstruction is found among 20–33 per cent of infertile couples. It may occur without any history of significant physical findings.

- Hysterosalpingography gives information about the uterine cavity and isthmus of the tube, that laparoscopy and dye cannot provide. Laparoscopy gives information about the presence of peritubal

Table 5.7 Causes of secondary amenorrhoea (0.8% of general population).

1 Uterine
Normal endocrine function
Intrauterine adhesions (previous evacuation, curettage)
Obliteration of the uterine cavity
Endometrial destruction
Previous endometritis or fibrosis following myomectomy, metroplasty,
    Caesarean section
Diagnosis – pass uterine sound

2 Polycystic ovary syndrome
Elevated LH levels
Elevated androgen levels
Functional hypothalamic amenorrhoea

3 CNS – hypothalamic causes
Interference with gonadotrophin-releasing hormone (GnRH) release
Craniopharyngiomas, granulomatous disease (tuberculosis and sarcoidosis),
    encephalitis

4 Pituitary causes
Non-neoplastic lesions – damage of pituitary cells due to anoxia, thrombosis or
    haemorrhage
Sheehan's syndrome – hypotensive episode in pregnancy

5 Drugs
Phenothiazines
Antihypertensive agents

6 Stress and exercise
Mechanism: low adipose tissue shifts the pathway of oestrogen metabolism
    towards 16-hydroxylation, forming catechol oestrogens. The competition
    between catecholamine and catechol oestrogens for catechol-O-
    methyltransferase may increase dopamine levels which in turn suppress the
    release of GnRH and hence LH.

7 Weight loss
Mechanism due to failure of normal GnRH release
Anorexia nervosa – 1 in 1000 white women

8 Ovarian causes
Hypogonadotrophic hypogonadism – failure of the ovary to secrete sufficient
    oestrogen to produce endometrial growth if the follicles are damaged as a
    result of infection, interference with blood supply or depletion caused by
    bilateral cystectomies
Premature ovarian failure – hypoparathyroidism, Hashimoto's thyroiditis,
    ovarian irradiation, Addison's disease
No evidence of autoimmune disease – antibodies to gonadotrophins as well as
    to thyroid and adrenal glands, e.g. non-organ-specific antibodies, mainly
    antinuclear antibodies or rheumatoid factor

5

5

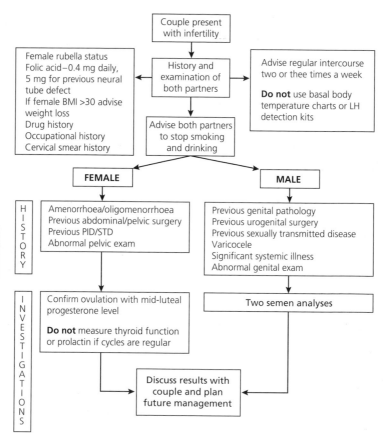

Fig. 5.5 The investigation of infertility. (RCOG (1998).) [16]

adhesions, endometriosis and ovarian pathology. It has a 1–2 per cent complication rate, including injury to bowel or blood vessels, post-operative infection and a mortality rate of 8 in 100 000.

Male partner

It is rare that any drugs can be given to improve sperm count. Therefore, use has to be made of what sperm are present. Normal

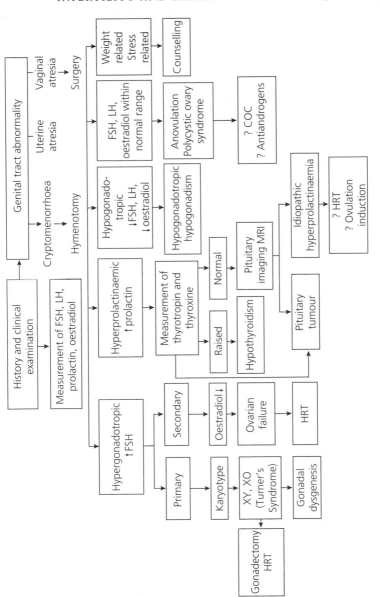

Fig. 5.6 Investigation and treatment of women with amenorrhoea. [Baird (1997),] [17]

5

sperm parameters are identified by defined criteria (WHO 1992) (Table 5.8). Semen characteristics can be further defined as to degrees of asthenozoospermia and oligozoospermia and types of morphology (Tables 5.8, 5.9) [18].

Treatment is in the form of

- Intrauterine insemination (IUI)
- *In vitro* fertilisation (IVF)
- Intracytoplasmic sperm injection (ICSI).

Obstructive azoospermia is not a common cause of infertility. Obstructive azoospermia and primary spermatogenic failure account for only about 2 per cent of infertility. The exception is vasectomy reversal where success rates range from 17 to 82 per cent, depending on the length of time since the operation and any other complicating factors.

TREATMENT OF MALE INFERTILITY

Where there are identifiable anatomical defects of sperm transport, anatomical reconstruction may be done [19–21] (Tables 5.9–5.13).

ART include:

Intrauterine insemination

The cervix, with ideal mucus, acts as a reservoir for sperm. Only about 10 per cent of sperm in the ejaculate will reach the uterus. Penetration of cervical mucus depends on vigorous sperm motility. Cervical mucus filters out morphologically abnormal sperm or

Table 5.8 Infertility investigation – WHO values for a normal semen analysis.

Appearance	Homogeneous, grey and opalescent
Volume	≥2 ml
Liquefaction time	Within 60 min at room temperature
Concentration	>20 million per ml
Motility	>50 per cent progressive motility
Morphology	>30 per cent normal forms
White blood cells	<1 million per ml
Viability	75 per cent or more viable
Immunobead test	<20 per cent spermatozoa with adherent particles

Table 5.9 Clinical categorisation of infertile men.

Untreatable sterility
Primary testicular failure
  Kleinfelter's syndrome
  Yq microdeletions
  Androgen receptor defects
  Postinflammatory mumps orchiditis
  Undescended testes (past or present)
  Past cytotoxic or X-ray therapy
  Idiopathic
Other
Total teratospermia (absent acrosomes, decapitate sperm)
  Zero sperm motility (immotile cilia syndrome)
  Specific defects of sperm–oocyte interaction (e.g. disordered zona pellucida
    induced acrosome reaction)

Treatable conditions
Genital tract obstruction
Gonadotrophin deficiency-suppression
Sperm autoimmunity
Coital disorders
Reversible toxin exposure – illness

Subfertility currently without proven effective treatment
Idiopathic oligospermia, asthenozoospermia, teratozoospermia or combinations
Associated conditions: varicocele, genital tract inflammation, adverse lifestyle
  factors

those coated with antisperm antibodies. If sperm concentration is low, or if many of the sperm are poorly motile, morphologically abnormal or coated with antibody, too few may penetrate the cervix and reach the fallopian tubes. Fertilisation is unlikely to occur.

- Sperm suitable for IUI can be separated by swim-up percoll density gradient into culture medium to obtain a specimen enriched in motile normal sperm.
- Washing the sperm reduces the sperm count to 10 per cent. At least 1 million are needed for successful fertilisation.
- The sperm is free of leukocytes.
- The chance of conception is enhanced by superovulating the partner and increasing the number of eggs with accurate timing of insemination.

Table 5.10 Effect of drugs on fertility. (With permission from RCOG (1998) [16].)

Drug	Effect on fertility
Male	
Sulphasalazine (when used to treat inflammatory bowel disease)	Decreases sperm concentration and motility and increases abnormal morphology
Nitrofurantoin	Spermatogenic arrest and decreased sperm counts at high dosage
Tetracyclines	Chlortetracycline and minocycline, in particular, bind to spermatozoa and interfere with sperm motility
Cimetidine	As a weak antiandrogen, it has been associated with seminal abnormalities as well as gynaecomastia and impotence
Ketoconazole	Single oral doses reduce serum testosterone concentrations although the clinical importance of this is unknown. Gynaecomastia, loss of libido and impotence have also been reported
Colchicine, allopurinol	Associated with defects of fertilisation capacity of sperm as demonstrated by abnormal sperm penetration tests
α-drenoreceptor blocking agents (e.g. methyldopa, clonidine, terazosin, phentolamine, phenoxybenzamine), tricyclic antidepressants (e.g. imipramine, amitryptyline, trimipramine), monoamine oxidase inhibitors (e.g. phenelzine, tranylcypromine), phenothiazines (e.g.chlorpromazine, thioridazine)	Ejaculatory dysfunction
Propranolol	Impotence
Chemotherapeutic agents, especially alkylating agents	Affect spermatogenesis through a direct effect on germinal epithelium. May also cause transient chromosomal aneuploidies in sperm
Cannabis	FSH and LH secretion is decreased leading to defective testicular function and spermatogenesis. Libido may also be decreased
Cocaine	Decreases sperm concentration and motility. Increases proportion of abnormal forms

Table 5.10 *Continued*

Drug	Effect on fertility
Anabolic steroids	Decreased secretion of FSH and LH via feedback inhibition of the hypothalamus and pituitary gland, which can lead to hypogonadotrophic hypogonadism. Sperm concentration, motility and normally formed sperm are all reduced but are reversible after stopping steroids. Azoospermia, gynaecomastia and reduced libido have also been reported
Female	
Non-steroidal anti-inflammatory drugs	Associated with an increased incidence of luteinised unruptured ovarian follicles
Chemotherapeutic agents, especially alkylating agents	Ovarian failure. Degree of reversibility dependent on drugs used and age of woman
Cannabis	Oligomenorrhoea and anovulation

5

- IUI is suitable for couples with mild to moderately impaired semen analysis. It is likely to be less successful than conventional IVF but cheaper per cycle.
- Where sperm dysfunction has been demonstrated, ICSI is the treatment of choice because success rates from IVF are decreased due to a decreased fertilisation rate and the chances of success by IUI are unknown.

Intracytoplasmic sperm injection

ICSI involves the injection of a single spermatozoon through the zona pellucida directly into the oocyte. ICSI is the procedure of choice when epididymal or testicular sperm is obtained surgically from patients with an obstructive or non-obstructive azoospermia, because fertility rates using sperm from the testis are poor in IVF.

Table 5.11 Effects of occupational factors on fertility. (RCOG (1998) [16].)

Occupation/exposure	Effect on fertility
Male	
Agricultural chemicals especially pesticides, e.g. dibromochloropropane (DBCP)	Oligozoospermia and azoospermia, some of which is reversible
X-ray exposure	High exposure may lead to reduced sperm count
Ethylene glycol ethers and their acetates, used in preparations containing solvents, especially paint products	May decrease sperm count but fertility not necessarily affected
Heavy metal exposure (e.g. mercury, arsenic, cadmium, lead, manganese). This can occur during the processes of smelting and welding, and in chemical factories	Lead, in particular, seems to be associated with decreased fertility in couples whilst the male partner is exposed. However, confounding factors such as concurrent exposure to heat need to be taken into account
Female	
VDU use	No effect detected
Anaesthetic gases	No effect proven for either male or female exposure
Environmental pollutants, e.g. polychlorinated biphenyls (PCBs) found in insecticides, fungicides and herbicides	Multiple exposure makes toxic effects of one individual compound difficult to evaluate. Possible detrimental effect on oocyte recovery during IVF in women with high follicular fluid concentrations of PCGs

Table 5.12 Patency rates and pregnancy rate (n = 1469) in microsurgical vasectomy reversal procedures. Microsurgical epididymal sperm aspiration and ICSI results in a 29% delivery rate. Epididymal sperm aspiration and ICSI should be reserved for failed surgery or causes not amenable to surgical reconstruction. (Belker *et al.* (1991) [20].)

Interval after vasectomy (years)	Patency rate (%)	Pregnancy rate (%)
3	97	76
3–8	88	53
9–14	79	44
15+	71	30

Table 5.13 Other causes of obstructive azoospermia. Obstructive lesions of the seminal tract should be suspected in azoospermia or severe oligospermia with normal-sized testes (>15–20 ml volume). (Hendry *et al.* (1990) [19].)

Conditions	Patency rate (%)	Pregnancy rate (%)
Epididymovasostomy (postinfective) blocks in the cordal part of the epididymis	52	38
Obstruction in the capital part of the epididymis (not due to an infective aetiology)	12	3
Postinfective obstruction in the vas (corrected by total anatomical reconstruction)	73	27
Transvasovasotomy	9	0

5

ICSI procedure [18]

A single motile spermatozoon is immobilised and aspirated, tail first, into the injection pipette. The oocyte is fixed with a holding pipette with the polar body situated at the 6 o'clock position. The injection pipette is put through the zona pellucida and the oolemma into the cytoplasm at the 3 o'clock position and the sperm is delivered with the smallest amount of medium. With the oocyte orientated in this way there is minimal risk from the injection pipette damaging the metaphase plate.

Oocytes are considered to be normally fertilised when two pronuclei are visible. Embryo cleavage of normally fertilised oocytes is assessed 24 hours after further *in vitro* culture. They are graded 1 (excellent, type A embryos with no anucleate fragments), 2 (good quality, type B embryos with between 1 and 20 per cent of the volume filled with anucleate fragments) and 3 (fair quality, type C embryos with between 21 and 50 per cent of the volume filled with anucleate fragments).

Delivery rates vary from 22 to 30 per cent per ICSI treatment cycle.

Complications for children born after ICSI

There is a statistically significant increase in sex chromosome aberrations compared with data in the literature on a normal neonatal population (about twice the rate of the non-ICSI population). However, it is clear that this increased incidence is related to the increased risk of chromosomal aberrations in the parents and the concomitant sperm abnormalities as a result of these. There is no increased risk with vasectomy reversal, cryptorchidism, major deformity of the vas, or obstructive azoospermia. There is no statistical difference in outcome measured in terms of prematurity, low birth weight, very low birth weight or loss of pregnancy.

Risk advice prior to treatment for infertility

Ovulation induction has an associated risk of ovarian hyperstimulation (Table 5.3 and Fig. 5.4) which can be a life-threatening situation if the woman gets pregnant [22]. Therefore she must be carefully counselled about the risks and the ovulatory dose of human chorionic gonadotrophin (hCG) withheld or the eggs retrieved, fertilised and embryos frozen to avoid pregnancy associated with ovarian hyperstimulation. The real risk of ART is the increased risk of multiple pregnancy with the associated risks of preterm labour and long-term complications. The perinatal mortality rate in 1995 of twins was 40 per 1000, in stillbirths 65.1 per 1000, compared with 8 in 1000 for singletons. The incidence of cerebral palsy in triplets is 47 times more than that of a singleton. The rate for cerebral palsy in twins is approximately 7 per 1000 births, and for triplets 27 in 1000 compared with 1.5 in 1000 for singletons [23].

Recently the risk of ovarian cancer associated with the use of fertility drugs has been reported [24–26].

OVULATION DISORDERS AND OVULATION INDUCTION

Ovulation induction is indicated for the treatment of anovulatory infertility, once pathological causes have been excluded.

Pharmacological induction of ovulation – clomiphene citrate (Clomid and Serophene) [27,28]

- Clomiphene citrate causes an increase in pituitary gonadotrophin release, stimulating maturation of the ovarian follicle.
- It has a half-life of 5–7 days and there is a slow rate of clearance, so clomiphene levels will increase in serum over time following successive monthly treatment cycles.

- It competes with endogenous circulating oestrogens for oestrogen-binding sites in the hypothalamus. It blocks normal negative feedback of the endogenous oestrogens and produces a significantly increased pulse frequency of GnRH. GnRH stimulates FSH and LH release with resulting oocyte maturation and an increase in oestradiol levels.

- Clomiphene citrate is given for 5 days beginning on day 2 after the start of menstruation or after a progesterone (10 mg Provera, 5 mg norethisterone)-induced withdrawal bleed if there is amenorrhoea.

- The dosage is 25–50 mg or 100 mg for 5 days. Clomiphene citrate should be commenced at as low a dose as 25–50 mg, especially with PCOS. If ovulation occurs this dose is maintained. Otherwise the dose may be increased to a maximum of 150 mg per day for 5 days. Cycles should be monitored with oestrogen levels to identify a response, and once levels are at 500 pmol/l ultrasound scans conducted to assess follicular growth and to avoid multiple pregnancy (if there are three or more follicles 18–22 mm sexual intercourse should be avoided unless the risk of multiple pregnancy is accepted). A serum progesterone on day 21 >20 IU/l is indicative of ovulation. The dose should only be increased if there is no response to 50 mg clomiphene after three cycles. Of those women who will respond to 50 mg, only two thirds will do so in the first cycle. Doses of ≥150 mg confer no benefit and only worsen the side effects, particularly of thickened cervical mucus.

- Some women who have troublesome side effects with clomiphene may benefit from tamoxifen (20–40 mg, days 2–6 of cycle). Side effects include visual disturbances (stop the drug immediately), multiple pregnancy (in approximately 10 per cent), abdominal tenderness, dizziness and nausea.

- Clomiphene is currently licensed for only 6 months' use in the UK because of the putative increased risk of ovarian cancer where an association was found between >12 months' use and incidence of ovarian cancer. It may be due to the indication (unexplained infertility) rather than the medication. The Committee on Safety in Medicine recommended recently that clomiphene should not be used for more than six cycles because of this link. The tendency is to use it for longer than that because often the dosage needs to be adjusted. Patients should be fully informed of the risk.

5

Results

Up to 85 per cent of conceptions occur during the first three ovulatory cycles. Nearly 50 per cent of women require increased dosages or longer treatment than 3 months. There is a positive correlation between the patient's weight and the dose of clomiphene needed to induce ovulation.

- Treatment induces ovulation in 70–80 per cent of women.
- The conception rate is 40–50 per cent.
- The multiple pregnancy rate is 8 per cent – 6.9 per cent twins, 0.5 per cent triplets, 0.3 per cent quadruplets, 0.13 per cent quintuplets.
- Clomiphene may have an anti-oestrogenic action causing thickening of the cervical mucus which may impede the passage of sperm through the cervix.
- When clomiphene is stopped oestrogen secretion continues, which produces a negative feedback control on the hypothalamus or release of GnRH. The exponential rise in the oestradiol produced by the dominant follicle has a positive feedback effect on the hypothalamus. GnRH release stimulates a surge of gonadotrophin output and ovulation occurs. Ovulation usually occurs 7 days after the last clomiphene tablet is ingested.
- Ovulation is indicated by a serum progesterone on day 21, i.e. 2 weeks after the ingestion of the last clomiphene tablet.
- The incidence of miscarriage is not increased with conceptions occurring after clomiphene treatment (15 per cent).
- The incidence of congenital anomalies is approximately 2.5 per cent, which is no higher than those that occur after spontaneous conception.
- Ovarian cysts occur in 5 per cent. Most will regress spontaneously within 4 weeks.

Side effects of clomiphene

- Side effects are uncommon and infrequently interfere with treatment. They are dose related and are more frequent and more severe when higher doses of clomiphene are given.
- The more common side effects are hot flushes (vasomotor symptoms similar to the menopause which disappear on discontinuation of the therapy, 10 per cent), abdominal discomfort due to distension, bloating, pain or soreness (5 per cent).
- Ovarian enlargement and visual blurring is also reported.

- Visual disturbances (1.5 per cent), described usually as blurring or spots or flashes (scintillating scotomata), increase in incidence with total dose and disappear within a few days or weeks after discontinuation.
- Other less frequently reported symptoms include nausea, vomiting, increased nervous tension, depression, fatigue, dizziness or lightheadedness, insomnia, headache, breast soreness, heavier menses, weight gain, urticaria (0.6 per cent), urinary frequency, and moderate reversible hair loss (0.3 per cent).
- In unresponsive women the dose of clomiphene may be increased to 10 days.

Tamoxifen is a similar drug to clomiphene. A triphenylethylene derivative, it appears to be as effective as clomiphene in inducing ovulation in anovulatory or oligo-ovulatory women. It may have less of an anti-oestrogenic effect on cervical mucus.

In the patient with PCOS, if clomiphene therapy fails there is the option of either laparoscopic ovarian diathermy or gonadotrophin therapy.

Laparoscopic ovarian diathermy has the advantage of a 50 per cent success rate in terms of pregnancy while avoiding the risk of multiple pregnancy associated with the use of gonadotrophins, and therefore is particularly useful in patients with PCOS. Ovarian diathermy or the use of gonadotrophins is indicated after a failure of conception with 9–12 treatment cycles of clomiphene.

Gonadotrophin therapy

Gonadotrophin therapy is indicated for women who have been treated with anti-oestrogens who have failed to ovulate or who have negative postcoital tests due to the anti-oestrogenic effect on cervical mucus [29].

It is also used for ovulation induction in those women who are anovulatory and failed to ovulate with clomiphene citrate or bromocriptine.

Gonadotrophins were initially urinary-derived human menopausal gonadotropins (hMGs or FSH). Modern FSH is made from recombinant technology. Gonadotrophins are glycoprotein hormones. Their activity can only be measured by bio-assay and not immunoassay. The cumulative live birth rate with gonadotrophin stimulation is 60 per cent, with multiple pregnancy rates of up to 20 per cent and miscarriage rates of up to 30 per cent, after 12 months. Down-regulation with GnRH agonists and subsequent gonadotrophin stimulation may result in a two-fold increase in the pregnancy rate.

Principles of treatment

The amount of medication and duration of therapy vary in different patients, but also in different treatment cycles in the same patient. A certain basic FSH threshold is necessary to initiate follicular development, and this varies from cycle to cycle. The patient is monitored to determine when one or more mature pre-ovulatory follicles have developed. Maximal diameter of the dominant follicle is correlated with serum oestradiol levels. The total volume of all developing follicles also correlates with oestradiol concentration. One mature pre-ovulatory follicle can be identified in association with a serum oestradiol level of approximately 500 pmol/l. If ultrasound imaging of the follicles is not done, serum oestradiol concentrations of 1000 pmol/l may be presumed to indicate that at least one or two follicles have reached pre-ovulatory status. hCG is given when there is a mature pre-ovulatory follicle shown on ultrasound scanning (≥18 mm).

Protocol for gonadotrophin administration

Hyperstimulation and multiple pregnancy ought to be avoided
Traditionally 75–150 IU of gonadotrophin was used and increased by 75 IU every 3–5 days. Low dose step-up regimens should now be used. Start with 37.5–50 IU FSH, which is increased after 14 days if there is no response, and then by 37.5–50 IU FSH every 7 days. Treatment cycles may be up to 28–35 days but the risk of multiple follicular growth is reduced. A 10–30 per cent increment in the dose of exogenous FSH is required for follicular growth. Ovulation is triggered with a single intramuscular injection of hCG (10 000 IU). It is given when there is at least one follicle ≥18 mm in diameter. It should not be given if there are three or more follicles larger than 16 mm in diameter or four follicles larger than 14 mm, as the risk of triplets is unacceptable.

After 3–5 days measure the serum oestradiol level. If the baseline concentration has doubled the same dose of gonadotrophin is given. If the oestradiol level is unchanged, the dose of gonadotrophin is increased by 50 per cent and the oestradiol level measured 3 days later. If the oestradiol level remains similar to the baseline level, the dose is increased by 50 per cent and the oestradiol level measured every 3 days until a response occurs. Whenever the oestradiol level has doubled, the new dose is maintained.

There is no value in increasing the initial dose before the fifth day because recruitment of follicles takes between 5 and 15 days. Further increases are made at 4–7 days. In subsequent cycles the starting dose is determined by the patient's previous response.

In subsequent treatment cycles, therapy begins at that level. An ultrasound scan is done when the oestradiol level reaches about 500 pmol/l. Scanning is repeated every 2–3 days until the mean diameter of the dominant follicle is 14 mm. After that scanning is done daily. When a follicle is ≥18 mm the gonadotrophin is discontinued and 10 000 IU hCG is given 24 hours later to cause ovum release. It should be withheld if there are three or more follicles 18 mm or more in diameter. This regimen should give ovulation rates approaching 100 per cent with 70 per cent conception rates. The pregnancy rate per cycle is approximately 18 per cent and the mean number of treatment cycles is three. Eight per cent of pregnancies are multiple. Ovarian enlargement may occur in up to 10 per cent of treatment cycles. Treatment should not be given for more than a year.

GnRH agonists

The use of GnRH agonists in addition to gonadotrophin therapy enables accurate timing of ovulation and hence either intercourse or intrauterine insemination.

Use of GnRH agonists (Table 5.14)

LH and FSH secretion is determined by the pulsatile secretion of luteinising hormone-releasing hormone (LHRH)/GnRH. The half-life of GnRH is 2–8 minutes. Intermittent pulsed administration of GnRH results in sustained release of FSH and LH, whereas continuous administration inhibits the secretion of both FSH and LH. Repeated pulses of GnRH stimulate an increase in the number of GnRH receptors, or modulate a post-receptor response leading to self-priming or up-regulation. In contrast, constant infusions of GnRH down-regulate by depleting receptors and therefore desensitising the post-receptor response.

Table 5.14 Types of GnRH analogues and recommended dose.

Generic name	Trade name	Half-life	Administration route	Recommended dose
Nonapeptides				
Buserelin	Suprefact, Suprecur	80 min	s.c., i.n.	200–500 µg/day 300–400 µg three to four times daily
Goserelin	Zoladex	4.5 hours	s.c. implant	3.6 mg/month
Nafarelin	Synarel	4 hours	i.n.	200–400 µg twice daily

s.c., subcutaneous; i.m., intramuscular; i.n., intranasally

GnRH agonists act as if a constant GnRH infusion was being given because of their high receptor affinity. After an initial flare effect there is down-regulation with a profound reduction in gonadotrophin secretion. By blocking the endogenous gonadotrophin secretion, especially the LH surge, agonists improve the predictability of the ovarian response in women with PCOS and in superovulation regimens for IVF.

GnRH agonists are given intranasally, subcutaneously or as a depo injection, either subcutaneously or intramuscularly.

GnRH agonists prevent the surge of pituitary gonadotrophin that occurs in response to the rising serum oestradiol levels produced by multiple ovarian follicles, thereby reducing the chance of spontaneous ovulation and where the cycle can be cancelled. They allow continuation of stimulation in cases of asynchronous follicular growth. The other advantage of GnRH agonists is to provide ovarian stimulation protocols that can be timed to a convenient time for oocyte collection and embryo transfer, thus coordinating the patient, laboratory staff and clinician.

Down-regulation of the pituitary gland

Pretreatment with a GnRH agonist alters the hormonal milieu and the ovarian response to gonadotrophin and the pregnancy rate among women with polycystic ovaries. The advantage of an agonist is that the frequency of spontaneous premature LH surges in women with polycystic ovary syndrome is lower. However, the dose of gonadotrophin needed to achieve adequate follicular development is increased by 30–50 per cent with a GnRH agonist. The GnRH agonist must be terminated with giving the hCG.

GnRH protocols [30]

1 Long protocol
- Commence the GnRH agonist either in the mid-luteal phase of the preceding cycle or in the early follicular phase of the treatment cycle.
- GnRH agonists are continued after pituitary suppression and continued until the day of hCG administration.

2 Short protocol
GnRH agonists and gonadotrophin are started in the early follicular phase of the treatment cycle and continued until the day of hCG administration.

3 Ultra-short protocol
The GnRH agonist is only administered for 3 days at the beginning of the treatment cycle.

Laparoscopic ovarian drilling to induce normal cyclicity

- The procedure involves four to ten ovarian punctures per ovary (8 mm depth at 40 W for 4 seconds) using insulated needle cautery.
- It is inserted perpendicularly to the ovarian surface.
- The hilum of the ovary and the ovarian blood supply should be avoided.
- The ovarian surface is lavaged: 50–100 ml of crystalloid solution may be left in the peritoneal cavity to minimise ovarian adhesion formation.

Endocrine changes after laparoscopic ovarian drilling
- Decrease in serum LH concentrations
- Decrease in serum androgen concentration due to destruction of androgen-producing ovarian stroma and drainage of follicles which have high androgen levels
- These endocrine changes may persist up to 72 months after surgery.

Results
- Ovulation rates up to 80 per cent.
- Cumulative pregnancy rates up to 55 per cent

- Normalisation of serum LH levels
- Low miscarriage rate – 14 per cent.

Pregnancy rates are higher after IVF in those previously treated with ovarian drilling. Women treated with ovarian drilling have a lower rate of hyperstimulation and cancellation of IVF cycles compared to those not treated.

Complications
- Periadnexal adhesion formation
- Premature ovarian failure
- Minimising injury to the ovarian surface minimises adhesion formation
- Washing out the peritoneal cavity decreases adhesion formation because it removes fibrin exudate from raw peritoneal surfaces. It is the fibrin surface that provides the matrix for fibroblast and capillary formation.

Hypogonadotrophic hypogonadism
- This may be at the level of the pituitary or the hypothalamus.
- Oestradiol levels are <100 pmol/l.
- Gonadotrophin levels are subnormal (5 IU/l).
- Ovulation can be optimally induced in women with intact pituitary function by application of pulsatile LHRH or GnRH, administered s.c. or i.v. by infusion pump.
- The injections are given at 90 minutes at a dose of either 15 μg s.c. or 5–10 μg i.v.
- This method of ovulation induction is physiological and runs very little risk of multiple pregnancy or ovarian hyperstimulation syndrome (OHSS).

Complications of ovarian stimulation with gonadotrophins – ovarian hyperstimulation syndrome

Hyperstimulation can occur in the polycystic ovary because of the role of vascular endothelial growth factor (VEGF). OHSS is a sudden increase in vascular permeability resulting in a massive extravascular exudate (manifesting ascites), and a corresponding profound depletion of intravascular volume, as shown by haemoconcentration and decreased urine output. Loss of protein into the third space causes a fall in plasma oncotic pressure which results in further loss of intravascular fluid (Tables 5.15 and 5.16).

Table 5.15 Ovarian hyperstimulation syndrome – symptoms and signs.

Marked ovarian enlargement (>10 cm)
Ascites
Pleural effusions
Haemoconcentration
Hypercoagulability
Oliguria

Table 5.16 Management of ovarian hyperstimulation.

Grade I	Advise the patient to weigh herself daily and take abundant fluid. Weight gain more than 5 kg or abdominal distension, nausea and vomiting should lead to hospitalisation
Grade II	Intravenous therapy, progesterone, TED stockings, analgesia, paracetamol and pethidine for severe pain. Avoid non-steroidal anti-inflammatory drugs
Grade III	Ascites, respiratory difficulty, decreased circulation and renal function. Admit to intensive care. Central venous pressure (CVP), renal function, input and output
	Check haemoconcentration by measuring haematocrit, intravascular volume depletion and blood viscosity
	Haematocrit greater than 45% is a serious sign, greater than 55% is life-threatening. Leucocytosis may be greater than $40\,000 \times 10^9$. Measure body weight, serum urea, creatinine, electrolytes, serum albumin, liver function tests, coagulation profile: infusion of colloid maintains intravascular volume. Human albumin 50–100 ml repeated as required, normal saline for rehydration. Consider abdominal paracentesis

5

Grade I (mild ovarian stimulation) – fluid accumulation, weight gain, abdominal distension and discomfort. Ultrasound shows enlarged ovaries with a diameter greater than 5 cm.

Grade II (moderate) – nausea and vomiting. Great abdominal distension and more discomfort and dyspnoea. Ascites is present.

Grade III (severe) – life-threatening condition where there is clinical evidence of contraction of the intravascular volume (subnormal central venous pressure with reduced cardiac output), severe expansion of the third space (tense ascites, pleural and pericardial effusions), severe haemoconcentration and hepatorenal failure. Intravascular thrombosis may occur, particularly cerebral.

Prevalence

Overall risk 4 per cent, severe form 0.25 per cent. With in vitro fertilisation 1–10 per cent, severe cases 0.25–2 per cent.

Risk factors

- Polycystic ovaries
- Younger women with greater ovarian responsiveness
- Use of gonadotrophins
- Development of multiple immature follicles during treatment
- The use of hCG when the ovaries have been overstimulated
- An oestradiol level greater than 8000–10000pmol/l
- Twenty or more oocytes.

Ovarian hyperstimulation syndrome can be avoided in the woman responding too much by stopping the treatment and avoiding giving the ovulatory dose of hCG. Oocytes may be collected and fertilised *in vitro* and the embryos inserted on a later cycle to avoid the risk of OHSS associated with any pregnancy that might get established.

Monitor the following

- Degree of ascites
- Oliguria
- Rise in serum creatinine
- Falling creatinine clearance
- Haemoconcentration unresponsive to medical therapy
- Severe oliguria or renal failure persisting – give dialysis. Careful cardiac assessment to avoid cardiac tamponade from pericardial effusion. Avoid hydrothorax – paracentesis for relief of dyspnoea.

IN VITRO FERTILISATION

Steptoe and Edwards published their dramatic achievement in unassuming style [31].

> 'We wish to report ... a 30-year-old nulliparous married woman, was safely delivered by caesarean section on July 25, 1978, of a normal

healthy infant girl ... The patient had been referred to one of us (PCS) in 1976 with a history of 9 years' infertility, tubal occlusions, and unsuccessful salpingostomies done in 1970 with excision of the ampullae of both oviducts followed by persistent tubal blockages. Laparoscopy in February, 1977, revealed grossly distorted tubal remnants with occlusion and peritubal adhesions. Laparotomy in August, 1977, was done with excision of the remains of both tubes, adhesiolysis, and suspension of the ovaries in good position for oocyte recovery.

'Pregnancy was established after laparoscopic recovery of an oocyte on Nov. 10, 1977, *in vitro* fertilisation and normal cleavage in culture media, and the reimplantation of the 8-cell embryo into the uterus $2\frac{1}{2}$ days later' (with permission, *The Lancet*).

5

And so was born the technique of *in vitro* fertilisation.

Embryology

Ova pick-up is timed for 35 hours after the hCG injection, which is the equivalent of the LH peak. Once the eggs are collected into Irvine's Human Tubal Fluid (HTF) media they are supplemented with a 10 per cent serum substitute protein source. On the day of egg collection, sperm are added. In IVF, washed sperm at a concentration of 50 000 sperm per egg are added to the tube. With ICSI, washed sperm are used and a single sperm is injected into each egg using a microscope specifically set up with a micromanipulator.

The next time the eggs are looked at is 16–18 hours after the sperm are added. At that stage, if fertilisation has occurred, two pronuclei are visible inside the egg. One of these contains the genetic material from the egg and the other the genetic material from the sperm. These pronuclei membranes will break down and the genetic material will combine and become the genetic material of the new zygote.

At this stage, the sorts of things that are seen with the eggs are those with no pronuclei because fertilisation has not occurred even though sperm has got in. Sometimes three or more pronuclei are present which means in IVF more than one sperm has got in. With ICSI, the majority of times this would represent disruption of the meiotic spindle as a result of the interference.

Over the next 24 hours the embryo will start to divide, initially to a two-cell embryo. Initial divisions of the embryo are programmed by the maternal DNA in the cytoplasm. The genetic material of the zygote is not activated at this point. After the eight-cell stage, the embryonic genome is activated and controls further embryonic development.

Around the fifth day after egg pick-up the embryo goes through quite a major structural change – the formation of the blastocyst. At this stage the cells migrate to the periphery of the zona pellucida (egg shell) and fluid enters from the culture medium.

Transfer of embryos may occur on days 2–3 at the cleavage stage (two- to eight-cell stage) or on day 5 (the blastocyst stage). At days 5–6 the zona pellucida either bursts, dissolves or ruptures and implantation occurs. Therefore, transfer must occur before this otherwise the opportunity for implantation is missed. (Transfer of zona-free embryos can be done successfully.)

Various locations around the world have different constraints regarding the number of embryos that are replaced. These are based on ethical, scientific and pragmatic considerations. In general, two embryos are replaced in those women younger than 37 years. There is an international move to transfer only one good quality blastocyst to avoid the morbidity and high costs of high order multiple pregnancy complications.

Pre-implantation genetic diagnosis

Pre-implantation genetic diagnosis for aneuploidy, sex chromosome status and DNA analysis can be done for recurrent genetic disease. Around the eight-cell stage a single cell is taken out of the embryo, the theory being that each single cell inside the embryo is identical. That single cell is fixed, i.e. attached to a slide, and a specific DNA probe is used to identify chromosomes or genes of interest.

Grading of embryos

A 'good embryo':
- Has even-sized cells

- Has no evidence of fragmentation of any of the cells
- Has a granular appearance to the cytoplasm within these cells
- Develops according to a strict timetable.

At the blastocyst stage a 'good blastocyst' has a large number of cells in the embryo with a distinct inner cell mass.

Freezing of embryos

Embryos may be frozen at the pronuclei stage, cleavage stage or blastocyst stage. Generally freezing/thawing at the pronuclei stage is more successful.

Propandiol and glycerol are the most commonly used cryoprotectants. These replace water within the cell. When freezing, the damage to cells is always from swelling with ice crystal formation within the cells which, when thawed, disrupts the integrity of the cell membrane. Embryos are transferred into a series of increasing concentrations of cryoprotectants to completely replace all the water in the cell. In general, it requires three concentrations (taking about 30–45 minutes) and at that point the freezing process takes place. The actual freezing process is run through a computer program. Starting at room temperature (22°C), the temperature is decreased by 2°C every minute down to −6°C, at which point the straw is 'seeded' to start crystallisation. It is held at −6°C for 10 minutes. The reduction from −6 to −30°C occurs at a rate of 0.3°C per minute. Then the reduction of temperature occurs at 2°C per minute down to −40°C, then the embryos are plunged into liquid nitrogen which is at −196°C. They are stored then until thawed for up to 5–10 years.

Thawing involves a reversal of the above process. The embryos are taken out of liquid nitrogen into air temperature for 15–30 seconds, then plunged into 30°C for 30–50 seconds and then they are put through a series of decreasing concentrations of sucrose in phosphate-buffered saline until the solution is all saline, which replaces the water in the cell. They are then kept in media until transfer to the woman (usually on the same day). Glycerol is used for the blastocyst stage and propandiol for the two- to eight-cell (cleavage) stage.

Freezing sperm

Sperm are a lot sturdier than embryos. Sperm are mixed with an equal quantity of human sperm preservation media. They are loaded into straws which are then cooled down and suspended just above the level of liquid nitrogen in a canister for 30 minutes. They are then plunged into the liquid nitrogen (–196°C).

To thaw, the straws are removed from the liquid nitrogen and left at room temperature. Thawing takes 5 minutes and then the sperm may be used for insemination/ICSI. A percentage of sperm are always lost in the freeze/thaw cycle. In general 40 per cent of motile sperm will survive freezing and thawing, but if it is used for IUI it needs to be washed, and if washed the yield is 10 per cent.

Maturation stage

Pregnancies are achieved with mature female gamete type and metaphase type II. The main safety mechanism is possible damage to the meiotic spindle in the induction of aneuploidy.

Cryopreservation of oocytes

No one has been able to grow *in vitro* a primordial follicle through to a mature oocyte. To be able to do this would be ideal. In animals the frozen ovarian tissue has been grafted back and it has taken. Freezing ovarian tissue is still not possible.

Oocytes may be preserved where fertility is likely to be impaired, mainly due to chemotherapy, and is indicated if the woman does not have a partner. For every 100 oocytes that are frozen there are 4 babies, compared with freezing 100 embryos, where there are 25 pregnancies. Therefore it is more appropriate where there is a partner to freeze embryos. The stages can be summarised as:

(1) Preliminary exposure to the cryoprotectants, which are substances that reduce cell damage from ice crystals.
(2) Progressive temperature reduction down to –196°C.
(3) Storage.
(4) A subsequent thawing after a variable length of time.
(5) Dilution and washing of the cryoprotectants to restore a physiological micro-environment and allow subsequent development.

The two most critical moments affecting cell survival are the phase of initial cooling and the return to physiological condition. When reducing the temperature between –5 and –15°C, the ice nucleation is first induced in the extracellular medium by a process called 'seeding'. As the temperature is gradually decreased, ice builds up in the solid concentrate in the extracellular medium. This determines an osmotic gradient: water moves out of the cytoplasm and cells shrink from the dehydration. If freezing is carried out slowly, water diffusion from the cell does not allow the formation of large ice crystals inside the cytoplasm. Two events that occur during thawing which can reduce cell survival are recrystallisation and osmotic shock. Recrystallisation means that water moves back inside the cell and solidifies around small ice crystals already formed, increasing their size. The likelihood of recrystallisation depends on both cooling and thawing rates. It is avoided by careful dehydration and rapid thawing of the cells.

Osmotic shock may occur if, after thawing, the cryoprotectant that penetrated the cell during cooling cannot diffuse out quickly enough to prevent the influx of water and swelling of the cells.

The main factors that influence the outcome of cryopreservation concern the oocyte – size, quality, age (should be picked up between 35 and 37 hours after administration of hCG), maturity, cumulus and the technique – type, temperature, concentration and exposure time of cryoprotectants, freezing and thawing rates. Oocytes must be cryopreserved the same day of collection, possibly within 8 hours.

TUBAL SURGERY

- Tubal surgery has not been made redundant by IVF. If the tubes are thin walled, with little muscle fibrosis and reasonable mucosa, over one third of women will achieve a live birth subsequently, and half of those will go on to have a second live birth.
- Microsurgery enables avoidance of damage to delicate serosal and coelomic surfaces.
- Magnification (by loupes (×10) or microscope – focal length 200–300 mm) is necessary for tubal surgery in dealing with a tubal diameter of 0.5 mm.
- The main indication for tubal surgery is tubal block caused by pelvic inflammatory disease, endometriosis (at the cornual end) or congenital anomalies.
- Salpingostomy is the opening of a totally blocked fimbrial end.
- Fimbrioplasty is used for fimbrial phimosis or when there is a fibrous ring partly obstructing the fimbrial end.
- Salpingolysis is the division of adhesions around the tube.

- Salpingotomy – incision in the tube wall and inspection of the lumen – is usually associated with ectopic pregnancy.
- Diathermy dissection gives clean results and can largely be bloodless. Cutting diathermy is by a fine needle of 4–5 W (monopolar).

Instruments

- Microsurgical instruments should be used, with needleholders to hold a suture of 140 μm in diameter (up to 8/0 non-absorbable nylon). Polypropylene amide (prolene) is also ideal because of its lack of tissue reaction.
- Fine probes made of Teflon or glass are useful for handling tissues and supporting them during dissection. They reduce abrasion or trauma that would be caused by handling with gloved fingers.
- The steridrape used has a 15 cm ring which can be inserted inside the wound at the start of laparotomy. It prevents leakage of blood into the abdominal cavity, reducing the risk of serious peritoneal abdominal wall adhesions after surgery.

The prognostic variables for reversal of sterilisation are maternal age and tubal length of >4 cm with intrauterine pregnancy.

REFERENCES

1 Collins, J.A., Burrows, E.A. & Willan, A.R. (1995) The prognosis for live birth among untreated infertile couples. *Fertility and Sterility*, **64**, 22–28.
2 Greenhall, E. & Vessey, M. (1990) The prevalence of subfertility: a review of current confusion and a report of two new studies. *Fertility and Sterility*, **54**, 978–983.
3 Te Velde, E.R., Eijkemans, R. & Habbema, H.D.F. (2000) Variation in couple fecundity and time to pregnancy, an essential concept in human reproduction. *The Lancet*, **355**, 1928–1929.
4 Menken, J., Trussell, J. & Larsen, U. (1986) Age and infertility. *Science*, **23**, 1389–1394.
5 Wichmann, L., Isola, J. & Tuohimaa, P. (1994) Prognostic variables in predicting pregnancy: a prospective follow-up study of 907 couples with an infertility problem. *Human Reproduction*, **9**, 1102–1108.
6 Wilcox, A.J., Wineburg, C.R. & Baird, D.D. (1995) Timing of sexual intercourse in relation to ovulation. Effects on the probability of conception, survival of the pregnancy and sex of the baby. *New England Journal of Medicine*, **333**, 1517–1521.

7 Hull, M.G.R., Glazener, C.M., Kelly, N.J. *et al.* (1985) Population study of causes, treatment, and outcome of infertility. *British Medical Journal*, **291**, 1693–1697.

8 Hughes, E.G. & Brennan, B.G. (1996) Does cigarette smoking impair natural or assisted fecundity? *Fertility and Sterility*, **66**, 679–689.

9 Vine, M.F., Margolin, B.H., Morrison, H.I. & Hulker, B.F. (1994) Cigarette smoking and sperm density: a meta-analysis. *Fertility and Sterility*, **61**, 35–43.

10 Health Education Authority (1996) *Think about drink, there's more to drink than you think.* HEA, London.

11 Garrow, J.S. (1991) Treating obesity. *British Medical Journal*, **302**, 803–804.

12 Mieusset, R. & Bujan, L. (1995) Testicular heating and its possible contributions to male infertility: a review. *International Journal of Andrology*, **18**, 169–184.

13 European Society for Human Reproduction and Embryology (1996) Guidelines to the prevalence, diagnosis, treatment and management of infertility. *Human Reproduction*, **11**, 1775–1807.

14 Oehninger, S. (1995) An update on the laboratory assessment of infertility. *Human Reproduction*, **10**, 38–43.

15 Van den Eed, E. (1995) Investigation treatment of infertile couples: ESHR guidelines for good clinical and laboratory practice. European Society for Human Reproduction and Embryology. *Human Reproduction*, **10**, 1246–1271.

16 Royal College of Obstetricians and Gynaecologists (1998) *Initial Investigation and Management of Infertile Couples.* Evidence-based clinical guidelines No. 2. RCOG, London.

17 Baird, D.T. (1997) Amenorrhoea. *The Lancet*, **350**, 275–279.

18 Fishel, S., Dowell, K., Timson, J., Green, S., Hall, J. & Klentzeris, L. (1993) Micro-assisted fertilisation with human gametes. *Human Reproduction*, **8**, 1780–1784.

19 Hendry, W.F., Levison, D.A., Parkinson, M.C., Parslow, J.M. & Royle, M.G. (1990) Testicular obstruction: clinicopathological studies. *Annals of the Royal College of Surgeons of England*, **72**, 396 407.

20 Belker, A.M., Thomas, A.J. Jr, Fuchs, E.F., Konnak, J.W. & Sharlip, I.D. (1991) Results of 1469 microsurgical vasectomy reversals by the Vasovasostomy Study Group. *Journal of Urology*, **145**, 505–511.

21 Matthews, G.J., Schledgel, P.N. & Goldstein, M. (1995) Patency following microsurgical vasoepididymostomy and vasovasostomy: temporal considerations. *Journal of Urology*, **154**, 2070–2073.

22 Brinsden, P.R., Wada, I., Tan, S.L. & Jacobs, H.S. (1995) Diagnosis, prevention and management of ovarian hyperstimulation syndrome. *British Journal of Obstetrics and Gynaecology*, **102**, 767–772.

23 Bryan, E.M. (1992) *Twins and Higher Order Births: a Guide to Their Nature and Nurture.* Edward Arnold, London.

24 Rossing, M.A., Daling, J.R., Weiss, N.S., Moore, D.E. & Self, S.G. (1994) Ovarian tumours in a cohort of infertile women. *New England Journal of Medicine*, **331**, 771–776.

25 Venn, A., Watson, L., Lumley, J., Giles, G., King, C. & Healey, D. (1995) Breast and ovarian cancer incidence after infertility and *in vitro* fertilisation. *The Lancet*, **346**, 995–1000.

26 Artini, P.G., Fasciani, A., Sellar, V. *et al.* (1997) Fertility drugs and ovarian cancer. *Gynaecological Oncology*, **11**, 59–68.

27 Balen, A.H. (1997) Anovulatory fertility and ovulation induction. Policy and Practice Subcommittee of the British Fertility Society. *Human Reproduction*, **12** (Suppl. II), 83–87.

28 Balen, A.H., Braat, D.D., West, C., Patel, A. & Jacobs, H.S. (1994) Cumulative conception and live birth rates after the treatment of anovulatory infertility: safety and efficacy of ovulation induction in 200 patients. *Human Reproduction*, **9**, 1563–1570.

29 Hamilton-Fairley, D., Kiddy, D., Watson, L., Sagle, M. & Franks, S. (1991) Low-dose gonadotrophin therapy for induction of ovulation in 100 women with polycystic ovary syndrome. *Human Reproduction*, **6**, 1095–1099.

30 Tan, S.L., Maconochie, N., Doyle, P. *et al.* (1994) Cumulative conception and live birth rates after *in vitro* fertilisation with and without the use of long, short, and ultrashort regimens of the gonadotrophin-releasing hormone agonist buserelin. *American Journal of Obstetrics and Gynecology*, **171**, 513–520.

31 Steptoe, P.C. & Edwards, R.G. (1978) Birth after the reimplantation of a human embryo (letter). *The Lancet*, **ii** (8085), 366.

5

6 Ultrasound and the Use of Imaging in Gynaecology

Wendy Hadden

PELVIC ULTRASOUND

Technique

The female pelvic organs are visualised through a full bladder, as a window to the pelvis (Fig. 6.1). This is the original technique, from the days of static scanning. There are problems associated with this technique.

- The organs of interest are pushed into the far field of the image.
- They will be out of the focal zone of the transducer.
- A lower frequency transducer will need to be used.

The result is a decrease in resolution of the uterus and ovaries, with the potential to misinterpret information obtained and lesions may be pushed out of the pelvis by the full bladder, hidden by bowel gas, and missed.

Graded compression of the pelvis

This is an acceptable technique with present generation ultrasound machines [1]. This brings the organs of interest into the near field and allows a higher frequency probe to be used.

- It obviates the need to fill the bladder – a bonus if an anaesthetic is contemplated. In fact, drinking and producing fluid-filled peristalsing bowel degrades the image and makes it more difficult to obtain.
- For optimal visualisation the bladder is empty and gentle pressure to the lower abdomen will allow the female pelvic organs to be seen.
- A coronal view of the uterus will be obtained (Fig. 6.2). This may be confusing for the operator in the first instance.
- The cervix is recognised as a hypoechoic area with echogenicity adjacent to the cervical canal.
- The ovaries may be seen. If not seen, it implies they are small.

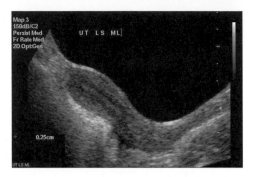

Fig. 6.1 Abdominal ultrasound. The uterus in the sagittal plane seen through a full bladder.

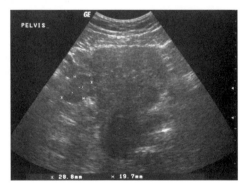

Fig. 6.2 Graded compression ultrasound of pelvis showing a coronal view of the uterus with hypoechoic cervix inferiorly, and with a small ovary to the right.

- If there is considerable pelvic fat the ovaries will stand out.
- Any fluid containing adnexal lesions can usually be detected.
- Significant pathology is not missed.
- A transvaginal ultrasound is not compromised by active bowel.

▪ A transvaginal ultrasound is necessary to evaluate the female pelvis properly.

Transvaginal ultrasound (TVS)

A full and proper assessment of the female pelvic organs cannot be made without performing a transvaginal ultrasound examination. Improved technology has made transvaginal transducers smaller and more acceptable to patients. A keyhole image of the pelvis is produced.

▪ With the transducer in the vagina, close to the organs of interest, a probe with a frequency higher than that for transabdominal ultrasound can be used, with consequent improvement in resolution of the uterus, and the ovaries.

▪ Wide-angle transducers, with angles approaching 270°, offer excellent coverage and spatial resolution in both the near and far fields, and much of the female pelvis can be imaged.

▪ By using the hand not holding the transducer for palpation on the abdomen, an examination similar to the bimanual examination can be performed.

▪ The periphery of the image, the pelvic side wall, that portion of the pelvis in the lower abdomen, and the bladder, are not well seen.

▪ Bone reflects sound and the bony pelvis is not seen. Thus the confines of the pelvis are not appreciated with transvaginal ultrasound.

▪ With colour Doppler or power imaging, colour-filled iliac vessels will be seen near the edge of the ultrasound image. This delineates the pelvis and helps with orientation.

▪ The vessels can be used as landmarks to find organs such as the ovary.

▪ The bladder and urethra can be seen and evaluated as the probe is removed.

▪ The rectum is not routinely imaged.

(See Tables 6.1, 6.2.)

Sensitivity of ultrasound

Skill in performing the examination has to be developed if accuracy of diagnosis is to be achieved with transvaginal ultrasound. The organs may not lie along the axes textbooks of anatomy suggest. Manoeuvres for finding organs when not readily visible will need to be learned.

Table 6.1 Requirements for pelvic ultrasound.

(1) Ultrasound machine
(2) Transabdominal probes – multifrequency convex array probes (2.5–7.5 MHz)
(3) Transvaginal probe – multifrequency (6–9.5 MHz) wide angle
(4) Colour flow power and duplex Doppler capability an advantage
(5) A facility for cleaning and disinfecting vaginal probes between patients is necessary
(6) Examination couch. The patient may be elevated with a bolster or scanned in a modified lithotomy position
(7) Means of recording procedure. Still capture or video recording

Table 6.2 How to perform a transvaginal ultrasound examination.

(1) Insert probe into the vagina
(2) Obtain a sagittal image of the uterus and the cervix for orientation
(3) Uterine fundus is to the right of the image and the cervix to the left
(4) Sweep the probe from side to side to view all of the uterus and cervix in the sagittal plane
(5) Check the appearance of the endometrium, myometrium and cavity
(6) Review and measure the endometrium in the sagittal plane
(7) Obtain additional information with use of colour flow or power Doppler
(8) Rotate the transducer through 90° and view the uterus in the transverse plane
(9) Sweep through the uterus from fundus to cervix in the transverse plane
(10) Check the endometrium, myometrium and the cavity again and correlate with the impression obtained from sagittal plane
(11) Use Doppler as necessary
(12) Return to the sagittal plane of the uterus and rotate and angle the probe to find the ovaries
(13) Use the internal iliac vein as a marker to the ovary if necessary
(14) Find the long axis of the ovary and plane at right angles and measure ovarian volume
(15) Review the appearance of each ovary
(16) Use colour flow or power Doppler to determine the periphery of the ovary and distinguish it and cysts from vessels in the adnexa
(17) Image the angle between the uterus and ovary – the 'ectopic angle' – and try to distinguish the fallopian tube as a separate structure
(18) Probe the isthmus portion of the tube. If pain is elicited this suggests endometriosis
(19) Use the hand not holding the transducer to palpate the abdomen as required to aid in finding structures and provide additional information about pain and fixation
(20) Check for free fluid in the pouch of Douglas and adnexa
(21) View the bladder and urethra as the probe is withdrawn
(22) Use a Valsalva manoeuvre to assess for incontinence and prolapse

6

- Ultrasound is totally operator dependent and relies on how the operator perceives what is being seen.
- Ultrasound is not as sensitive an imaging modality as many believe.
- Some ultrasound appearances are distinctive, but there is overlap with different conditions producing similar ultrasound appearances and lesions may not be recognised for what they are.
- Sensitivity for detecting abnormality depends on what abnormality is being detected.
- Sensitivities of 60 to 85 per cent for detection of abnormality with ultrasound are the norm.
- Other imaging modalities such as computerised tomography (CT) and magnetic resonance (MR) produce images that are more easily interpreted. They perform better in detection of abnormalities than ultrasound. Sensitivities for these modalities range from 90 to 98 per cent.
- Ultrasound is a good screening test but once malignancy is detected, CT and MR are required because of greater accuracy.
- Important diagnoses have the potential to be overlooked if transabdominal evaluation of the pelvis is not performed. Parts of the abdomen may need to be examined to make a diagnosis. The kidneys should always be examined. Hydronephrosis, if present, particularly if bilateral, is a very strong indicator of pelvic malignancy. Ascites, if present, is also suggestive of malignancy. Lymphadenopathy may be present.
- A normal ultrasound examination does not preclude a problem.

Problems

Wrong or missed diagnoses are possible.
- Transvaginal ultrasound is non-specific.
- An examination may not produce all the information required even in the ideal situation.
- In a certain percentage of patients, organs such as ovaries, and parts of organs such as the endometrium, may not be visualised.
Some patients are just not good candidates for ultrasound.
- Obesity is a problem. Fat reflects and attenuates sound. Fat is deposited in the pelvis just as it is elsewhere in the body and it compromises visualisation.
- Bowel in the pelvis can have confusing appearances. The gas in the bowel reflects sound and this can obscure lesions.
- The reflection by gas-filled loops of bowel can appear as a noisy artefact and can be mistaken for a cyst.

- In women after the menopause, visualisation of the pelvis can be difficult. The size of all the organs is reduced and because of increased fibrosis, the organs and their internal architecture become similar to surrounding structures.
- As age advances the uterus increasingly attenuates the sound beam. More especially in the nulliparous older woman, the myometrium and the endometrium become increasingly difficult to discriminate. The ovaries will be difficult to find as they become smaller and lose the follicular activity that is a guide to position.

Conduct of the ultrasound examination of the pelvis

The examination is an intimate one for the patient. Discussion of the procedure is necessary. Many women will not understand what is required of them when they come to have a pelvic ultrasound. Before commencing the transvaginal portion of the examination, the woman should be asked to empty her bladder to avoid discomfort during the procedure. Cooperation for the examination can often be obtained by suggesting the woman may like to introduce the probe herself. During the examination, talking to the patient and informing them about what is happening is reassuring. At all times the aim is to relax the patient. As a clinician there is also the opportunity to gather information, such as relevant history, during the procedure.

The examination can be performed on a regular examination couch. Using a bolster under the buttocks or merely using the patient's clenched fists to elevate the pelvis may facilitate manipulation of the probe. Asking the patient to roll and lift one side of the pelvis can also help to image the adnexa. Legs can be rolled or bent outwards or used for support.

Risk for infection

With a vaginal ultrasound, there is a greater risk for infection than with a transabdominal ultrasound. Every patient must be regarded as a potential source of infection and appropriate precautions should be taken to prevent cross-infection between patients and operators. Manufacturers' recommendations should be used with respect to disinfecting the probe. Soaking in sodium hypochloride solution (diluted to 500 parts per million) for 2 minutes is a satisfactory method. Cleaning of the probe, with soap and water if necessary, and removing gels from the transducer after each use are important measures of cleanliness. Covering the probe prior to each examination is important. Commercial probe covers containing gel are very convenient and easy to use. Probe covers are barriers for patient protection but are not infallible. There is a certain incidence of perforation. All air must be removed from the area between the cover and the transducer face to enable full sound transmission. The operator is advised to use gloves for their own protection.

Measurements

- Structures identified should be measured.
- An idea of size is often a clue as to whether an organ is normal or not.
- The size of an organ is not always appreciated at the time of the examination unless measured.

On-screen callipers are available for measuring with most machines. Machines that calculate volumes are useful and will produce volumes while the examination is in progress (Fig. 6.3). For example, this will allow a large ovary to be recognised as large and thus more attention can be paid to the appearance of the ovary to determine why it is large.

6

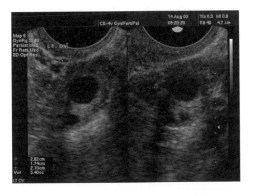

Fig. 6.3 An ovary measured at vaginal ultrasound with the ultrasound machine producing an on-screen volume of the ovary.

- Accuracy to 0.1 of a millimetre may be suggested by the readout from an ultrasound machine but this level of discrimination is not possible.
- Accuracy to 1–1.5 mm is to be expected but may be difficult to achieve.
- True orthogonal planes at right angles to one another are difficult to obtain at transvaginal examination.
- Except in a very few situations, there is no consistency between end points for measuring structures. Even the same operator can use different end points between examinations.
- Repeatability from one examination to the next is unreliable.
- Average diameters and volumes are recommended for comparing various examinations for size of organs or pathology over time.
- Multiple measurements of size convey little of the impression of size.
- A single measurement gives rapid understanding of size for clinical correlation. A 7 cm length uterus will be normal in a premenopausal nulliparous woman and a 10 cm length uterus will be enlarged. A postmenopausal uterus should be small, 5–6 cm in length. If larger than this pathology should be suspected.
- A film record is desirable. Measurements may need to be repeated or used to assess changes over time and over a number of examinations. A record will help with replication of measurements and help assess change.

Anatomy and normal appearances

The uterus

The uterus is a somewhat pear-shaped structure in the central lower pelvis. It lies posterior to the bladder. The myometrium contributes most to the ultrasound appearance of the uterus. Three layers of myometrium can be distinguished with the middle, an even and moderately echogenic layer, accounting for most of the uterus. A thin subendometrial anechoic layer can be seen. This is the junctional zone on MR imaging (Fig. 6.4). The outer subserosal layer is distinguished by the presence of vessels that can be seen as small hypoechoic areas within the myometrium at the periphery of the uterus, or as vessels with colour Doppler. The uterus is best imaged in sagittal and transverse planes.

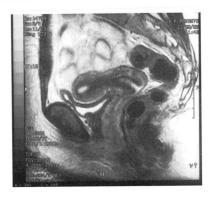

Fig. 6.4 MR image of the uterus. In this sagittal image the uterus is anteverted, the endometrium is a bright high signal centrally, the myometrium is the intermediate signal, and the junctional zone between the two is seen as a black low signal line 2–3 mm in thickness that is continuous into the cervix.

The overall uterine length in a premenopausal woman is 7–9 cm, the width 4 cm and the depth 3 cm, when measured abdominally and including the cervix. The cavity is a strong specular reflector that is seen as an echogenic line running the length of the uterus and continuing into the cervix where it represents the endocervical canal.

The uterus and the cavity are usually difficult to image in the coronal plane and the shape of the cavity is usually not appreciated. It can be seen when the uterus is anteverted and when transabdominal imaging with an empty bladder is used. Where assessment of the shape of the cavity is important, e.g. in imaging of congenital abnormalities, there are difficulties because the appropriate plane to image the cavity cannot be readily obtained. Three-dimensional imaging will allow easier imaging in the coronal plane and will offer improvement over the current two-dimensional imaging for assessment of uterine anomalies.

The endometrium

The endometrium is echogenic and lies adjacent to the cavity. It can be measured accurately (Fig. 6.5). Although one study suggests an interobserver error of 1.5 mm^2, other studies have suggested better

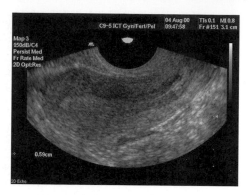

Fig. 6.5 Vaginal ultrasound of the uterus showing the endometrium measured in the sagittal plane.

correlation. The appearance and thickness of the endometrium vary according to the age of the patient and the stage of the menstrual cycle. In the postmenopausal patient the endometrium is seen as a thin echogenic line very little different from the cavity echo. The uterus and endometrium are not normally particularly vascular, but the subserosal vessels can be particularly prominent and when filled with colour they can be used to assess whether colour flow Doppler is being applied correctly to the uterus.

The ovaries

The ovaries are two ovoid structures lying medial to the internal iliac artery and vein and lateral to the uterus. The ovarian artery is seen entering the superior pole confirming the nature of the structure as an ovary. The ovaries are less echogenic than the uterus and they have a somewhat heterogeneous appearance from the small follicles present. Size varies according to age. A normal ovary in a woman in the reproductive age group will have a volume of around 9 ml. Postmenopausal women will have an average ovarian volume of 2–3 ml and premenarche females will have ovaries of 3 ml. Volume (length × breadth × depth × 0.523) is the most reliable method of measuring size.

The fallopian tubes are more difficult to image. They are not seen abdominally unless dilated and fluid filled. Normal tubes can be

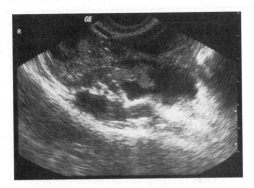

Fig. 6.6 The fimbrial end of the fallopian tube is readily imaged at vaginal ultrasound when surrounded by fluid.

identified transvaginally. They are two tubular structures of similar echotexture to the uterus arising from the uterine cornu and extending laterally. They will be better seen when surrounded by fluid (Fig. 6.6). An attempt should be made to visualise them at all times to exclude pathology.

Hormonal status

The appearance of the female pelvic organs is closely related to the hormonal environment. In the premenopausal woman the cyclical changes in the levels of oestrogen and progesterone will alter the appearances of the endometrium and the ovaries. The endometrium is thin following the menses but thickens as the cycle progresses. By mid-cycle it will have a prominent hypoechoic layer, giving it a tri-layered appearance. It will become progressively thicker and more echogenic in the second secretory half of the cycle. The developing follicle will be seen in one or other ovary as a simple cyst that is rounded, anechoic, thin walled and that will reach a size of about 22 mm before it ruptures (Fig. 6.7). It will be replaced by a corpus luteum (Fig. 6.8). This may have a very similar appearance to the preceding follicle.

Circumferential blood flow around a corpus luteum as demonstrated by colour flow Doppler can often be the distinguishing

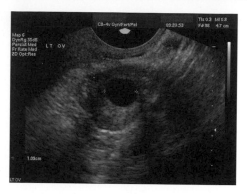

Fig. 6.7 A developing follicle (measured) seen with the ovary at vaginal ultrasound.

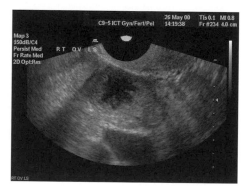

Fig. 6.8 A corpus luteum is seen in this ovary as an irregular cyst with contained echoes.

feature. At all times the appearance of the endometrium and ovaries should be correlated with the stage of the menstrual cycle, and if there is inconsistency, pathology can be suspected.

The oral contraceptive pill suppresses ovarian function and the ovaries will become smaller and the follicles much less obvious. The uterus also becomes smaller with size approaching the lower limit of normal with a length of 6–7 cm. The endometrium is often reduced to a thin echogenic line. Similarly in the postmenopausal woman, oestrogen withdrawal correlates with a small uterus and ovaries. As follicles are no longer present the ovaries become harder to identify. Although in the early postmenopausal period, follicular activity may be identified within the ovaries and small simple cysts around 20–30 mm are not unusual, they may need to be followed until they disappear to exclude pathology. They tend to become much less common over time.

Small ovaries – less than 2 ml in volume, without follicles and with absence of blood flow – in a woman in the reproductive age group will indicate premature menopause.

Hormone replacement therapy affects the appearance of the uterus, endometrium and ovaries. Appearances will differ depending on the nature of the hormone replacement used. Sequential therapy mimics the menstrual cycle. The thickness of the endometrium will depend on the stage of the induced cycle. Unopposed oestrogen will thicken the endometrium considerably.

EARLY PREGNANCY – FIRST TRIMESTER ULTRASOUND (see Chapter 2)

6

Note that the first sign of pregnancy is thickening of the endometrium. This may not be recognised for what it is.

Pregnancy-related gynaecological problems

Fetal abnormality in the first trimester

There is increasing emphasis on recognising fetal abnormality (Fig. 6.9), particularly in the late first trimester, so that an early termination can be performed if necessary. The entire fetus needs to be imaged and normal appearances recognised so that fetal early abnormality is not missed. Anencephaly is one abnormality that may have a different appearance to later in pregnancy and is not recognised for what it is. A whole new range of fetal abnormality appearances has to be learned by those practising early ultrasound assessment.

Nuchal translucency

Measurement of the nuchal translucency (NT) is a screening test and an indicator of age-adjusted risk for trisomy 21 or Down's syndrome

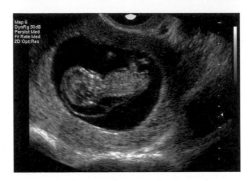

Fig. 6.9 Fetus with Turner's syndrome.

[3]. Rigorous guidelines have been developed for measurement of the tissues behind the fetal neck in fetuses ranging from a crown rump length (CRL) of 45 mm to a CRL of 84 mm (11 to 13 +6 weeks gestational age). Graphs for values for increasing thickness indicating increasing age-adjusted risk have been developed [4] (Fig. 6.10). A computer program based on the data simplifies the process and provides a more accurate age-adjusted risk assessment [5]. This is not so important for young women, where age is a lesser factor, but in the older women aged 36 years and up a high risk from age may be reduced by a normal NT measurement and obviate the need for karyotyping with its associated risk.

As a guide for measurement: an NT less than 3 mm suggests the fetus is at low risk for Down's syndrome. At age 40 years the risk for Down's syndrome can be reduced four times from 1 in 50 to 1 in 200 if the NT measurement is less than 2.5 mm.

Retained products of conception

- Either postpartum or post-miscarriage/termination echogenic thickening of the central echogenicity/endometrial complex of the uterus, or an echogenic mass within the uterus, suggests retained products of conception.
- Heterogeneous thickening or the presence of fluid in the uterine cavity is less certainly retained placental tissue. It is more likely to represent blood clots and/or necrotic material.

RISKS FOR TRISOMY 21

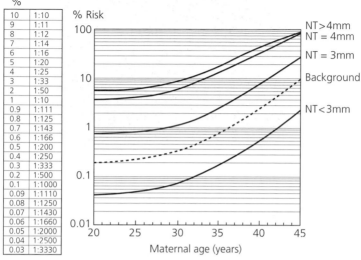

Adjusted risk for trisomy 21 with maternal age according to nuchal translucency (NT) thickness measurements of <3mm, 3mm, 4mm and more than 4mm

Fig. 6.10 Graph illustrating estimated risks for trisomy 21 at 10 to 14 weeks of gestation on the basis of maternal age alone (background) and maternal age with nuchal translucency thickness measurements of 3 mm, 4 mm and greater than 4 mm. (Snijders *et al.* (1996) [4].)

6

- A small amount of fluid is normally seen in the post-termination uterus at 7–10 days.
- Although gas in the uterine cavity may be indicative of infection and endometritis, it may be a normal finding postpartum from 3 days to 3 weeks.

An unusual occurrence postpartum is dehiscence of a Caesarean section scar. The scar will be widened, the uterine muscle thinned and complex echogenic fluid will be present and continuous with fluid in the uterine cavity (Figs 6.11 and 6.12). This should not be confused with retained products of conception.

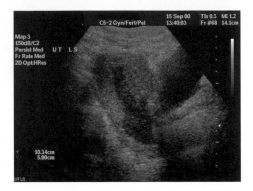

Fig. 6.11 Abdominal and transvaginal appearances of dehiscence of a Caesarean section scan producing an appearance similar to retained products of conception but distinguished by a deficiency in the uterine wall anteriorly.

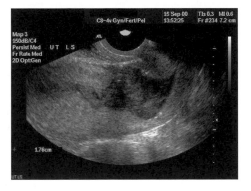

Fig. 6.12 The vaginal ultrasound shows the defect in Fig. 6.11 to advantage.

Ectopic pregnancy

In the appropriate setting ectopic pregnancy can have suggestive or definitive sonographic findings. It should also be considered as a cause for any adnexal lesion in a premenopausal woman.

Definitive sonographic findings include:
- An echogenic thick-walled ring structure, of an appearance similar to an intrauterine gestational sac, in an extrauterine position. This

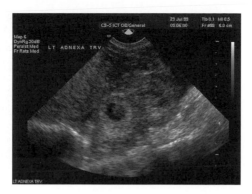

Fig. 6.13 An ectopic pregnancy demonstrated at vaginal ultrasound, showing a thick-walled echogenic ring structure of an appearance strongly suggestive of a gestational sac in an extrauterine position between the uterus and ovary in the 'ectopic angle'.

will lie in the ectopic angle between uterus and ovary (Fig. 6.13). Size is often smaller for a given gestational age than when intrauterine.

- It may contain a yolk sac, and fetal parts with or without fetal heart activity.
- A 'ring of fire' produced by the high velocity, low impedance blood flow on colour Doppler or power ultrasound can aid detection of trophoblast [6] and confirmation of an ectopic pregnancy (Fig. 6.14).
- An adnexal mass on its own is less convincing of an ectopic pregnancy. It is evidence of an embryo or trophoblast that makes the diagnosis.
- In a patient with a positive pregnancy test, an empty uterus, and the isolated finding of free intraperitoneal fluid, there is 69 per cent sensitivity for an extrauterine gestation [7]. If the free peritoneal fluid is echogenic, the specificity is improved for detection of an ectopic pregnancy. Echogenic fluid has a positive predictive value of 93 per cent. It is due to the presence of a bleeding or ruptured ectopic pregnancy.

Trophoblastic disease

Typically there is a 'snowstorm' appearance of multiple vesicles of the hydatidiform mole within the uterus (Fig. 6.15). It is mimicked

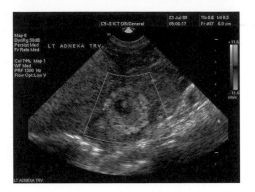

Fig. 6.14 Interrogation with colour flow Doppler showing a 'ring of fire' appearance, confirming the presence of trophoblast and showing that echoes seen within the sac are produced by an embryo with cardiac activity.

6

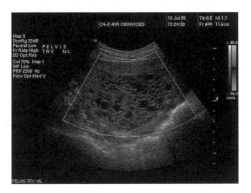

Fig. 6.15 The 'snowstorm' appearance of a hydatidiform mole.

only by some uterine dysgerminomas, sarcomas or lymphomas. These tumours do not usually produce the hormonal markers, β human chorionic gonadotrophin (βhCG) or α-feto protein (αFP), and can be distinguished. Transvaginal ultrasound may have an ancillary role to serial βhCGs (which measure cure, possible persistent trophoblast disease, or metastases) in diagnosis and in monitoring treatment. Nodules of residual gestational trophoblastic disease show evidence of angiogenesis with frequent arterio-venous anastomoses. This produces a characteristic ultrasound appearance with striking blood flow on colour or power Doppler imaging. **Arteriovenous malformations** secondary to uterine curettage may have a similar appearance. Both will produce an ultrasound angiogram of bizarre vascularity, irregular vessels of varying sizes, turbulent high blood flow and aliasing. Ultrasonically they are indistinguishable.

UTERINE PATHOLOGY

Fibroids

- The classic ultrasound appearance is of a large rounded mass within the uterus of low to moderate echogenicity with a heterogeneous echotexture.
- The echogenicity of the fibroid depends on the ratio of smooth muscle to fibrosis, with the more echogenic fibroids containing more fibrous tissue.
- Alternatively they may be quite hypoechoic, almost cystic.
- They can usually be distinguished from a cyst by the fact that they are strongly attenuating of sound, such that there is either posterior shadowing or there is poor definition of the structures posterior to the fibroid.
- Fibroids may be submucous, mural, subserosal or pedunculated.
- Ultrasound will identify fibroids but may not give an accurate idea of size, number or location of the fibroid in relation to the uterine cavity. This may be relevant in fertility patients or prior to surgical treatment of the fibroids.
- For a fibroid uterus greater than 12-week size, a transabdominal ultrasound will be more informative as to number, size and location of the fibroids.
- There is often prominent peripheral blood flow and only a little internal flow on colour Doppler interrogation.
- Calcification within a fibroid may be seen as bright echogenic foci within the fibroid.
- Malignant change may not be appreciated.
- The various patterns of degeneration are usually not able to be determined at ultrasound although red degeneration of pregnancy or

6

haemorrhagic infarction of a fibroid may be seen as fluid within a fibroid, allowing recognition.

Submucous fibroids

Of all types of fibroids, the submucous type is the one that should be recognised as it is more often implicated as a likely cause of fertility problems or excessive bleeding. If there is a view to operative intervention, the proportion of the fibroid that is related to the uterine cavity should be assessed and an idea of the depth of penetration of the fibroid into the myometrium made.

Saline infusion sonography (SIS)

Saline introduced into the uterine cavity, via a fine catheter, improves the specificity of the diagnosis of submucous fibroids [8]. It defines the relationship of fibroid to uterine cavity (Fig. 6.16). Both transvaginal ultrasound alone and with saline in the uterine cavity are more sensitive than hysteroscopy for diagnosing fibroids [9]. The discomfort from the distension of the uterine cavity by saline is minimal. The procedure takes only a little longer than a regular vaginal ultrasound. Infective complications are rare. Submucous fibroids characteristically have an overlying rim of endometrial

6

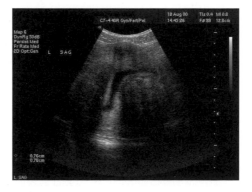

Fig. 6.16 The submucous position of a fibroid is demonstrated more clearly when the uterine cavity is distended with saline. There is a thin rim of endometrial tissue over the fibroid with more normal thickness endometrium elsewhere in the cavity.

tissue that aids recognition and confirms the submucous location. If SIS identifies fibroids, hysteroscopy could be avoided.

Subserosal fibroids

These are of lesser importance than submucous fibroids, but if they become exophytic and pedunculated they may be difficult to distinguish from an ovarian mass such as a solid ovarian neoplasm. In this situation a connection between the mass and uterus should be looked for. Colour flow Doppler may identify blood flow showing the connection between the two.

When there is difficulty with ultrasound imaging in determining the number, size and location of fibroids, MR imaging should be considered [10]. MR is preferable to CT as it has superior contrast resolution and can resolve the internal architecture of structures in the female pelvis. Sarcomatous change within a fibroid is difficult to detect with ultrasound. It is rare and occurs in less than 1 per cent of women with fibroids. It is more common with intramural and cervical fibroids. No imaging modality, even MR, is reliable in the detection of uterine malignancy. A change in size or appearance of the fibroids may be the only clue to aggressive pathology.

6

Adenomyosis

The appearances at imaging are varied and relate to the distribution of the heterotopic endometrial tissue, the degree of associated muscle hypertrophy, and to the presence of cysts within the heterotopic endometrial tissue. Adenomyosis is often poorly recognised at ultrasound, even at transvaginal ultrasound. In one series where hysterectomy was performed and the prevalence of adenomyosis was 28 per cent, preoperative transvaginal ultrasound assessment yielded a sensitivity of 83 per cent and a specificity of 67 per cent for detection [11]. An *in vitro* study of uteri suggests good intra- and interobserver error in the detection of adenomyosis [12]. Once ultrasound criteria are well established and recognised, high resolution transvaginal ultrasound should allow greater detection of adenomyosis.

MR imaging for adenomyosis has a higher sensitivity and specificity for detecting adenomyosis with an overall accuracy of 85–90.5 per cent [13]. It also defines the endometrium and the layers of the myometrium to greater advantage than ultrasound. The junctional zone on MR, the innermost myometrium is composed of a compact cellular layer. The irregular thickening of this band allows the diagnosis of **diffuse adenomyosis** to be made on MR.

On ultrasound adenomyosis is more difficult to detect and is not seen as widening of the hypoechoic junctional layer. Small subendometriotic cysts when present give a definitive diagnosis for adenomyosis, but they are rarely seen. Heterogeneity of the echotexture of the myometrium is a clue to diagnosis. High resolution imaging may allow detection of more specific changes such as subendometrial linear striations, echogenic nodules, poor definition of the endometrial–myometrial junction and asymmetric myometrial thickening for a more accurate diagnosis (Fig. 6.17).

Focal adenomyosis is often not distinguishable from a uterine fibroid. Subtle differences between the two may allow differentiation. The adenomyoma will be hypoechoic with poorly defined margins, will blend imperceptibly with the myometrium, and will produce a mass effect on the uterine cavity that is smaller than the size would suggest or it will wrap around the endometrium rather than bulging into the cavity of the uterus. An increase in blood to the region on colour Doppler interrogation (Fig. 6.18) may aid diagnosis, particularly as most fibroids will show peripheral flow. Difficulties will occur when both adenomyosis and fibroids are present together in a uterus. However in this situation distinction may not be clinically relevant.

6

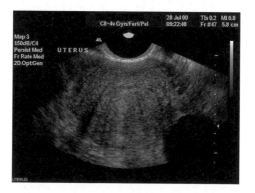

Fig. 6.17 Adenomyosis, showing heterogeneity of the echotexture of the myometrium and asymmetric myometrial wall thickening.

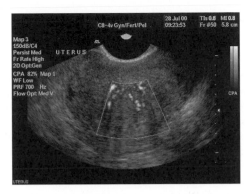

Fig. 6.18 Increased blood flow in the myometrium demonstrated by colour flow Doppler suggests the presence of adenomyosis.

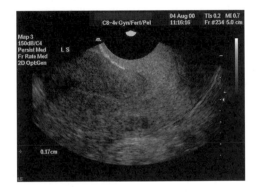

Fig. 6.19 A normal thin endometrium shown at vaginal ultrasound in a postmenopausal woman.

ULTRASOUND ASSESSMENT OF THE ENDOMETRIUM

Transvaginal ultrasound allows accurate assessment of the endometrium (Fig. 6.19). It can be used to evaluate symptomatic women with postmenopausal bleeding or pre- or perimenopausal women with spotting, irregular or heavy bleeding. Accuracy is greater in postmenopausal women.

Data from a meta-analysis of 35 studies that included 5892 women, aimed at determining the accuracy of transvaginal ultrasound to detect endometrial disease, including endometrial cancer, in postmenopausal women with vaginal bleeding, by assessing endometrial thickness, found that transvaginal ultrasound had a high sensitivity for detecting endometrial cancer and other endometrial diseases [14]. Using a 5 mm threshold to define abnormal endometrial thickness, 96 per cent of women with cancer had an abnormal result; 92 per cent of women with endometrial disease including cancer polyp or atypical hyperplasia had an abnormal result.

This did not vary with hormone replacement use. However, 23 per cent of women using hormone replacement therapy (HRT) had a thickened endometrium at ultrasound but a normal endometrium at histology, compared with 8 per cent of woman on no HRT who had an abnormal ultrasound result but normal histology. There will be more intervention in women on HRT but they are more likely to have a normal result.

The study also suggested that a measured endometrial thickness of less than or equal to 5 mm thickness can exclude endometrial disease including endometrial cancer in the majority of postmenopausal women with vaginal bleeding, regardless of hormonal use. For a postmenopausal woman with vaginal bleeding with a 10 per cent pretest probability of endometrial cancer, the probability of cancer would be 1 per cent following a normal transvaginal ultrasound. The Nordic study, where the data from 1168 women were analysed, suggests that if a value of 5 mm is used as the cut-off, two endometrial cancers would be missed [15]. If a 4 mm cut-off is used then the sensitivity is increased to 96 per cent for detecting any endometrial abnormality, but the specificity is reduced to 68 per cent. With a sensitivity of 94 per cent and a specificity of 78 per cent for diagnosing endometrial abnormality using 5 mm for endometrial thickness, there is still reliability of the measurement for detecting cancer. The probability of missing a pathological diagnosis is 6.1 per cent.

In practical terms it means that a postmenopausal woman with an isolated episode of vaginal bleeding and an endometrial thickness of 5 mm or less is unlikely to have endometrial pathology.

Endometrial thickness may be increased up to 8 mm and still be normal in postmenopausal women:

- Who are of heavier build (i.e. greater body mass index (BMI))
- Those on combined oestrogen – progesterone HRT
- Asymptomatic women on calcium channel antagonists to control hypertension.

Other problems of using this method to diagnose endometrial pathology relate to the fact that a single linear measurement is used to assess the entire endometrium. The accuracy of the measurement can be unreliable if the true anteroposterior (AP) diameter is not taken, if fibroids distort the endometrium, or if the endometrium cannot be measured. One study of 182 women showed that where the endometrium could not be defined, one of five women had endometrial cancer.

Morphological assessment of the endometrium may increase sensitivity and specificity of diagnosis. When combined with the use of intracavity saline instillation in the presence of a thickened endometrium there is an improvement in sensitivity and specificity.

Saline sonohysterography or saline infusion sonography (Table 6.3)

SIS is a great advance in the assessment of the endometrium [16]. It competes favourably with office hysteroscopy. A small 5F catheter is inserted into the uterus and sterile saline instilled under real-time ultrasound visualisation (Fig. 6.20). The uterus and the endometrium are viewed systematically in two planes. The cavity is best seen in the sagittal plane and in the same plane the endometrium can be

Table 6.3 Uses of saline infusion sonography.

(1) Abnormal uterine bleeding in premenopausal women
(2) Postmenopausal bleeding
(3) Irregular bleeding in women on hormone replacement therapy
(4) Abnormal thickening of the endometrium shown at TVS or MR
(5) Assessing women on tamoxifen
(6) Assessment of uterine masses prior to surgery, e.g. hysteroscopic resection of fibroids
(7) Recurrent pregnancy losses
(8) Prior to endometrial ablation

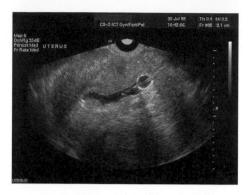

Fig. 6.20 Saline sonohysterography. A small balloon catheter is shown within the uterine cavity after instillation of saline.

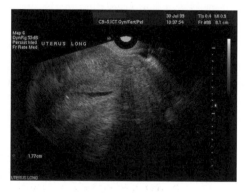

Fig. 6.21 Irregular thickening of the endometrium is well shown when the uterine cavity is distended with fluid.

measured accurately by adding together both layers of the endometrium from the anterior and posterior uterine walls (Fig. 6.21). The hypoechoic subendometrial line should not be included as it is part of the myometrium.

Although the procedure can be performed at any time in the menstrual cycle, it is best carried out in the early proliferative stage of the menstrual cycle when the endometrium is of intermediate thickness. The procedure is not particularly painful and is essentially without risk. Caution may be necessary if pelvic infection is suspected. If the fallopian tubes are patent then the saline will spill into the peritoneal cavity. The likelihood of flushing endometrial cancer cells into the peritoneal cavity is speculative. With the use of small amounts of fluid and low pressure of injection the risk is minimal.

Findings at SIS

Intracavity lesions of the uterus can be evaluated. Pathological causes of endometrial thickening can be differentiated. Uterine polyps and submucous fibroids (see above) should be distinguishable [17].

Polyps

- The endometrial echo is thickened at transvaginal ultrasound.
- Simple polyps are homogeneous, evenly echogenic and blend with the endometrium (Fig. 6.22).
- Complex polyps will be more heterogeneous with hypoechoic areas (Fig. 6.23). These polyps will have more complex histology with areas of infarction, haemorrhage or hyperplasia.
- Small cystic spaces due to dilated glands within the endometrium at transvaginal ultrasound often indicate the presence of a polyp (Fig. 6.24).

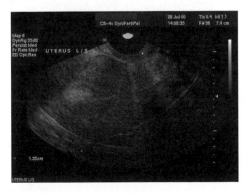

Fig. 6.22 Small echogenic endometrial polyp within the uterine cavity.

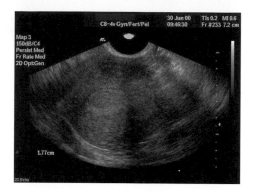

Fig. 6.23 Thickened heterogeneous endometrium due to the presence of a large endometrial polyp, which is not shown as a separate structure without the use of intracavity saline.

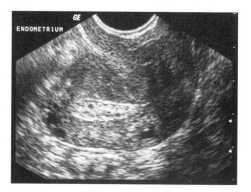

Fig. 6.24 Thickened endometrium containing microcysts suggests the presence of an endometrial polyp.

- A hyperechoic line partially around the thickened endometrium is a reliable sign for the presence of a polyp.
- Blood flow within the polyp may be identified.
- When saline is introduced into the cavity the polyps can be readily seen to be within the cavity (Fig. 6.25).

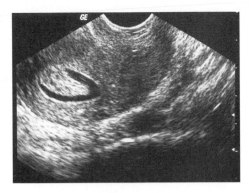

Fig. 6.25 The endometrial polyp is clearly seen when saline is instilled into the uterus. Same case as Fig. 6.24.

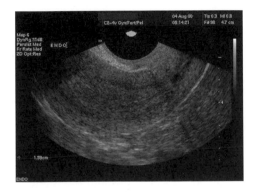

Fig. 6.26 A hyperplastic endometrium seen at vaginal ultrasound in a woman with polycystic ovaries.

6

- The attachment of the stalk and the location of the polyp can be identified.
- The endometrium can be assessed and measured separately from the polyp.
- The endometrium is usually of normal thickness.

Endometrial hyperplasia
- Most hyperplasias present as thickened endometrium (Fig. 6.26).

- In the postmenopausal patient this will measure between 6 and 13 mm with a mean thickness of 10 mm.
- It is a diffuse process usually involving all of the endometrium.
- It can be a focal process or it can be present in a broad-based polyp.
- At transvaginal ultrasound the endometrium is hyperechogenic.
- With saline, the irregular asymmetric endometrium is clearly demonstrated against the saline-filled cavity.
- Rather than involving the whole endometrium, there may be multifocal areas of irregular endometrium.
- The endometrial–myometrial interface will be intact.
- Transvaginal ultrasound, even with the introduction of saline into the cavity, cannot make the diagnosis [18]. Histology is needed for a definitive diagnosis.

Endometrial cancer

- Carcinoma can be difficult to distinguish from hyperplasia.
- The endometrium is thickened at both transvaginal ultrasound and when saline is introduced.
- On average the endometrium is thicker and usually greater than 47 mm (Fig. 6.27).
- The endometrium is irregular and of mixed echogenicity.

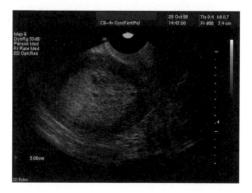

Fig. 6.27 Endometrial cancer with a thickened endometrium of mixed echogenicity. Histologically this was a FIGO grade 1 endometrioid adenocarcinoma of the endometrium, Stage 1c.

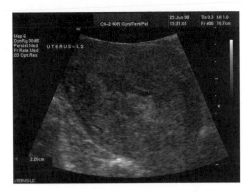

Fig. 6.28 Endometrial carcinoma with complex endometrial echoes, with irregular bands of tissue bridging the cavity and with disruption of the endometrial–myometrial interface.

- The borders are irregular and there is disruption of the endometrial–myometrial interface (Fig. 6.28).
- The cavity of the uterus may be bridged.
- Endometrial carcinoma should be strongly suspected if it is difficult to distend the cavity at SIS.
- In postmenopausal patients, if the endometrial thickness is less than 5 mm, but still identifiable, carcinoma is rare.
- As the endometrium increases in thickness the risk for carcinoma increases.
- Interrogation of the endometrium with colour flow or power Doppler ultrasound has increased specificity only marginally.
- It has been found that in the presence of malignant tissue the impedance to uterine blood flow is significantly reduced compared to controls. Resistive index (RI) values of 0.26 and 0.31 have been found at the periphery of the malignant endometrial echo. Markedly lowered pulsatility index (PI) values of 1.00 have been found compared to atrophic endometrium with a PI value of 3.80.
- A histological diagnosis is necessary to confirm the ultrasound findings.

Endometritis

A thickened endometrium can be due to an infective process.

Atrophic endometrium

When the endometrium measures less than 5 mm in thickness it can be considered to be an atrophic endometrium. It is usually seen as an echogenic line bordering the saline-filled cavity at SIS. Histologically there is sclerosis and dilatation of glands within the atrophic endometrium and occasionally cystic spaces relating to the glands can be seen on ultrasound.

Tamoxifen

Tamoxifen has both oestrogenic and anti-oestrogenic effects on the endometrium and is used to treat breast cancer in postmenopausal patients. Women on tamoxifen need surveillance, as there is an increased risk for endometrial cancer with an incidence of 2 to 3 cases per 1000 women treated. Screening for endometrial carcinoma in women on tamoxifen with TVS may be indicated.

- Appearances at TVS are often unusual.
- Tamoxifen causes changes in the ultrasound appearances of both the endometrium and the myometrium.
- Endometrial thickening with cysts that may indicate endometrial carcinoma needs to be distinguished from myometrial cysts.
- Typically myometrial cysts are quite large cystic spaces surrounded by strong echoes that fill the central cavity region of the uterus (Fig. 6.29).

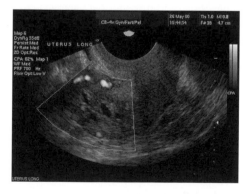

Fig. 6.29 Tamoxifen changes in the uterus with the typical large myometrial cystic spaces associated with marked atrophy of the endometrium. The endometrium is not visualised.

- Most long-term users of tamoxifen have an atrophic endometrium. The cysts seen are usually myometrial cysts rather than endometrial cysts.
- There is the potential at vaginal ultrasound for over-reporting of change towards endometrial malignancy.
- Saline introduced into the uterine cavity can show these changes to be within the myometrium rather than in the endometrium.
- The changes are probably related to endometrial atrophy and formation of microcysts, with the junction between the endometrium and the myometrium becoming irregular and non-linear.
- Alternatively tamoxifen can increase uterine size and thicken the endometrium.
- There is an increased incidence of adenomatous polyps of 36 per cent versus 10 per cent as well as carcinoma.

Adhesions

These can be identified within the uterus at SIS as either thin or thick bridging bands distorting the endometrium. They can be seen to move with saline.

SIS for assessment before endometrial ablation

Because SIS shows intrauterine pathology to advantage, particularly deep location of fibroids, that may preclude the technique of endometrial ablation, it should be considered prior to surgery. If submucous fibroids are demonstrated, hysteroscopy may be used to remove them before endometrial ablation. Adenomyosis is a contraindication to endometrial ablation but it is shown rather better at MR imaging than ultrasound imaging, even TVS.

SIS for infertility patients

For infertility patients or recurrent miscarriage patients, the traditional imaging technique is the contrast hysterosalpingogram. However, it has a high false-positive rate of 10–30 per cent for detecting uterine abnormalities. As hysteroscopy does not evaluate the fallopian tubes, it is of lesser use in infertility patients. SIS may be a practical alternative. It can clearly demonstrate submucous fibroids and endometrial polyps.

Problems in performing SIS

If the uterus is greater than 12–14 weeks' size, the technique is usually unable to be performed. Similarly submucous fibroids of greater than 4–5 cm in diameter will prevent adequate visualisation of the cavity. Large or transmural fibroids will attenuate the sound and reduce visualisation. If the uterus is difficult to catheterise, dilatation of the cervix may be necessary. Problems may be encountered in the retroverted uterus, if synechia are present or if there is cervical stenosis. A uterus with a septum may also be difficult. Kinking of the catheter and air bubbles are additional problems. A patulous cervix and an inability to distend the cavity can be overcome by using a balloon catheter.

Intrauterine contraceptive device (IUD)

An IUD should be readily identifiable in the uterine cavity as a double strong linear echo produced by the front and back walls of the device. The crosspiece of the device should lie across the fundus of the uterus. An attempt at recognising the device is often beneficial in ascertaining that it is correctly positioned. Incorrectly positioned IUDs may be seen traversing the uterine muscle but once extrauterine, they are almost impossible to detect with ultrasound and will need radiography to ascertain whether they are still present within the pelvis or have been passed.

The Mirena is the hardest to see ultrasonically. It has two sets of strong echoes at either end of the device. One group should be detectable in the fundus and the other lower in the body of the uterus if the device is correctly positioned.

THE ADNEXA – OVARIAN LESIONS

Pelvic ultrasound is more sensitive than pelvic examination for the detection of ovarian tumours. Vaginal ultrasound was used to evaluate 52 postmenopausal women before gynaecological surgery unrelated to adnexal disease. None had palpable ovaries. Of 104 ovaries, 85 were visualised with ultrasound and 9 of 10 ovaries with pathological conditions were detected.

Cysts

Cysts are common lesions.
- Because they contain fluid and this is echo-free, cysts are easy to see at ultrasound (Figs 6.30–6.32).

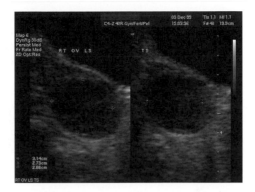

Fig. 6.30 Apparently simple ovarian cyst at abdominal ultrasound.

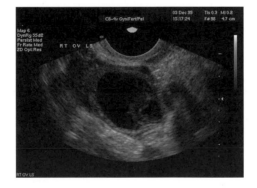

Fig. 6.31 Shown to be a more complex cystic lesion at vaginal ultrasound. This cyst did not resolve over time and was a recurrence of a borderline mucinous cystadenoma.

- They are either simple cysts or they may be more complex lesions with the appearance of multiple cysts within the ovary. Most are ovarian, follicular and physiologic and will resolve given time.
- Typically they are anechoic, round or oval, have smooth thin walls, and are increased through transmission of sound.
- Excess importance should not be placed on the finding of a cyst. A simple cyst is virtually always benign.

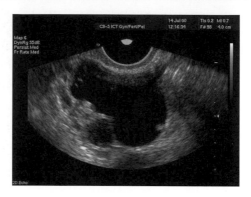

Fig. 6.32 Complex adnexal cyst with a solid tissue and a papillary component. This was a recurrence of a struma ovarii at surgery.

- Simple cysts can be ignored unless they are large, greater than 5 cm.
- They are not uncommon, even in postmenopausal women.
- The problem with the larger cyst is overlooking a feature indicative of malignancy such as an internal papillary projection.
- Cysts can be followed. They should resolve completely over a short time.
- Assessment of cancer cell surface antigen 125 (CA125) may be helpful in determining whether malignancy is likely.
- Haemorrhage into a cyst is the most common complication. The haemorrhagic corpus luteum has a fairly typical ultrasound appearance with contained low level echoes and multiple thin septa producing almost a spoke wheel appearance (see below).

If a cyst does not resolve, has thick septa, or there is a papillary projection, it may be neoplastic (Fig. 6.33). The ovary is often stretched and difficult to recognise when adjacent to a cyst. Care is needed to distinguish ovarian tissue adjacent to a cyst from replacement of the ovary by a cystic and solid neoplasm. Ideally, ultrasound is performed within the first half of the cycle so that a corpus luteum is not misinterpreted as pathology.

Torsion, rupture and haemorrhage into a cyst are acute problems and usually present with pain.

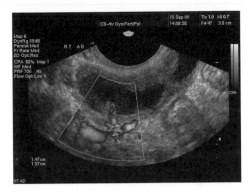

Fig. 6.33 Papillary projection with evidence of blood flow within the stalk. Thought to be a cystic neoplasm but at surgery found to be part of a complex chronic inflammatory process of adhesions and loculated fluid. It is a major difficulty distinguishing between neoplasia and chronic inflammation at ultrasound.

6

Ovarian malignancy

Screening by ultrasound for ovarian malignancy has not produced a reduction in mortality in the same way mammography has in screening for breast cancer [19]. Rather than population screening, regular ultrasound in high risk groups such as the nulliparous, the infertile and those women with one or more first degree relatives with ovarian cancer may be helpful in detecting ovarian cancer early. A cautious approach is necessary. The fact that innocent cysts are common, particularly in the premenopausal patient, may produce considerable anxiety for women being screened. Although ultrasound is useful for diagnosing adnexal lesions, the accuracy or the specificity, particularly for separating benign from malignant lesions, is limited.

Distinguishing benign from malignant lesions

This includes serous and mucinous cystadenomas and cyst adenocarcinomas and carcinomas of low malignant potential.

- The most reliable method of distinguishing benign from malignant lesions is morphological assessment at grey scale ultrasound.

Table 6.4 Ovarian masses: major criteria for increased risk of malignancy.

---

(1) Size greater than 5cm[1]
(2) Complex cystic and solid lesions
(3) Persistence over time

---

[1] Size is questionable as a small lesion can still be malignant.

6

- A cystic component is present in about 50–60 per cent of ovarian neoplasms, making them easily recognised at ultrasound. **Benign** serous cystadenomas are usually large, grossly cystic, often multi-locular and contain simple fluid. **Malignant tumours** are more often complex cystic and solid masses.
- The likelihood of malignancy increases with the size of the lesion detected (Table 6.4): 56 per cent will be malignant if the lesion is greater than 15 cm, 40 per cent will be malignant in the 5–15 cm range, and only 3.9 per cent will be malignant if they are smaller than 5 cm.
- Adding size to the morphological appearances of a lesion does not improve the sensitivity or the specificity for detecting malignancy.
- If an ovary can be identified separate from a lesion, the lesion is more likely to be benign. It may be a pedunculated or degenerating fibroid. If it has a tubulocystic appearance it may be a hydrosalpinx.
- Ovarian size varies and a large ovary per se should not be considered malignant.
- Detection of one or more **papillary projections** arising from the wall of a cyst can identify a serous tumour of low malignant potential, about 15 per cent of all.
- If the papillary projections are numerous and cover much of the surface of the tumour, the tumour will be frankly malignant.
- Thick septations (greater than 2–3 mm thick) increase the chance of malignancy.
- Blood flow patterns may aid in differentiation.
- If there is a significant amount of free intraperitoneal fluid, malignancy should be suspected.

A dermoid does not follow these criteria but can often be recognised for what it is at ultrasound (see below).

Table 6.5 Definitions of spectral display indices.

Name	Abbreviation	Expression[1]
Pulsatility index	PI	A-B/mean
Resistive index	RI	A-B/A
Systolic diastolic ratio	SDR	A/B

[1] A represents the maximum value at peak systole, and B represents the minimum value at end diastole.

Blood flow patterns in ovarian lesions

Doppler evaluation of the blood flow is helpful but not discriminating in distinguishing benign from malignant lesions. There will be higher diastolic flow in a malignant tumour. Tumour vessels do not have muscular walls so they produce less resistance to blood flow. Where there is considerable angiogenesis, i.e. in the more malignant lesions, arteriovenous shunting with aliasing and turbulence of blood flow will be evident. Colour flow Doppler detects vessels, but duplex Doppler is needed to evaluate the blood flow pattern properly.

Measurements of PI and RI indices (Table 6.5) aid categorisation of lesions. PI and RI values will be lower in malignant lesions. Various statements about cut-off values have been made.

- A PI of less than 1 indicates malignancy.
- An RI of less than 0.4 is discriminatory for malignancy.
- The indices are variable and overlap quite widely between benign and malignant.

What is most likely is that there is no single cut-off value but rather a range of values that can be a guide to interpretation as to the nature of a detected lesion. Benign lesions may have low PI and RI values, for example a corpus luteum in the second half of the menstrual cycle, but malignant lesions seldom have high values. If the blood flow pattern is particularly resistive with high PI and RI values and the waveform trace has a dicrotic notch in the diastolic phase, the lesion is almost certainly benign.

Solid ovarian tumours

These are usually benign lesions that can be detected ultrasonically both abdominally and transvaginally, but they may be difficult to separate from other lesions, such as pedunculated fibroids, and they may be difficult to distinguish from bowel. Thecomas, fibromas, thecofibromas and Brenner cell tumours all have a similar ultrasound appearance. They present as a solid, ill-defined, rounded, hypoechoic, strongly attenuating mass. Size may allow distinction between the three lesions, with thecomas being the smallest in the 2–5 cm range, thecofibromas the largest, reaching as much as 16 cm in diameter. Brenner cell tumours are often intermediate at 2–8 cm in diameter. Fibromas may be multiple. The rim of some of the tumours, particularly the Brenner cell tumours, may calcify and give quite a distinctive appearance that has an echogenic rim, as well as attenuation, and on transabdominal ultrasound this is particularly confusing with normal appearance of bowel. Although adnexal they are mostly benign and they seldom obstruct ureters. They can obstruct the venous return from the ovary and occasionally pelvic ascites (Meig's syndrome) will be seen.

Metastatic lesions to the ovaries and adnexa (Krukenberg's tumours) are usually irregular, echogenic solid lesions that do not attenuate the sound and are prone to obstruct ureters. Occasionally haematogenous metastases to the ovaries may infiltrate and enlarge the ovary. Typically it is late stage breast carcinoma that spreads in this way, producing a large hypoechoic ovary. Particularly, abdominally the appearance may suggest a polycystic ovary. If there is ureteric obstruction and an enlarged ovary there is likely to be a malignant process. In the appropriate clinical setting, ureteric obstruction should always raise the possibility of malignancy.

Benign cystic teratoma of the ovary/dermoid cyst

A dermoid cyst may be an incidental finding on ultrasound of the pelvis. It can have a wide-ranging but distinctive ultrasound appearance such that a specific diagnosis can often be made. The range of appearance reflects the components of the tumour (Fig. 6.34). The lesion is usually unilocular but may be multilocular. Arising from the cyst wall and projecting into the lumen is a solid component, the dermoid plug. This can be composed of a variety of different tissues. It is usually seen as one or more highly echogenic nodules in the cyst. The size of the plug can vary from small to large, and can occupy a small or large portion of the cyst. More specifically, and allowing a confident diagnosis of a dermoid cyst on ultrasound, is the presence

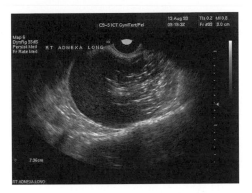

Fig. 6.34 Ovarian dermoid cyst.

of teeth or bone within the plug. These structures will produce an echogenic focus with distal acoustic shadowing. The cystic portion of the dermoid usually contains echoes. Occasionally the echoes will be arranged as hypoechoic lines and dots in the fluid. Echoes of various intensities and anechoic fluid can produce one or more fluid levels within the cyst. In distinction to a haemorrhagic cyst, a dermoid cyst usually attenuates sound. If the dermoid cyst lies at the periphery of the image and strongly attenuates sound, it may be mistaken for bowel. It may not be recognised for what it is. If there is a strong clinical suspicion of an adnexal lesion, and there is a palpable abnormality that is not demonstrated on ultrasound, serious consideration should be given to repeating the ultrasound examination, specifically directed towards detecting an ovarian dermoid.

Haemorrhagic or functional haemorrhagic cyst

This can be mistaken for a dermoid. Particularly in the acute stage the haemorrhage into the cyst can be echogenic and closely resemble a dermoid. In time as the haemorrhage resolves, the cyst becomes hypoechoic and the contained bands and strands of echoes produce a fairly typical appearance. Because the haemorrhagic cyst is basically fluid, there will be increased through transmission of sound and enhancement of the tissues behind the cyst. With time the haemorrhagic cyst will involute and decrease in size.

A follow-up ultrasound examination to see that the cyst resolves is suggested.

Embryological duct remnant cysts

Simple cysts derived from the ducts are often identified on ultrasound but are often not recognised for what they are unless they can be seen as separate from the ovary and distinguished from functional cysts. Para-ovarian cysts are usually oval simple cysts lying between uterus and ovary. A para-ovarian cyst adenoma is a possibility and will be manifested as a cyst with mural nodules and/or septations within a para-ovarian cyst.

A hydatid of Morgagni cyst is by far the most common Müllerian duct cyst identified, usually rounded, 2–10 mm in diameter and often seen when there is pelvic fluid. It arises from the fimbri of the fallopian tube.

The other localised fluid collection within the pelvis that will have a cystic appearance is a **peritoneal inclusion cyst**. These are usually closely related to the ovary and are associated with the presence of adhesions from previous surgery or endometriosis. They will have very thin filmy septations, and the ovary may be included in the cyst. The cyst is an unusual shape with straight sides as it conforms to adjacent structures such as the pelvic wall.

Improvements to diagnosis of ovarian abnormalities

Using a combination of grey scale ultrasound, colour flow and pulsed Doppler ultrasound, an informed judgement as to the nature of an ovarian lesion can be made. All factors should be used to reach a diagnostic decision. Multivariate logistic regression and artificial neural network analysis of these factors may in the future allow improved discrimination between lesions [20]. Three-dimensional volume ultrasound has been suggested for assessing morphological features of ovarian cystic tumours, and alone or in association with 3D power Doppler to show the architecture of the vascularity may also aid early ovarian cancer detection [21].

POLYCYSTIC OVARIES

Polycystic ovaries (Figs 6.35–6.37) are found in 23 per cent of the population and can almost be considered a normal variant. The

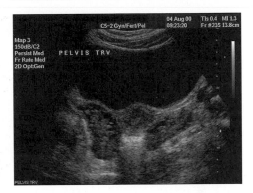

Fig. 6.35 Polycystic ovaries at abdominal ultrasound.

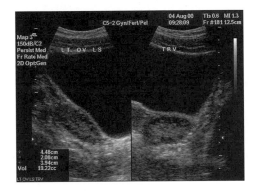

Fig. 6.36 As Fig. 6.36. Measurements show these are large ovaries, one with a volume of 19 ml.

typical ultrasound features are bilaterally enlarged ovaries, echogenic central stroma and multiple small peripheral follicles [22] (Table 6.6). There may be a difficulty in making the diagnosis. Approximately one third of women with polycystic ovaries will have normal ovarian volume. At transabdominal ultrasound only 39 per cent of polycystic ovaries have a typical appearance [23].

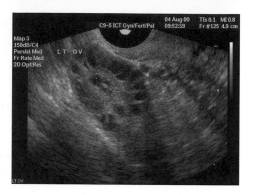

Fig. 6.37 Vaginal ultrasound shows the echogenic stroma and the multiple follicles, mainly peripherally distributed, of the polycystic ovary to advantage.

Table 6.6 Characteristic appearances of polycystic ovaries.

Large size
Echogenic stroma centrally located
Multiple small peripheral follicles, or
Multiple small follicles spread throughout the stroma

Transvaginal ultrasound is necessary to see the small cysts and to make the diagnosis. The major diagnostic criteria are:

- Ten or more small cysts present in any one plane or section. Small cysts or follicles are fairly uniform in size and range from 5 to 8 mm.

- Peripheral distribution of the cysts.

- The appearance of the ovarian stroma is subjective but is probably a better discriminator for distinguishing normal from polycystic ovaries.

- Stroma that is either moderately or considerably increased in echogenicity has 94 per cent sensitivity for diagnosing polycystic ovaries.

- A multivariate analysis suggests that adding in follicular size and ovarian volume gives the best discrimination.

- No additional predictive value is given by adding in the number of follicles present.

Absence of a dominant follicle is a helpful sign, but the converse – the presence of a large follicle – is less discriminatory. A large irregular follicle or cyst often approaching 3 cm is not uncommon in association with otherwise polycystic-appearing ovaries.

Uterine appearances in polycystic ovaries reflect the amount of oestrogen being produced and the absence of progesterone. Usually the uterus will be normal sized to small, with a considerably thickened echogenic proliferative endometrium. Hyperplasia of the endometrium is not uncommon.

At times the small follicles may be spread throughout the ovarian stroma. This variant, sometimes called multifollicular ovaries, is often associated with hypothalamic origin polycystic ovaries. In the multifollicular ovary, there is an overall decrease in oestrogen production. The uterus is usually small and the endometrium thin.

Because many patients with polycystic ovaries are obese, on occasion the ovaries may not be identifiable, even at transvaginal ultrasound. For some women TVS may not be an option. In both situations, MR imaging of the ovaries can be considered [24]. Diagnostic criteria for MR are similar to ultrasound. The multiple small peripheral follicles are clearly imaged on T2 sequences as fluid-filled cysts and make the diagnosis.

More recently blood flow patterns in the polycystic ovaries have been studied, particularly with regard to infertility and treatment for infertility. There is the suggestion that there may be a specific blood flow pattern for polycystic ovaries that can be detected by either colour flow or power Doppler. At this stage it would appear that the subjective assessment of increased intensity and quantity of colour relating to increased blood flow in the ovarian stroma is indicative of polycystic ovaries. There is the suggestion that the peak systolic blood velocity is increased nearly two times normal and that there is a trend towards lower RIs and PIs (RI = 0.52).

Adolescent females with a history of irregular periods and who have either multifollicular ovaries or polycystic ovaries are more likely to go on to the typical appearance of polycystic ovaries than revert to normal. This casts doubt on the suggestion that multifollicular ovaries are a normal finding in many adolescents.

6

ADNEXAL ABNORMALITIES

Infection – pelvic inflammatory disease

Ultrasound diagnosis of pelvic inflammatory disease is confusing and contradictory. Much of the problem is the confusion surrounding the clinical diagnosis of tubal inflammatory disease and the variety of names used to describe the condition. It would be helpful if sonographic markers of the disease could be placed in the context of the pathogenesis of the infective process, and if there could be reliable differentiation between the acute and chronic forms of the inflammatory process [25]. In making the diagnosis of the chronic inflammatory process, the ultrasound appearances need to be reliably distinguishable from the appearance of ovarian cystic neoplasms. In the appropriate clinical setting where inflammatory disease is suspected, sonographic markers of tubal infection include:

- Dilated fluid-filled tubulocystic structure seen at vaginal ultrasound as a pear-shaped, ovoid, or a retort-shaped structure.
- The fluid can be sonolucent or contain low level echoes.
- All of the tube may have one or more of what are relatively reliable signs of tubal infection.
- Incomplete septa.
- An echogenic structure that projects from the wall but does not touch the opposite wall.
- A 'cog wheel' appearance. A specific appearance, a cross-section through a thick-walled tube.
- 'Beads on a string' sign. Echogenic nodules 2–3 mm in diameter on a cross-sectional view of a distended fluid-filled tube.
- The wall thickness reliably differentiates between acute and chronic inflammation. If the wall is thickened greater than 5 mm, it suggests acute inflammation. Less than 5 mm, i.e. thin, is in keeping with chronic infection.

When the infection is confined to the tube the ovary will appear normal. At the tubo-ovarian complex stage the ovary and possibly the tube may be seen as identifiable structures, and may be able to be separated by pressure of the transvaginal probe. At the stage of the tubo-ovarian abscess the patient will be acutely ill, there will be marked tenderness to transducer pressure and the normal architecture of one or both adnexa will be lost. There will be formation of a conglomerate in which neither ovary or tube can be recognised as such. Free fluid is often seen.

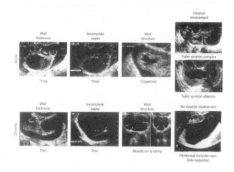

Fig. 6.38 Images demonstrating the various appearances of both acute and chronic pelvic inflammatory disease. (With permission from Timor-Tritsch *et al.* (1999) [25].)

Thus in acute pelvic inflammatory disease (PID), while the infection is confined to the tube, there will be a pear-shaped fluid-filled structure, with thick walls to within 5 mm, incomplete thick septa, and there may be a 'cog wheel' appearance at least in one plane. If it spreads to the ovary and the tubo-ovarian complex develops, initially the tube and ovary should still be recognisable but with progression to the tubo-ovarian abscess there will be a bizarre appearance to the fluid-filled structures, and the ovary will no longer be recognisable as such.

In the chronic stage, PID is suggested by a sonolucent dilated tubulocystic structure, with thin walls, of less than 5 mm thickness, and incomplete thin septa. The 'beads on a string' sign of stretched and flattened endoluminal folds can be seen.

Encysted fluid or a peritoneal inclusion cyst, where there is contained fluid adjacent to a pelvic wall, is a non-specific sign, but may be an indicator or late sequelae of PID. In the chronic stage there should be little or no tenderness to transducer pressure. In 10 per cent of cases of chronic PID, free fluid will be present in the pouch of Douglas (Fig. 6.38).

Endometriosis

Ultrasound plays no part in the diagnosis of endometriosis, as it cannot detect the endometriotic implants. Endometriosis is

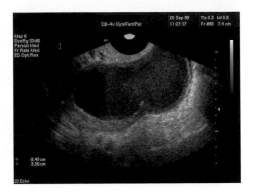

Fig. 6.39 Endometrioma. This vaginal ultrasound shows the distinctive appearance of endometriosis with cysts containing multiple low level echoes of varying intensities between cysts.

6

diagnosed by laparoscopy. However, endometriomas are readily and reliably detected at both transabdominal and transvaginal ultrasound [26]. Eighty to ninety per cent of endometriomas have a characteristic appearance on transvaginal ultrasound of a cystic mass, with multiple homogeneous low level echoes (Fig. 6.39). The rest will be anechoic cysts, cysts with low level echoes and a solid component, or a solid-appearing mass.

Functional haemorrhagic cysts, dermoid cysts and fibroids can be mistaken for endometriomas. If there is difficulty differentiating between the lesions, the presence of thick walls, homogeneity of the echo contents and multiplicity of cysts may help to suggest an endometrioma.

The presence of punctate or linear bright echogenic foci in the wall of the cyst favours the diagnosis of endometrioma. If there is a solid component then it should be avascular. A fluid level in an endometrioma is rare but can occur (Fig. 6.40).

For women with known endometriosis, ultrasound may be a means of assessing the pelvis, particularly if there is recurrent pain, but MR imaging may be a better option than ultrasound for evaluating the pelvis in a woman with known endometriosis and recurrent pain. Although not as accurate as laparoscopy for showing the extent of the disease, it is more accurate than ultrasound.

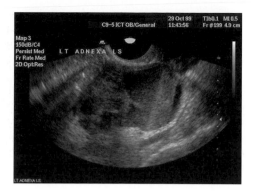

Fig. 6.40 Endometrioma with a fluid level.

If a malignancy such as a clear cell carcinoma relating to endometriosis is suspected then it is likely to be better evaluated by MR than ultrasound. Endometriosis of the bladder may be detected at ultrasound as small mucosal cysts in the bladder. When endometriosis involves other organs such as the bladder it may not be considered in the diagnosis.

FALLOPIAN TUBE PATHOLOGY

Fallopian tube carcinoma

Preoperative diagnosis of carcinoma of the fallopian tube is a sonographic challenge. Incidence of the disease is low, the appearance is not pathognomonic and there is overlap of the appearance with both cystic tumours of the ovary and pelvic inflammatory disease. The stage of the disease and identification of the spread of the tumour may also make distinction difficult. In advanced cases where the uterus and ovary cannot be identified separately, distinction is not possible.

Transvaginal ultrasound, colour and duplex Doppler help in making the diagnosis. Three-dimensional ultrasound, particularly aided by 3D colour Doppler and power ultrasound, may improve preoperative detection of this tumour in the future [27]. It usually presents as a complex dominantly cystic adnexal mass. Because it is derived from a dilated tube it often has a sausage-shaped appearance with associated solid tissue with papillary projections into the cyst. Abnormal blood flow can usually be identified either within the wall within the solid component or within the papillary projections. It should be seen separate from uterus and ovary to make the diagnosis. If there is abnormal vasculature, it will often consist of chaotic randomly dispersed vessels. Microaneurisms, arteriovenous shunts, tumoural lakes and disproportionate calibre vessels suggestive of malignant vasculature will be identified. Duplex interrogation of this vasculature should demonstrate a low RI of less than 0.4. It is suggested that 3D, with more precise depiction of tumour wall irregularities and blood flow patterns, would allow the diagnosis to be made more frequently.

PELVIC PAIN

Pelvic pain is a common problem and transabdominal and transvaginal ultrasound with colour or power Doppler are an effective means of detecting the location and source of pelvic pain. Ectopic pregnancy should be sought in all women of reproductive age with acute pain, particularly those where there is a positive pregnancy test. Occasionally the cause of pelvic pain can be detected by imaging techniques. In many women the cause of the pain will not be found despite full investigation.

Ovarian abnormalities, frequently haemorrhage into a cyst, account for about 10 per cent of women with pelvic pain. About 3 per cent of women will have an unsuspected endometrioma detected. Pelvic inflammatory disease and adhesions account for a large number of women but many will have little in the way of ultrasound findings.

Adhesions may be seen if there is fluid present; or assumed, if the uterus and ovaries do not move independently when the probe is introduced (sliding organ sign).

Adnexal torsion

Adnexal torsion as a cause of pain should be recognised with a careful ultrasound examination if the vascularity of the ovary is assessed with Doppler, but it is not as simple as documenting the presence or absence of blood flow to the ovary, because of the dual blood supply to the ovary. Occasionally the torsion itself can be visualised, but often the torsion is intermittent or chronic, with reduction in venous flow, and the arterial flow will be maintained either via the ovarian artery or the adnexal branch of the uterine artery. The signals from the intraovarian vessels will change and become high impedance with low, absent or reversed diastolic flow. They may become non-pulsatile and mimic a venous waveform. With obstruction to the venous flow the ovary will often enlarge. It usually remains recognisable as an ovary but the oedema may make the stroma echogenic and the peripheral follicles will stand out. An adnexal lesion that has contributed to the torsion may be identified. Haemorrhage usually produces a hypoechoic centre to the ovary. Punctate echoes or bands and strands of echoes may be seen within the hypoechoic centre. Comparison with the other ovary is essential to make the diagnosis.

Ovarian remnant syndrome

After a difficult oopherectomy, remaining remnants of the cortex may continue to function and may produce pain, particularly if there are associated adhesions. A small cyst or a haemorrhagic cystic space in the ovarian fossa with low impedance blood flow that is corpus luteal in nature will be detected.

Pelvic congestion syndrome

Pelvic congestion syndrome can produce chronic pelvic pain. It can be seen on vaginal ultrasound as dilated arcuate, ovarian and uterine veins greater than 3–4 mm in diameter. These will show slow, to-and-fro flow, of less than 3 cm/second. There should be no variation in size with respiration and the vessels will increase in size with a Valsalva manoeuvre. The condition is often seen with a retroverted uterus. It is more common on the left than on the right.

Ovarian vein thrombosis may be an underlying cause of pelvic congestion. The ovarian vein should measure no more than 5 mm in diameter.

MIMICS OF GYNAECOLOGICAL DISEASE

Gastrointestinal disease can mimic gynaecological disease. Ultrasound appearances may allow gastrointestinal disease to be recognised for what it is. Hypoechoic thickening of the wall of an aperistaltic loop of bowel is suggestive of an abnormal segment of bowel. Inflammatory processes such as Crohn's disease and diverticulitis can give this appearance. The inflamed appendix of appendicitis can be detected as a blind-ending non-peristaltic hypoechoic tubular structure in the right iliac fossa (RIF) with a diameter of greater than 6 mm. Enlarged lymph nodes, with the typical appearance of a hypoechoic ring with an echogenic centre, seen in the RIF may indicate inflammation (adenitis).

Abscesses related to inflammatory bowel disease may produce complex fluid collections indistinguishable from tubo-ovarian abscesses. At times strongly echogenic foci, shadowing and reverberatory artefacts from gas in the bowel may allow distinction.

Lymphoma and other neoplastic processes can produce marked hypoechoic thickening of the bowel wall.

Renal calculi may be seen as echogenicities in a dilated distal ureter and ureteric obstruction. Detection or lack of detection of a ureteric jet into the bladder with colour flow Doppler may aid this diagnosis.

6

PAEDIATRIC AGE GROUP

This age group covers right from the neonate to adolescent with a range of diseases and problems. Ultrasound, mainly transabdominal, is used to screen for abnormality and if abnormality is found consideration should be given that it may be gynaecological in origin. Most paediatric gynaecological pathology has a similar ultrasound appearance to the same condition in the adult. Ovarian cysts are common at all ages: 68–80 per cent of imaged ovaries in the paediatric problem will contain cysts or follicles. Even larger cysts up to 4 cm may be benign. If there is a change between ultrasound examinations from side to side, or if there is echogenic debris, or blood clot within a cyst, torsion needs consideration.

Ovarian neoplasms are uncommon. They are likely to be germ cell in origin. They may look like large dermoids or have a dermoid-like component. They are often large, solid and obviously malignant at the time of diagnosis with ultrasound.

In the teenager presenting with primary or secondary amenor-rhoea, ultrasound is the screening method of choice. Findings need to be correlated with hormonal status but there are helpful ultra-sound clues.

▪ An infantile pear-shaped appearance to the uterus with the cervix large and the uterus small and tubular suggests hypo-oestrogenism.

▪ Testicular feminisation syndrome, a male intersex condition, may present at puberty with primary amenorrhoea, and at ultrasound there will be no evidence of uterus or ovaries. A study of the groins may reveal inguinal masses (testes).

▪ Virilisation in teenage years is usually a result of polycystic ovaries.

▪ Tumours, more particularly Leydig-Sertoli tumours (Fig. 6.41) may need consideration. These may be seen as an enlarged ovary with a focal area of altered echotexture and should be considered in any adolescent with suspected polycystic ovaries.

▪ Uterine and vaginal obstruction may be identified as a complex cystic pelvic mass either from bleeding into the uterus or the vagina with production of a haematometra or haematometrocolpos. In these cases ultrasound may not identify the structures correctly, especially where the situation is complex.

6

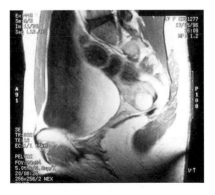

Fig. 6.41 A Leydig-Sertoli neoplasm of low grade malignant potential shown as a rounded area of high signal within the ovary post-injection of gadolinium. This 14-year-old girl presented with hirsuitism and this was originally thought to be due to polycystic ovaries.

- MR imaging is indicated as it gives greater anatomic detail and allows a more precise diagnosis of the complex abnormalities. MR has an accuracy rate approaching 100 per cent for classification for Müllerian duct anomalies and should be considered when doubt arises from either ultrasound or other imaging modality.

FERTILITY

Bicornuate and septate uteri can be identified on ultrasound. The type of imaging used in assessing uterine anomalies and distinguishing between the bicornuate and septate uterus needs to be accurate because prognosis and therapy differ in the two groups. Ultrasound, using a combination of abdominal and vaginal approaches, has the ability to image in multiple planes and evaluate the external contour of the uterus and the relationship with the internal cavity. It performs better than the hysterosalpingogram (HSG) examination [28]. HSG is limited in the planes it can demonstrate and by the fact that it demonstrates only the uterine cavity. It is better able to demonstrate tubal patency than ultrasound. Whether an HSG using oil contrast media for tubal inflation will improve fertility is still under investigation.

Meta-analysis shows that there is a point estimate of 0.65 for sensitivity for detecting tubal patency with a specificity of 0.85 for the regular HSG examination. Ultrasound demonstration of tubal patency, to be useful, must have similar sensitivities and specificities. There are a number of ultrasound microsphere-containing contrast agents that can be instilled into the uterine cavity. They are extremely echogenic and can be visualised as they pass through the fallopian tubes. With time the spheres rupture and the echogenicity is lost. A clear fluid is obtained and can be seen surrounding the tubal fimbria, confirming patency. The rate of passage through the interstitial portion of the tube is taken as a guide to patency. Turbulence and spill from the fimbrial end of the tube is not always visible. Concordance rates vary in different hands but are similar to the hysterosalpingogram, with specificities between 86 and 96 per cent (it is not a technique for the infrequent operator).

MR imaging does not demonstrate the tubes or tubal patency.

CERVICAL ABNORMALITIES

The cervix tends to be ignored at pelvic ultrasound. As it is readily accessible, diagnosis of a problem is usually done by direct visualisation. However, it is seen at ultrasound and wide angle transvaginal probes show the internal echo structure well.

Nabothian cysts are the most common finding. These vary considerably in size and number. They are of no significance. Similarly glands containing fluid and mucous can also be seen as echo-free spaces adjacent to the cervical canal.

Tumours can be seen but ultrasound plays no part in determining the extent of the lesion or in assessing the parametrial or vaginal extension of cervical cancer (Figs 6.42 and 6.43). MR promises greater accuracy and is being increasingly used in evaluating recently diagnosed cases for staging and spread. CT has been regarded as accurate (96 per cent specificity) for assessing nodal spread but MR is equally accurate and may obviate the need for CT. Two techniques, intraluminal ultrasound and rectal ultrasound, have been evaluated for staging carcinoma of the cervix but sensitivity is poor and they are not in widespread use.

6

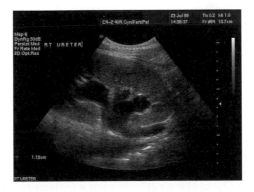

Fig. 6.42 Dilatation of the collecting system and ureter of the right kidney, raising the possibility of an obstructing lesion in the pelvis.

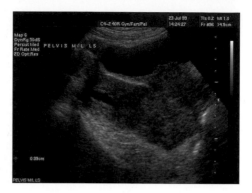

Fig. 6.43 Carcinoma of the cervix causing the ureteric obstruction.

UROGYNAECOLOGICAL ULTRASOUND

The bladder, urethra and vagina can be seen clearly at transperineal ultrasound and assessment of position and movement of the bladder neck, strength of the pelvic floor and uterovaginal prolapse can be quantified [29]. Criteria developed for radiography of the bladder can be applied to perineal ultrasound. Inverting the ultrasound image produces a similar appearance to a cystogram examination. The symphysis pubis can be used as a fixed point. The patient can be supine, the bladder is better empty than full and the position of the bladder neck can be noted at rest and on straining.

In the normal continent female the bladder neck should not descend more than 1–2 cm. Marked descent of the bladder neck, posterior inferior rotation and widening of the angle between the proximal urethra and bladder trigone are markers of stress incontinence. If colour Doppler is used, leakage of urine into the urethra may be detected as a flash of colour. Funnelling of the proximal urethra can also be seen but is non-specific for stress incontinence and can be seen in urge incontinence as well.

The examination is also able to show what is happening in prolapse. Urethral kinking and other unusual appearances of the urethra can be seen if the retrovesical angle is preserved. Strengthening of pelvic floor musculature for continence training can be visualised and provide patient feedback. Following colposuspension proce-

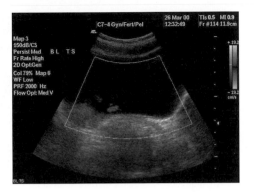

Fig. 6.44 Bladder tumour seen as a thickening of the bladder wall next to the ureteric jet at vaginal ultrasound in a woman presenting with menorrhagia.

dures, ultrasound can be used to show the degree of elevation and distortion of the bladder neck and slings can be visualised, as can other fixation materials. Urethral diverticula can be detected and distinguished from anterior vaginal wall prolapse. A bladder neoplasm or bladder involvement by a neoplasm can be seen (Fig. 6.44).

Even if an ultrasound examination is not directed towards a urogynaecological assessment, vaginal ultrasound in postmenopausal women can be concluded with a quick examination of the bladder neck region. As the transvaginal probe is withdrawn into the lower vagina, the region is visualised. If the patient is asked to strain, in a very short time an assessment of the pelvic floor and continence or otherwise can be established.

ULTRASOUND AND THE DIAGNOSIS OF BREAST DISEASE

Screening for breast cancer

Mammography is the accepted imaging modality used in screening asymptomatic women for breast cancer. There is unequivocal evidence from randomised controlled clinical trials that population-based screening of women between the ages of 40 and 74 can reduce the mortality from breast cancer by approximately 30 per cent [30]. Screening programmes are in place in a number of countries. Age range and frequency of mammograms vary from country to country. Mostly, two-view mammography is offered to women in the 50–65 year age group on a 2- to 3-yearly basis. In this age group there is a high sensitivity and specificity for detecting breast cancer at an early stage when it is most likely to be cured. For most countries, undertaking population-based screening in this age group will be a cost-effective public health measure.

While screening is recommended in the 40–49 year age group, the data for a mortality benefit for these women are less robust. Meta-analyses of the trial data show varying mortality reductions from 10 per cent to 18–29 per cent [31]. The incidence of breast cancer is lower in younger women and there appears to be a relationship between increasing age and increasing sensitivity of mammography for detecting breast cancer. Women 65 years and older stand to gain as much from screening mammography as women in the 50–64 year age group. The gain persists until the compliance is reduced or other health problems intervene. Woman can continue to have regular screening mammography for their lifetime.

For women younger than 35 years, screening mammography is not recommended. Whether there is a role for ultrasound in younger women with significantly increased risk for developing breast cancer is debatable. These women are few in number and there is no demonstrable benefit for them. Most women overestimate their risk of developing breast cancer. Even if there is a family history the risk may not be as great as imagined (Table 6.7). For young women, personalised risk assessment, with the possibility of looking for *BRCA1* and *BRCA2* genes, and individualising a screening protocol would be appropriate.

Breast ultrasound

Ultrasound is not a screening modality [32]. It should be reserved for evaluating women with mammographic abnormalities and breast symptoms. Ultrasound can and will detect breast cancer at a rate of about 3 per 1000 cases. Its use is limited by the fact that it is significantly operator dependent. Targeted to a problem it has excellent sensitivity and specificity for detecting cancer. Sensitivity is independent of age, performing equally in the young woman as in the older

Table 6.7 Specific risk factors for developing breast cancer.

Women should be given an **absolute risk**, not a **relative risk**

Age-related absolute risk of developing breast cancer

Age group	25–44	45–54	55–79	>80
5-year absolute risk (%)	<0.5	0.5–1.0	1–1.5	1.5–2

High risk factors (multiply by 4–10 the above risks for age)
A strong family history:
- Three or more first or second degree relatives on the same side of the family diagnosed with breast or ovarian cancer
- Two or more first or second degree relatives on the same side of the family with breast or ovarian cancer including any of the high risk factors such as bilateral breast cancer, breast cancer diagnosed at less than 40 years of age, breast and ovarian cancer in one individual, breast cancer in a male relative
- One first or second degree relative diagnosed with breast cancer at less than 45 years of age and another first or second degree relative on the same side, less than 45 years of age with carcinoma or sarcoma of the breast

Genetic factors (e.g. *BRCA1* genes). Women with *BRCA1* and *BRCA2* have a one in four lifetime risk of developing breast cancer
High grade ductal carcinoma in situ (DCIS)
Atypical ductal hyperplasia with a family history of breast cancer
Previous breast cancer, particularly in women under 45 years of age at diagnosis
Previous treatment for a childhood cancer (×20 age-related risk), or Hodgkin's disease (×10 age-related risk)

Moderate risks (multiply age-related risk by 2)
A moderate family history of breast cancer:
- One or two first degree relatives diagnosed with breast cancer before the age of 50 without the high risk factors above
- Two first or second degree relatives on the same side of the family diagnosed with breast or ovarian cancer without the high risk factors above

Previous personal history of breast cancer including DCIS
Previous personal history of ovarian cancer
Gross cystic disease of the breast
Atypical ductal hyperplasia with no family history of breast cancer

6

woman, in distinction to mammography. When a cancer has been detected by mammography, ultrasound can act as a guide for various types of needle biopsy for a cellular diagnosis. Fine needle aspiration or core needle biopsy under ultrasound are often more acceptable to a woman than using mammographic guidance.

For breast ultrasound to be successful a high frequency linear transducer of the order of 7–12 MHz should be used. High quality equipment with high digital resolution is a necessity if small cancers are to be found and the interior architecture of a lesion determined, so that a distinction between benign and malignant lesions can be made.

It is no longer sufficient to provide a distinction between cystic and solid lesions. Many ultrasound machines will do this, but there is considerable risk with less than optimal equipment of calling a small hypoechoic cancer a simple cyst. Correlation of clinical and ultrasound findings with any palpable abnormality is essential. The palpable lesion and the ultrasound abnormality must correlate. The technique of the hand not guiding the transducer palpating the breast ahead of the transducer is particularly helpful. Apart from palpating lumps it smoothes the breast and lets the transducer slide more easily over the breast. It gives the operator a good idea of overall breast texture.

Breast cancer

6

Breast cancer at mammography is usually identified as a spiculated area of dense breast tissue – a 'white star'. The larger the lesion the easier it is to detect. A cancer is easier to detect in breasts that are composed of fat and more difficult to detect in dense breasts where a lot of fibroglandular tissue is present. Younger women often have dense breasts. Consequently, a breast cancer can be obscured and not as readily detected. Breast cancer is often multiple and the number of cancers present may not be detected in a dense breast.

Where the breasts are dense, ultrasound can be used to advantage. A breast cancer is usually a hypoechoic lesion that attenuates sound resulting in decreased through transmission. This may be marked and seen as refractory shadowing behind the lesion. Where this is present it is typical of a breast cancer and it allows the breast cancer to be readily recognised (Fig. 6.45). By contrast some hypoechoic lesions will have little or no refractory shadowing and will be difficult to distinguish from benign lesions.

Differentiation of malignant from benign lesions uses the following signs:
- The irregular outline
- Distortion of the tissues around a lesion

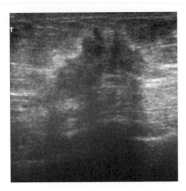

Fig. 6.45 Breast carcinoma. The typical appearance of a large cancer with irregular margins to the lesion, distortion of the surrounding tissue, increased echogenicity anteriorly and acoustic shadowing posteriorly.

- A lesion that is higher than it is wide
- Heterogeneity of the internal architecture
- The appearance of the vasculature associated with the lesion.

If there is uncertainty as to whether a lesion is benign or malignant, biopsy is mandatory.

Calcifications on a mammogram may suggest malignancy, either invasive cancer or ductal carcinoma in situ (DCIS). They may be within an obvious cancer or they may be in breast tissue. Malignant calcifications are typically irregular, of varying size, shape and density, and often have linear and branching forms. Not all calcifications are typical. The calcifications of low grade DCIS are particularly difficult to distinguish from benign calcifications. Calcifications are difficult to detect with ultrasound, and if biopsy is necessary to make a diagnosis this will need to be done under mammographic guidance. There are two ways of doing this – stereotactic core biopsy or open hook wire biopsy.

Benign breast lesions

Cysts

Benign lesions are usually seen on mammograms as circumscribed, well-defined rounded areas of density. The density is similar to that of the fibroglandular tissue in the breast. A margin or a halo around the lesion may allow it to be detectable as a separate lesion. If there are multiple similar lesions and if they are present in both breasts, a benign diagnosis can be made with mammography. However, ultrasound is particularly useful in distinguishing cystic from solid and if there is only one lesion present or the lesions are confined to one breast, ultrasound is particularly useful in distinguishing cysts from solid lesions.

- A cyst on ultrasound will have a similar appearance to cysts elsewhere in the body.
- It will be rounded, anechoic, and will have increased through transmission of sound.
- Aspiration of fluid contents is confirmatory but not always required.

It can be difficult to be confident about the nature of small cysts. They may have thick contents. They may no longer be simple on ultrasonic criteria. They will present diagnostic difficulties, being indistinguishable from other benign but solid lesions and from small cancers.

Fibroadenomas

Fibroadenomas will have the same mammographic appearance as cysts but will be solid lesions, i.e. containing echoes on ultrasound (Fig. 6.46). They are usually:

- Oval
- Hypoechoic, but they can be isoechoic or echogenic compared to the rest of the breast
- Wider than high
- Have homogeneous internal echo architecture
- Increased through transmission of sound
- The surrounding tissues are not distorted
- Mobile – they can move with or be deformed by the transducer and a twisting motion with the free hand can rotate them.

Biopsy or excision is required if there is any doubt or if they are larger than 3 cm, as malignancy is not reliably excluded.

There is a large fibroadenoma often called a giant fibroadenoma. It is a benign tumour. There is also the Phylloides tumour that has an appearance similar to a giant fibroadenoma but has varying malignant potential that is not detectable by imaging methods. All need excision biopsy for diagnosis.

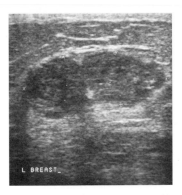

Fig. 6.46 A benign fibroadenoma of the breast. This oval hypoechoic lesion has a well-defined margin and increased through transmission of sound consistent with a benign lesion, but it is large and there is inhomogeneity of the echotexture such that biopsy is warranted to exclude malignancy. Core biopsy can be used to advantage in this type of lesion.

Inflammation and breast abscess

Inflammation due to bacterial infection, producing a cellulitis, will thicken the skin and increase the echogenicity of the tissues of the breast. The tissue planes, particularly the plane between the subcutaneous fat and the glandular tissue within the breast, will become indistinct. There may be shadowing. On ultrasound appearances alone it is indistinguishable from inflammatory cancer.

If abscess formation occurs a fluid-containing lesion will develop in the breast. This will have irregular thick walls. The contained fluid will vary in appearance from anechoic fluid to fluid containing low level or strong echoes. There will be a solid tissue component present as bands or clumps of echoes. There is usually increased through transmission of sound from the fluid component. Hyperaemia may be shown by increased vascularity on colour flow Doppler interrogation with many vessels in the wall of the lesion. There should be no vascularity within the fluid centre of the lesion.

CONCLUSION

This chapter makes imaging, particularly ultrasound of the female pelvis, sound easy, but it is fraught with traps for the unwary and there are pitfalls even for the most experienced operator. Those involved with ultrasound welcome the challenge it produces. However, as many important clinical decisions are based on ultrasound findings alone, the clinician responsible for the patient needs to exercise caution and continuously question whether the imaging diagnosis is appropriate in any given clinical setting.

REFERENCES

1 Benacerraf, B.R., Shipp, T.D. & Bromley, B. (2000) Is a full bladder still necessary for pelvic sonography? *Journal of Ultrasound in Medicine*, **19**, 237–241.

2 Bourne, T., Hamberger, L., Hahlin, M. & Granberg, S. (1997) Ultrasound in gynecology: endometrium. Review article. *International Journal of Gynecology and Obstetrics*, **56**, 115–127.

3 Pandya, P.P., Snijders, R.J.M., Johnson, S.P., De Lourdes Brizot, M. & Nicolaides, K.H. (1995) Screening for fetal trisomies by maternal age and fetal nuchal translucency thickness at 10–14 weeks of gestation. *British Journal Obstetrics and Gynaecology*, **102**, 957–962.

4 Snijders, R.J.M., Pandya, P., Brizot, M.L. & Nicolaides, K.H. (1996) First trimester fetal nuchal translucency. In: *Ultrasound Markers for Fetal Chromosomal Defects*, p. 133. *Frontiers in Fetal Medicine Series*. Parthenon Publishing Group, Carnforth, Lancashire.

5 Snijders, R.J.M., Noble, P., Sebire, N., Souka, A. & Nicolaides, K.H. (1998) UK multicentre project on assessment of risk of trisomy 21 by maternal age and fetal nuchal translucency thickness at 10–14 weeks of gestation. *Lancet*, **351**, 343–346.

6 Frates, M.C. & Laing, F.C. (1995) Sonographic evaluation of ectopic pregnancy update. *American Journal of Roentgenology*, **165**, 251–259.

7 Kaakaji, Y., Nghiem, N.V., Nodell, C. & Winter, T.C. (2000) Sonography of obstetric and gynaecologic emergencies: Part I: obstetric emergencies *American Journal of Roent-genology*, **174**, 641–649.

8 Bradley, L.D., Falcone, T. & Magen, A.B. (2000) Radiographic imaging techniques for the diagnosis of abnormal uterine bleeding. *Obstetrics and Gynecology Clinics of North America*, **27**, 245–276.

9 Vercellini, P., Cortesi, I., Oldani, S., Moschetta, M., De Giorgi, O. & Crosignani, P.G. (1997) The role of transvaginal ultrasonography in outwoman diagnostic hysteroscopy in the evaluation of women with menorrhagia. *Human Reproduction*, **12**, 1768–1771.

10 Ueda, H., Togashi, K., Konishi, I. *et al.* (1999) Unusual appearances of uterine leiomyomas: MR imaging findings and their histopathologic backgrounds. *RadioGraphics*, **19**, S131–S145.

11 Vercellini, P., Cortesi, I., De Giorgi, O., Merlo, D., Carinelli, S.G. & Crosignani, P.G. (1998) Transvaginal ultrasonography versus uterine needle biopsy in the diagnosis of diffuse adenomyosis. *Human Reproduction*, **13**, 2884–2887.

12 Atri, M., Reinhold, C., Mehio, A.R., Chapman, W.B. & Bret, P.M. (2000) Adenomyosis: US features with histologic correlation in an *in vitro* study. *Radiology*, **215**, 783–790.

13 Reinhold, C., Tafazoli, F., Mehio, A. *et al.* (1999) Uterine adenomyosis: endovaginal US and MR imaging features with histopathologic correlation. *RadioGraphics*, **19**, S147–S160.

14 Smith-Bindman, R., Kerlikowske, K., Feldstein, V.A. *et al.* (1998) Endovaginal ultrasound to exclude endometrial cancer and other endometrial abnormalities. *Journal of the American Medical Association*, **280**, 1510–1517.

15 Karlsson, B., Granberg, S., Wikland, M. *et al.* (1995) Transvaginal ultrasonography of the endometrium in women with postmenopausal bleeding: a Nordic multicentre study. *American Journal of Obstetrics and Gynecology*, **172**, 1488–1494.

16 Cullinan, J.A., Fleischer, A.C., Kepple, D.M. & Arnold, A.L. (1995) Sonohysterography: a technique for endometrial evaluation. *RadioGraphics*, **15**, 501–514.

17 Jorizzo, J.R., Riccio, G.J., Chen, M.Y.M. & Carr, J.J. (1999) Sonohysterography: the next step in the evaluation of the abnormal endometrium. *RadioGraphics*, **19**, S117–S130.

18 Dubinsky, T.J., Stroehlein, K., Abu-Ghazzeh, Y., Parvey, H.R. & Maklad, N. (1999) Prediction of benign and malignant endometrial disease: hysterosonographic–pathologic correlation. *Radiology*, **210**, 393–397.

19 Menon, U. & Jacobs, I. (2000) Ovarian cancer screening in the general population. *Ultrasound in Obstetrics and Gynecology*, **15**, 350–353.

20 Biagiotti, R., Desii, C., Vanzi, E. & Gacci, G. (1999) Predicting ovarian malignancy: application of artificial neural networks to transvaginal and color Doppler flow US. *Radiology*, **210**, 399–403.

21 Kurjak, A., Kupesic, S., Breyer, B., Sparac, V. & Jukic, S. (1998) The assessment of ovarian tumor angiogenesis: what does three-dimensional power Doppler add? *Ultrasound in Obstetrics and Gynecology*, **12**, 136–146.

22 Adams, J., Polson, D.W. & Franks, S. (1986) Prevalence of polycystic ovaries in women with anovulation and idiopathic hirsutism. *British Medical Journal*, **293**, 355–359.

23 Pache, T.D., Wladimirroff, J.W., Hop, W.C.J. & Fauser, B.C.J.M. (1992) How to discriminate between normal and polycystic ovaries: transvaginal US study. *Radiology*, **183**, 421–423.

24 Mitchell, D.G., Gefter, W.B., Spritzer, C.E. *et al.* (1986) Polycystic ovaries: MR imaging. *Radiology*, **160**, 425–429.

6

25 Timor-Tritsch, I.E., Lerner, J.P., Monteagudo, A., Murphy, K.E. & Heller, D.S. (1998) Transvaginal sonographic markers of tubal inflammatory disease. *Ultrasound in Obstetrics and Gynecology*, **12**, 56–66.

26 Patel, M.D., Feldstein, V.A., Chen, D.C., Lipson, S.D. & Filly, R.A. (1999) Endometriomas: diagnostic performance of US. *Radiology*, **210**, 739–745.

27 Kurjak, A., Kupesic, S. & Jacobs, I. (2000) Preoperative diagnosis of the primary fallopian tube carcinoma by three-dimensional static and power Doppler sonography. *Ultrasound in Obstetrics and Gynecology*, **15**, 246–251.

28 Pellerito, J.S., McCarthy, S.M., Doyle, M.B., Glickman, M.G. & DeCherney, A.H. (1992) Diagnosis of uterine anomalies: relative accuracy of MR imaging, endovaginal sonography, and hysterosalpingography. *Radiology*, **183**, 795–800.

29 Dietz, H.P. (2000) Ultrasound imaging in urogynaecology: a review. *ASUM Bulletin*, **3**, 9–15.

30 Tabar, L., Fagerberg, G., Chen, H.H. *et al.* (1995) Efficacy of breast cancer screening by age. New results from the Swedish two county trial. *Cancer*, **75**, 2507–2517.

31 Smart, C.R. & Hendrick, R.E. (1995) Benefit of screening mammography in women aged 40 to 49 years. *Cancer*, **75**, 1619–1626.

32 Teh, W. & Wilson, A.R. (1998) The role of ultrasound in breast cancer screening: a consensus statement for the European group for breast cancer screening. *European Journal of Cancer*, **34**, 449–450.

6

7   Menorrhagia

Menorrhagia affects approximately 20 per cent of otherwise healthy women (i.e. it adversely affects lifestyle) and approximately 5 per cent of women of reproductive age will consult their general practitioner with menstrual dysfunction. Up to 20 per cent of women have a hysterectomy by the age of 60 and in 50 per cent a normal uterus is removed. The 90th centile for blood loss during menstruation is 80 ml [1] and anaemia is significantly increased in women with a loss of greater than 60 ml. However, there are perceptual difficulties with the degree of menstrual loss, with 25 per cent of women with measured blood loss in the normal range considering it to be 'heavy' and 40 per cent of those with documented menorrhagia describing their loss as 'light' (Tables 7.1 and 7.2) [2].

Pathophysiology of menstrual loss

Immediately prior to menstruation intense spiral arteriole vasoconstriction occurs. The spiral arterioles dilate and menstrual bleeding occurs. Platelet adhesion in endometrial vessels is initially suppressed, but with increased blood extravasation, damaged vessel ends are sealed by intravascular plugs of platelets and fibrin. By 20 hours after the onset of menses, when most of the endometrial shedding has occurred, haemostasis occurs by intense spiral arteriole vasoconstriction. Endometrial regeneration begins within 36 hours of the onset of menses, while some shedding is still occurring.

Evaluation of women with abnormal uterine bleeding

History
- Onset
- Frequency
- Duration
- Severity of the bleeding (ask about number of pads used)
- Cyclic or acyclic
- Change of pattern
- Pain

Table 7.1 Definitions applied to abnormal uterine bleeding.

Dysfunctional uterine bleeding – abnormal uterine bleeding with no demonstrable organic cause from the reproductive tract

Menorrhagia – bleeding greater than 80 ml occurring at regular intervals

Metrorrhagia – irregular uterine bleeding at frequent intervals that is variable

Menometrorrhagia – uterine bleeding that is prolonged and occurs at completely irregular intervals

Polymenorrhoea – uterine bleeding occurring at regular intervals less than 21 days

Intermenstrual bleeding – bleeding between periods of variable amounts

Postmenopausal bleeding – bleeding occurring at more than 1 year after the last menses in a woman with ovarian failure

Postcoital bleeding – bleeding occurring after intercourse

Premenstrual spotting – scanty bleeding that occurs a few days to a week before menses

Table 7.2 The normal menstrual cycle.

Length	28 ± 7 days
Duration of menstrual flow	4 ± 2 days
Menstrual blood loss:	40 ± 20 ml[1]
Average iron loss	16 mg

[1] 95% of normal women lose less than 60 ml of blood with each menses. Loss >80 ml is correlated with a lower mean haemoglobin, haematocrit and serum iron level.

- Age
- Parity
- Partner status
- Sexual history
- Contraceptive history
- Medications
- Dates of past pregnancies
- Any symptoms of pregnancy and amount of medication taken.

Physical examination
- Clinical signs of anaemia
- Hypothroidism
- Pelvic examination
- Uterine size

- Shape
- Adenexal masses
- Appearance of cervix
- Cytology of recent cervical smear result.

DYSFUNCTIONAL UTERINE BLEEDING

Dysfunctional uterine bleeding (DUB) is abnormal uterine bleeding with no demonstrable organic cause occurring from the reproductive tract. Twenty per cent of cases occur immediately post-menarche. Fifty per cent of women with DUB are 40–50 years old. It is usually associated with chronic anovulation, but it can occur in ovulatory cycles. The diagnosis is made after excluding pathological causes of genital bleeding or coagulation diatheses.

Investigation of DUB

Haemoglobin (Hb) measurement (abnormal less than 11 g/dl) should be done on all women with menorrhagia because symptoms and signs of anaemia do not correlate well with the haemoglobin level until the patient is moderately to severely anaemic. An Hb level is a non-specific test for iron deficiency. A serum ferritin of less than 65 mmol/l has the best specificity, sensitivity, positive and negative predictive values of any test for iron deficiency anaemia [3]. Serum ferritin is a quantitative measure of the amount of stored iron in the body and is the first parameter to decrease in iron deficiency. An iron deficiency anaemia includes both iron deficiency plus a low haemoglobin.

An endometrial biopsy is not necessary at the initial assessment of women with menorrhagia. Endometrial cancer is uncommon in women under 40 years of age (incidence 0.85 per cent) [4]. The incidence of endometrial cancer is 0.66 per 100 000 women aged 30–34; 3000–4000 D&Cs would have to be done to detect one endometrial cancer in women aged under 35. This is the reason for the advice for endometrial sampling only in women aged 40 and over.

Most endometrial cancers in women under 40 present with irregular bleeding, rather than heavy regular bleeding. However, careful account should be taken of risk factors for endometrial carcinoma because 50 per cent of endometrial cancers occur in women with

Table 7.3 Risk factors for endometrial carcinoma.

Oligo-ovulatory or anovulatory cycles (PCOS)
Nulliparity
Obesity
Endometrial hyperplasia
Diabetes

Pathological features of the endometrium and percentage that become malignant [5]

Endometrial hyperplasia	Progression to endometrial cancer (%)
Simple hyperplasia without atypia	1
Complex hyperplasia without atypia	3
Simple hyperplasia with atypia	8
Complex hyperplasia with atypia	29
Systemic disease	1

PCOS, polycystic ovary syndrome.

risk factors (Table 7.3). If a woman with menorrhagia has not improved with drug therapy, a further assessment of the uterine cavity with transvaginal ultrasound or diagnostic hysteroscopy and endometrial biopsy is indicated (Table 7.4).

Coagulation disorders to be excluded

Von Willebrand's disease

This is the most common inherited coagulopathy.

- Von Willebrand's disease (vWD) is a deficiency of, or defect in, von Willebrand's factor (vWF), i.e. 'the platelet glue' which forms a platelet plug and also transports other clotting factors. Some people will also be low in factor VIII.

- Von Willebrand's factor serves as a bridge between platelets and damaged endothelium and it prevents the degradation of clotting factor VIII which is vital to the normal coagulation process.

- There are three major types of the disorder:

  Type 1 – deficiency in the levels of normally functioning vWF: 80 per cent

  Type 2 – the levels of vWF may be near normal but there are abnormalities in function

Table 7.4 Abnormal uterine bleeding: differential diagnosis for dysfunctional uterine bleeding – organic causes.

(1) Complications of pregnancy
    (a) Threatened, inevitable, incomplete or missed miscarriage
    (b) Retained products of conception
    (c) Trophoblastic disease
(2) Benign pelvic lesions
    (a) Leiomyomata (fibroids) – submucous fibroids (pedunculated fibroids usually cause intermenstrual bleeding)
    (b) Endometrial or endocervical polyps
    (c) Adenomyosis or endometriosis
    (d) Infection
    (e) Traumatic lesions of the vagina
    (f) Foreign body
(3) Cervical or endometrial polyps
(4) Malignant tumour – endometrial, cervical, vaginal, vulval and fallopian tube

Type 3 – there is a complete or almost complete absence of vWF in the circulation: rare.

- Up to 1 per cent of the general population and 20 per cent of adolescents hospitalised due to menorrhagia have von Willebrand's disease or another blood dyscrasia.
- Up to 95 per cent of women with von Willebrand's disease are unaware of their condition.
- Von Willebrand's disease is an autosomal dominant form of haemophilia – incidence 1 per cent. Only 10 per cent have the severe form.
- Even in mild forms of vWD women are at an increased risk for impaired clotting and heavy bleeding.
- Early recognition of vWD allows for management with a synthetic analogue of vasopressin.

Screen patients for von Willebrand's disease who:

- Bruise easily
- Have prolonged or heavy menstrual bleeding
- Have prolonged bleeds after surgery, trauma, dental work or childbirth
- Have frequent nosebleeds.

Screening tests for von Willebrand's disease
- Von Willebrand's factor antigen

- Ristocetin cofactor
- Collagen binding assays factor VIII levels.

Treatment for moderate sufferers is a non-blood product, desmo-pressin (DDAVP), injected or delivered as a high potency nasal spray which releases von Willebrand's factor from body storage sites. Others have to take a clotting factor concentrate in factor VIII.

Intraoperative cover for women with von Willebrand's disease
- Avoid all drugs likely to affect platelet function such as aspirin, other anti-inflammatory drugs, tricyclic antidepressants, phenothiazine-based drugs, including antiemetics and possibly halothane anaesthesia.
- Prophylactic antibiotics should be used to avoid infection and subsequent secondary haemorrhage.
- Give DDAVP at a dose of $0.4\,\mu g/kg$ given as an infusion over 15–30 minutes, the first part given approximately an hour to an hour and a half prior to surgery and repeated 12 hours later if there is any bleeding.
- Give tranexamic acid at a dose of 1 g (two tablets) three times daily, commencing 24 hours prior to surgery and continuing for 4–5 days postoperatively.
- Freeze-dried plasma should be available as a precaution, in case there is a poor response to the above regimen.

7

Medical conditions to be excluded as a cause of menorrhagia

Hypothyroidism

Hypothyroidism may be associated with abnormal uterine bleeding. With normalisation of the thyroid-stimulating hormone (TSH) women become euthyroid and abnormal uterine bleeding resolves.

Liver disease

Cirrhosis of the liver interferes with the ability to metabolise and conjugate oestrogens. Thus the levels of free oestrogen are increased, causing hyperstimulation of the endometrium and uterine bleeding.

Iatrogenic causes

These include steroids used for contraception, hormone replacement therapy, corticosteroids, anticoagulants, tranquillizers, antidepressants, digitalis, dilantin and intrauterine devices.

Treatment of dysfunctional uterine bleeding

The aim of treatment is to control the bleeding, prevent recurrences, correct associated conditions, preserve fertility and induce ovulation in patients who wish to conceive. Medical treatment is indicated to preserve fertility and if there is no associated pelvic pathology. Women on tamoxifen need special consideration (Fig. 7.1).

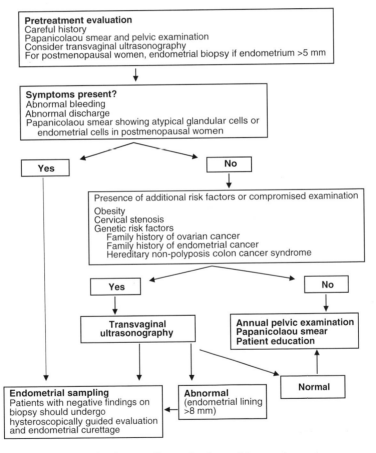

Fig. 7.1 Algorithm for surveillance of endometrial cancer in women receiving tamoxifen. (With permission from Suh-Burgmann and Goodman (1999) [6].)

Acute bleeding

Oestrogen controls acute bleeding because it promotes rapid regrowth of the endometrium over denuded epithelial surfaces.

It causes proliferation of the endometrial ground substance and stabilisation of lysosomal membranes.

Therapy for acute bleeding

- **Conjugated equine oestrogen (CEE)**, 10 mg/day in four divided doses. Continue for 21–25 days. Give medroxyprogesterone acetate (MPA), 10 mg, with the oestrogen for the last 7 days;
- or **CEE**, 15–25 mg intravenously every 6–12 hours for 24 hours, or until bleeding is controlled. Bleeding usually stops within 6 hours. After bleeding is controlled, oral CEE, 10 mg/day for 15 days, followed by 10 mg/day oral CEE and 10 mg/day MPA for another 7 days. All medication is then stopped and withdrawal bleed occurs;
- or **high dose oestrogen/progesterone** therapy: combined oral contraceptive pill containing 35 μg or less of ethinyloestradiol per tablet – give four tablets per day, one tablet every 6 hours. This may not be as effective as oestrogen alone because the progestogens may interfere with the rapid growth-promoting effects of unopposed high dose oestrogen;
- or **high dose oral MPA**, 60–120 mg on the first day followed by 20 mg/day for the following 10 days.

Uterine currettage is not indicated when the ultrasound scan is normal. This should only be done if the ultrasound indicates intrauterine pathology.

In adolescence, the use of progestogens or the combined oral contraceptive pill does not interfere with the maturation process of the hypothalamus. Where heavy dysfunctional bleeding occurs (due to anovulatory cycles), therapy should be instituted for 6 months to a year and then stopped to see whether or not the normal menstrual cycle has been established.

MEDICAL MANAGEMENT OF MENORRHAGIA [7]

1 Antifibrinolytic agents

Excessive fibrinolytic activity has been demonstrated in the endometrium of women with menorrhagia, and increased levels of plasminogen activator is found during the menstrual phase of women with menorrhagia.

Tranexamic acid – an antifibrinolytic [8]

Dosage: 1–1.5 g orally three to four times daily for the period of bleeding.

This is the first line of therapy.

- The action of tranexamic acid is via a strong inhibitory effect on the activation of plasminogen, i.e. the conversion of plasminogen to plasmin in the fibrinolytic system. It is excreted unchanged in the urine. Maximal levels are achieved within 2–3 hours.
- It results in a 50 per cent reduction in menstrual blood loss (MBL).
- Success is greatest in women with the greatest loss of menstrual blood.
- Side effects (mainly gastrointestinal – nausea, vomiting, diarrhoea – and dose dependent) are reported in about one third of women.
- There is no increase in the incidence of thromboembolic disease in over 20 years with using antifibrinolytics, as studied in Scandanavia.
- There are no known drug interactions. If there is evidence of compromised renal function, the dose should be reduced because of the risk of accumulation.

  Contraindications of tranexamic acid include a history of previous thromboembolic disease.

2 ε-Aminocaproic acid

Dosage: 3 g four times a day. It reduces menstrual blood loss by up to 60 per cent of women compared with pretreatment values. The reduction in menstrual loss does not persist after stopping treatment.

3 The combined oral contraceptive pill

- Reduces average MBL by 40–50 per cent
- 70–80 per cent of patients benefit
- Few side effects
- Avoid in women aged >35 who are cigarette smokers
- Avoid in those with a body mass index (BMI) of >30

• Consider and investigate with a family history of thrombo-embolism or relative risk factor for venous thromboembolism.

4 Non-steroidal anti-inflammatory drugs (NSAIDs)

Levels of the prostaglandins PGE_2 (a vasodilator) and $PGF_{2\alpha}$ (a vaso-constrictor) are increased in women with increased menstrual blood loss. NSAIDs block both the prostacyclin and thromboxane biosynthetic pathways and are effective in reducing menstrual blood loss in women with menorrhagia.

Mefenamic acid

Dosage: 500 mg three times a day with meals from the onset of menses and continued as necessary. In general it does not need to be used for more than 7 days each cycle.

• Mefenamic acid inhibits the enzymes of prostaglandin synthetase and also antagonises the action of prostaglandin at the receptor site. It is therefore effective for the treatment of primary dysmenorrhoea as well as menorrhagia.

• It is contraindicated in women with evidence of gastrointestinal inflammation and/or ulceration, and in women in whom aspirin and other NSAIDs induce symptoms of bronchospasm, allergic rhinitis or urticaria.

• It should be avoided in women with impaired renal function.

• It may induce diarrhoea (approximately 5 per cent).

• It causes lowering of the prothrombin concentration.

Alternative NSAIDS: ibuprofen, 400 mg q.i.d.; diclofenac sodium, 100 mg t.d.s.; naproxen sodium, 275 mg 6-hourly; sulindac, 100–200 mg b.i.d.

Give on the first 3 days (since over 90 per cent of bleeding occurs in the first 3 days in both normal menstruation and menorrhagia) or throughout the period of bleeding. NSAIDs control menstrual blood losses at least as well as oral contraceptives or antifibrinolytic agents. They may be combined with oral contraceptives or progestogens (from days 5 to 26) to achieve a greater reduction in menstrual blood loss. Measured blood loss decreases by up to 25 per cent sustained over long-term treatment.

Table 7.5 Potency of various progestogens.

	Norethisterone (mg)	Levonorgestrel (mg)	Desogestrel (mg)	Gestodene (mg)
Transformation from proliferative to secretory endometrium Dosage (per day from day 14 of the cycle)	10–15	0.5	0.05–0.25	0.25
Dosage for menstrual delay (per day)	10–15	0.25–1.0	0.25	0.25
Dosage of progesterone that inhibits ovulation (per day)	0.5	0.5–1	0.06	40 µg

5 Oral progestogens (Table 7.5)

Norethisterone

Norethisterone has an inhibitory effect on the secretion of gonadotrophins in the anterior lobe of the pituitary. It is partially metabolised to ethinyloestradiol.

Dosage: 5 mg t.d.s. from days 5 to 26 of the cycle.

Medroxyprogesterone acetate

Dosage: 10 mg daily from days 5 to 26 of the cycle. MPA works by transforming proliferative endometrium into secretory endometrium.

- Side effects include fatigue, mood changes, weight gain and deleterious changes to the lipid profile.
- 30–50 per cent reduction in MBL.
- 20–70 per cent of patients benefit.

Potencies of different progestogens vary (see Table 7.5 for the effects of different progestogens on endometrial transformation from proliferative to secretory) for the control of bleeding and the dosage that inhibits ovulation. Progestogens can be used to extend the luteal phase. To reduce the degree of menorrhagia treatment should be from days 5 to 26, especially in an anovulatory cycle. They may be given for shorter periods, but usually for at least 10–14 days.

▪ Depo-medroxyprogesterone acetate produces amenorrhoea or infrequent hypomenorrhoea in the majority of women. MPA is more potent than progesterone and has a long duration of action. It suppresses the secretion of pituitary gonadotrophins which prevent follicular maturation. Therefore long-term anovulation occurs. A single dose of 50 mg parenteral MPA has the equivalent effect of 20 mg oral progesterone given daily for 10 days in its effects of producing secretory change in an oestrogen-primed endometrium. It is given in a formulation of 150 mg/ml which reaches half its initial concentration in about 27 days. It is slowly absorbed from the injection site.

▪ The dose of 150 mg is given every 3 months by deep intramuscular injection.

▪ MPA is contraindicated in women with thromboembolic disorders, cerebrovascular disease or liver dysfunction.

▪ MPA has a prolonged contraceptive effect. The medium time to conception for those who do conceive is 10 months after the last injection (range 4–31 months). Decreased glucose tolerance may occur. Following repeated injections, amenorrhoea and anovulation may persist for up to 18 months or longer.

▪ Adverse effects (reported in less than 1 per cent of women in trials) include menstrual irregularity, decreased libido, leukorrhoea, vaginitis, pelvic pain, headache, nervousness, dizziness, depression, insomnia, abdominal pain or discomfort, nausea, bloating, skin and mucous membrane changes, breast discomfort and weight gain.

▪ MPA may produce troublesome episodes of frequent, prolonged or erratic spotting or bleeding during the early months of use due to increased fragility of superficial venules.

▪ Side effects include erratic bleeding and an unpredictable delay in the return of fertility after use.

6 The levonorgestrel intrauterine releasing system
(LNG-IUS) (Mirena)

This is the most effective medical therapy for menorrhagia when there is no underlying pathology, particularly fibroids [9,10].

The Mirena intrauterine device (IUD) is a T-shaped polyethylene frame with a bar comprising a mixture of polydimethylsiloxane and levonorgestrel moulded around its vertical arm. The device is 32 mm in length. The bar contains 53 mg levonorgestrel, coated with a poly-dimethylsiloxane membrane regulating the release of levonorgestrel to 20 µg per 24 hours, for 5 years. This gives a stable plasma levo-norgestrel concentration which, after the first week following inser-tion, levels off at 0.4–0.6 nmol/l in women of fertile age. It is effective for 5 years.

Amenorrhoeic women still ovulate with it. The endometrium is exposed to the levonorgestrel IUD and therefore is insensitive to ovarian oestradiol stimulation. This may be due to the reduction of oestrogen and progestogen receptors. Bleeding patterns may vary from regular scanty menstruation in some women to oligo-/amen-orrhoea. During the first months of use, up to 20 per cent of women may experience prolonged bleeding which decreases to 3 per cent during the first 3 months of use. The menstrual pattern is the result of the direct action of the levonorgestrel on the endometrium and does not reflect the ovarian cycle. There is no clear difference in fol-licle development, ovulation or oestradiol and progesterone levels in women with different bleeding patterns. Ovarian function is normal and oestradiol levels are maintained even when users of Mirena are amenorrhoeic. The volume of menstrual bleeding is decreased by nearly 60 per cent in menorrhagic women by the end of 3 months' use, and by 97 per cent after 12 months of use [9,11]. Up to 30 per cent of women are amenorrhoeic after 1 year's use. There is a con-comitant increase in the haemoglobin concentration.

Dysmenorrhoea is also alleviated. Because of the low drug levels in plasma the systemic effects of the progestogen are minimised. In women of fertile age, the Mirena should be inserted into the uterine cavity within 7 days of the onset of menstruation to enable time for its contraceptive effect.

Insertion of the LNG-IUS

The steroid reservoir requires a wider (4.8 mm) insertion tube. Although cervical dilators should be available, they are not really necessary in parous women under the age of 45. If dilatation of the cervix is required (using Hegar dilators, size 3–6, since the insertion tube is wider at 4.8 mm) then it should be done under local paracer-vical anaesthetic block with 1 per cent lignocaine. Routine premedi-cation should be given (mefenamic acid, 500 mg) half an hour before the insertion.

Insertion technique of the LNG-IUS

Pre-insertion visit
- Take swabs (endocervical and ureteral) to exclude *Chlamydia trachomatis*. If identified, treat with doxycycline (100 mg twice daily for 7 days) or azithromycin 1 g stat). Take an endocervical swab for gonorrhoea (see Chapter 10 for treatment).
- Check uterine size bimanually and identify its size, shape and position (anteverted or retroverted) and any tenderness.
- Arrange insertion within 7 days of the start of menstruation if contraception is required.

At insertion
(1) Visualize the cervix and clean with antiseptic.
(2) Apply local anaesthetic to the 12 o'clock position of the cervix where the tenaculum is placed. A paracervical block may be necessary.
(3) Put traction on the tenaculum and check uterine length with uterine sound.
(4) Adjust the flange to length of the uterine cavity measured.
(5) Make sure the rounded edge of the inserter is just protruding outside of the tube.
(6) Insert the loaded system by introducing the insertion tube into the uterine cavity, until the flange touches the cervix.
(7) Pull the tube back and plunge up.
(8) Push gently to make sure the device is at the top of the uterus. The arms will be out so the risk of perforation is negligible. The device needs to be in the high fundal position.
(9) Remove the tube completely together with the plunger, making sure the threads run freely.
(10) Cut the threads 2 cm outside of the cervix.

Follow-up at 7–14 days post-insertion, 3 months and yearly for 5 years
- Signs of infection – pain, discharge
- Bleeding pattern
- Check threads.

Results of use

These results are superior to any current pharmacological methods of treatment. Oral contraceptive prostaglandin inhibitors and antifibrinolytics reduce menstrual loss by <50 per cent. Danazol and gonadotrophin-releasing hormone (GnRH) agonists are effective in producing oligo-/amenorrhoea, but unlike that occurring while using the LNG-IUS there is definite hypo-oestrogenism and systemic side effects. On this basis they may not be used for more than 6 months.

The LNG-IUS is a simple, effective and cheap treatment for dysfunctional uterine bleeding as an alternative to both hysterectomy and endometrial ablation, with the advantage of preserving fertility. It has the advantage that it usually treats menstrual pain effectively.

Benefits of the LNG-IUS

- It reduces the amount and duration of menstrual bleeding by rendering the endometrium inactive and insensitive to the proliferative effects of oestradiol. There is an increase in mean haemoglobin concentration amounting to 1–1.5 g/dl after 5 years. The Mirena IUD compared with transcervical resection of the endometrium (TCRE) has a significantly greater reduction in blood loss.
- Reduced incidence in growth of uterine fibroids (after 6–18 months of use). This may be due to levonorgestrel-induced effects on insulin-like endometrial growth factors and their binding protein.
- Reduction in the risk of ectopic pregnancy. The absolute rate of ectopic pregnancy with the LNG-IUS is 0.02 per 100 women years, which is an 80–90 per cent reduction in risk compared with those not using any contraceptive method (estimated as 0.12–0.26 per 100 women years).
- It is an extremely effective form of contraception.
- The removal for infection is 0.5 per 100 users by 3 years of use.
- There is an increase in haemoglobin and serum ferritin levels. It has no effect on carbohydrate metabolism, coagulation parameters, liver enzymes or lipid levels.
- The action of the LNG-IUS is mainly local but not exclusively so. There is individual variation but in general the mean blood level of levonorgestrel is one quarter of the peak level after taking a standard 30 µg levonorgestrel progesterone-only pill. Prolonged light bleeding and spotting may occur. The first few months are characterised by a definite increase in total bleeding days but after 3 months a monthly mean of only 7 days of spotting or bleeding is usual. From the fifth month onwards there is a profound reduction in the duration of bleeding. A significant number of women are amenorrhoeic after the first year of use (due to the localised effect on the endometrium, not serum oestradiol levels). Oestradiol levels in women

without bleeding are similar to those of normal fertile women. With long-term use, over two thirds of cycles are ovulatory. Women should be reassured that using the LNG-IUS produces a reduction or absence of bleeding, primarily as a direct result of the levonorgestrel on the endometrium. It is not a signal of ovarian dysfunction and does not need treatment. It is the benefit of the method.

7 Danazol

Dosage: 200–400 mg daily.

▪ Danazol may reduce MBL by more than 200 ml per cycle (up to 87 per cent).

▪ It is associated with androgenic side effects – weight gain (a statistically significant increase of 4.5 kg above pretreatment values on 400 mg daily), muscle cramps and acne. 100 mg is not effective. The incidence of side effects is high and therefore discontinuation with it is high.

8 Gestrinone (Dimetriose)

▪ An advantage is a dose of one 2.5 mg capsule twice a week.

▪ Gestrinone is a synthetic steroid hormone with antiprogestogenic and anti-oestrogenic activity. It has weak androgen and progestogen activity. Its main action is on the hypothalamic–pituitary axis where it inhibits gonadotrophin release with a weak inhibitory effect on synthesis. The suppression of the ovular gonadotrophin peak is observed after the first month of treatment. Ovarian oestrogen secretion stops, leading to endometrial atrophy. Its antiprogestogenic activity is on cell receptors in both the endometrium and extrauterine ectopic implant.

▪ The first dose should always be taken on the first day of the menstrual cycle. The second dose should be taken 3 days later. The capsules are then taken on the same two days of the week, preferably at the same time every week, for the duration of treatment which should be only 6 months in view of its effects in decreasing bone density.

▪ Gestrinone does inhibit ovulation in many women, but pregnancies can occur so it must not be relied on for contraception. It can cause some degree of fluid retention and so patients with cardiac or renal dysfunction require close monitoring.

• Adverse effects include acne, seborrhoea, fluid retention, weight gain, hirsutism, hair loss, decrease in breast size, voice change and other androgen-type effects. Other undesirable effects are headaches, irritability, gastrointestinal disorders, change in libido, hot flushes, cramps, arthralgia and increase in liver transaminases.

9 GnRH agonists

▪ GnRH agonists are highly effective at producing amenorrhoea. They need to be balanced by 'add back therapy' (hormone replacement therapy (HRT) – see Chapter 9) to minimise bone loss and their use is only recommended for 6 months because of hypo-oestrogenic side effects, particularly osteoporosis.

▪ They are expensive and therefore impractical for most cases of menorrhagia.

The antifibrinolytic ethamsylate is not an effective treatment for menorrhagia.

SURGICAL TREATMENT FOR MENORRHAGIA

Up to 50 per cent of hysterectomies are done for dysfunctional uterine bleeding. Mortality for hysterectomy is 6–11 per 10 000 procedures and morbidity is 3–40 per cent. Operative complications from ablation may occur in up to 6 per cent for first time procedures, and 15 per cent for repeat ablation. Patient satisfaction with endometrial ablative techniques, including transcervical resection of the endometrium, is high at 55–90 per cent with amenorrhoea rates of 10–75 per cent [12] and avoidance of hysterectomy in 76 per cent after 4–6 years' follow-up [13].

Post menopausal HRT after endometrial ablation requires a progestogen.

Minimal access surgery – endometrial ablation [14–18]

TCRE gives excellent relief of symptoms and better health postsurgically in those initially managed medically [19]. Therefore those who do not have a treatment preference can be allocated to endometrial ablation before a therapeutic trial. Over 80 per cent of those managed by TCRE at the outset avoid further surgical treatment.

Nevertheless, 40 per cent of women treated medically will not undergo surgical treatment.

Preoperative medical endometrial thinning should be used in order to achieve a satisfactory depth of destruction. A thin or atrophic endometrium should increase the likelihood of destruction of the basal layer. MPA (150 mg) is given intramuscularly on the day of the procedure to maintain a hypo-oestrogenic state and facilitate adhesion formation. The rate of amenorrhoea is twice as high (70 versus 40 per cent) if Depo-Provera is administered on the day of surgery. Danazol, 400 mg twice daily for four weeks [20], or GnRH analogues for 4–6 weeks may be used before treatment [21]. Prior to laser ablation endometrial thinning is considered essential.

Endometrial laser ablation

Surgical destruction of the endometrium with the neodymium: yttrium–aluminium garnet (Nd:YAG) laser results in a satisfactory outcome for 80 per cent of women and a hysterectomy in up to 20 per cent after 5 years. Laser energy is set at 80 W delivered through a 600 mm quartz fibre. Focal lesions of the endometrial cavity may be excised at the same time. A single prophylactic dose of antibiotics may be given and 10 ml of 0.25 per cent bupivacaine and 1 : 200 000 adrenalin may be injected radially into the cervix at the end of the procedure for postoperative pain relief [22].

Uterine thermal balloon therapy (Thermachoice)

The concept of the thermal uterine balloon therapy system for endometrial ablation was introduced as a potentially safer and simpler technique [23]. Improved results are obtained with increasing age, higher balloon pressure, smaller uterine cavity and a lesser degree of preprocedure menorrhagia.

Anaesthesia may be given using either general anaesthesia, paracervical block, intravenous sedation with paracervical block, intravenous sedation alone or regional anaesthesia.

The uterine balloon therapy system consists of a 16 cm long by 4.5 mm diameter catheter with a latex balloon at its distal end housing a heating element. The controller unit continuously monitors, displays and controls preset intraballoon pressure, temperature and duration of treatment. The balloon is inserted into the uterus and filled with a variable volume of 5 per cent dextrose water until a starting pressure between 140 and 180 mmHg is achieved. The treatment cycle is commenced when the fluid temperature reaches 87 ± 5°C and continued for 8 minutes. At the conclusion of the treatment the balloon is emptied, removed and checked again for any leaks.

For safety, the balloon automatically deactivates when the pressure falls below 45 mmHg or reaches 200 mmHg and above. Pressures <140 mmHg have been demonstrated to be inadequate for optimal treatment. There is an overall minor complication rate mainly due to endometritis and haematometra, treated with uterine sounding and antibiotics. The balloon catheter has up to a 90 per cent success rate, and therefore compares favourably to operative endometrial ablation [24].

Contraindications to balloon therapy
- Pathology distorting the uterine cavity
- Atypical endometrial hyperplasia
- Suspected genital tract infection or malignancy
- Uterine cavity >12 cm
- Previous endometrial ablation
- Desire for preservation of fertility.

Patient dissatisfaction may not be related to the blood loss. There will be an average decrease of slightly more than 50 per cent in blood loss but this may not satisfy all women. Women who received one or two doses of depot GnRH agonist before balloon treatment have been found to have statistically higher rates of post-procedure amenorrhoea and spotting.

Microwave endometrial ablation (Microsulis PLC) [25]

This has also been subject to randomised controlled trial [26]. It uses an 8 mm diameter probe emitting microwaves with a frequency of 9.2 GHz. At this frequency, penetration is restricted to a maximum of 6 mm. It is faster than TCRE, requiring less operator skill.

Radiofrequency for thermal destruction of tissue

This was introduced as a treatment originally for prostatic hypertrophy. Postoperative pain is temporary but substantial and complications include:

- Vesicovaginal fistula (0.01 per cent), usually due to the probe slipping down the endocervical canal where there was no guard.
- Bowel injury due to a false passage of the probe through the wall of a retroverted uterus. Although described with some success [27], the above methods are associated with fewer and less severe complications.

Complications of ablation

- Distorted uterine cavity due to fibrosis
- Haematometra, pyometra endometriosis
- Abdominal pain
- Pregnancies after endometrial ablation have been reported.

Endometrial resection and the MISTLETOE Study [28]

The MISTLETOE Study (minimally invasive surgical techniques – laser, endothermal or endoresection survey) was an audit of 10 686 women who had had endometrial resection and ablation for menstrual disturbances from April 1993 to October 1994 in the UK. It included the minimally invasive surgical techniques: combined (diathermy loop and rollerball used together), resection (diathermy loop used alone), rollerball (rollerball diathermy used alone), laser ablation (laser energy used), radiofrequency ablation (radiothermal energy used) and cryoablation (freezing used).

Main outcome measures which included perioperative, postoperative and delayed complications were analysed by method of surgery and experience of the operator.

Women having laser or rollerball ablation had consistently fewer immediate operative complications. There were fewer occasions where additional emergency surgery was needed. The combined diathermy group produced significantly fewer total immediate operative complications than the loop alone. This was a combined effect of reduced haemorrhage and uterine perforations, but individually they were only statistically significant at the 5 per cent level. Laser ablation was significantly less likely to result in emergency hysterectomy than the loop alone. Endometrial thinning agents did not significantly decrease the complication rates or emergency surgery rate.

Intraoperative and postoperative complications of endometrial ablation

- Fluid overload – hyponatraemia
- Uterine perforation
- Haemorrhage
- Thermal damage to visceral and vascular structures
- Heavy bleeding
- Abdominal pain
- Urinary retention, urinary tract infection, haematuria
- Hypotension
- Nausea and vomiting
- Bradycardia
- Chest pain
- Cervical shock
- Hyponatraemia
- Pyrexia
- Deep vein thrombosis
- Death.

Complications of endometrial ablation from the MISTLETOE survey

- Rates ranged between 0.77 and 2.86 per cent and there were no significant differences between methods at the 1 per cent level.
- Laser and rollerball ablations were associated with the fewest operative and postoperative complications.
- Combined loop and rollerball diathermy was associated with a higher rate, but fewer immediate operative complications than loop resection alone.
- Complications at 6 weeks (1.25–4.58 per cent) post-procedure included endometritis, septicaemia, pneumonia, peritonitis, hysterectomy, laparotomy and bowel repair and pulmonary embolism.
- Ten deaths were reported but only two appeared to be directly related to the ablation/resection procedure. Direct mortality rates were 2 in 10000 for the combined procedure (TCRE and rollerball) and 3 in 10000 for resection alone.

The conclusions of the MISTLETOE Study were that low complication rates were associated with laser treatment. The resection loop should be combined with an ablation technique, as the complication rates for the resection alone group were significantly greater. The use of hormonal endometrial preparations does not significantly decrease the complication rates or risk of emergency surgery. It is therefore doubtful whether it is necessary, apart from those using radiofrequency.

Endometrial ablation techniques have a high patient satisfaction and acceptability. Premenstrual symptoms and dysmenorrhoea improve following endometrial ablation.

Postoperative complications occur in 3 per cent of first time patients. The MISTLETOE audit reported 7.2 per cent of cases with serious complications.

REFERENCES

1 Hallberg, L. & Nilsson, L. (1964) Determination of menstrual blood loss. *Scandinavian Journal of Clinical Laboratory Investigation*, **16**, 244–248.

2 Rees, M.C.P. (1991) Role of menstrual blood loss measurements in management of complaints of excessive menstrual bleeding. *British Journal of Obstetrics and Gynaecology*, **98**, 327–328.

3 Guyatt, G.H., Oxman, A.D., Ali, M., Willan, A., McIlroy, W. & Patterson, C. (1992) Laboratory diagnosis of iron-deficiency anaemia: an overview. *Journal of General Internal Medicine*, **7**, 145–153.

4 Vessey, M., Clark, J. & McKenzie, I. (1979) Dilatation and curettage in young women. *Health Bulletin*, **39**, 59–62.

5 Kurman, R.J., Kaminski, P.F. & Norris, H.J. (1985) The behaviour of endometrial hyperplasia. A long-term study of 'untreated hyperplasia' in 170 patients. *Cancer*, **56**, 403–412.

6 Suh-Burgmann, E.J. & Goodman, A. (1999) Surveillance for endometrial cancer in women receiving tamoxifen. *Annals of Internal Medicine*, **131**, 127–135.

7 Coulter, A., Kelland, J., Peto, V. & Rees, M.C. (1995) Treating menorrhagia in primary care. An overview of drug trials and a survey of prescribing practice. *International Journal of Technology Assessment in Health Care*, **11**, 456–471.

8 Bonnar, J. & Sheppard, B.L. (1996) Treatment of menorrhagia during menstruation: randomised control trial of ethamsylate, mefenamic acid and tranexamic acid. *British Medical Journal*, **313**, 579–582.

9 Milsom, I., Andersson, K., Andersch, B. & Rybo, G. (1991) A comparison of flurbiprofen, tranexamic acid, and a levonorgestrel-releasing intrauterine contraceptive device in the treatment of idiopathic menorrhagia. *American Journal of Obstetrics and Gynecology*, **164**, 879–883.

10 Kittelson, N. & Istre, O. (1998) A randomised study comparing the levonorgestrel intrauterine system (LNG-IUS) and transcervical resection of the endometrium (TCRE) in the treatment of menorrhagia: preliminary results. *Gynaecological Endoscopy*, **7**, 61–65.

11 Andersson, J.K. & Rybo, G. (1990) Levonorgestrel releasing intrauterine system in the treatment of menorrhagia. *British Journal of Obstetrics and Gynaecology*, **97**, 690–694.

12 Scottish Hysteroscopy Audit Group (1995) A Scottish audit of hysteroscopic surgery for menorrhagia: complications and follow-up. *British Journal of Obstetrics and Gynaecology*, **102**, 249–254.

13 Aberdeen Endometrial Ablation Trials Group (1999) A randomised trial of endometrial ablation versus hysterectomy for the treatment of dysfunctional uterine bleeding: outcome at 4 years. *British Journal of Obstetrics and Gynaecology*, **106**, 601–607.

14 Dwyer, N., Hutton, J. & Stirrat, G. (1993) Randomised controlled trial comparing endometrial resection with abdominal hysterectomy for the surgical treatment of menorrhagia. *British Journal of Obstetrics and Gynaecology*, **100**, 237–243.

15 Baggish, M.S. & Szeeh, M. (1996) Endometrial ablation: a series of 568 patients treated over an 11-year period. *American Journal of Obstetrics and Gynecology*, **174**, 908–913.

16 Lalonde, A. (1994) Evaluation of surgical options in menorrhagia. *British Journal of Obstetrics and Gynaecology*, **101** (Suppl. 11), 8–14.

17 O'Connor, H., Broadbent, J.A.M., Magos, A.L. & McPherson, K. (1997) Medical Research Council randomised trial of endometrial resection versus hysterectomy in management of menorrhagia. *The Lancet*, **349**, 897–901.

18 O'Connor, H. & Magos, A. (1996) Endometrial resection for the treatment of menorrhagia. *New England Journal of Medicine*, **335**, 151–156.

19 Cooper, K.G., Parkin, D.E., Garratt, A.M. & Grant, A.M. (1997) A randomised comparison of medical and hysteroscopic management in women consulting a gynaecologist for the treatment of heavy menstrual loss. *British Journal of Obstetrics and Gynaecology*, **104**, 1360–1366.

20 Goldrath, M.H. (1990) Use of danazol in hysteroscopic surgery for menorrhagia. *Journal of Reproductive Medicine*, **35**, 91–96.

21 Sculpher, M., Thompson, E., Brown, J. & Garry, R. (2000) A cost-effectiveness analysis of goserelin compared with danazol as endometrial thinning agents. *British Journal of Obstetrics and Gynaecology*, **107**, 340–346.

22 Phillips, G., Chien, P.W.F. & Garry, R. (1998) Risk of hysterectomy after 1000 consecutive endometrial laser ablations. *British Journal of Obstetrics and Gynaecology*, **105**, 897–903.

23 Neuwirth, R.S., Duran, A.A., Singer, A., MacDonald, R. & Bolduc, I. (1994) The endometrial ablator: a new instrument. *Obstetrics and Gynecology*, **83**, 792–796.

7

24 Amso, N.N., Strabinsky, S.A., McFaul, P., Blanc, B., Pendley, L. & Neuwirth, R. (1998) Uterine thermal balloon therapy for the treatment of menorrhagia: the first 300 patients from a multicentre study. *British Journal of Obstetrics and Gynaecology*, **105**, 517–523.

25 Sharp, N.C., Cronin, N., Feldberg, I., Evans, N., Hodgson, D. & Ellis, S. (1995) Microwaves for menorrhagia: a new fast technique for endometrial ablation. *The Lancet*, **346**, 1003–1004.

26 Cooper, K.G., Bain, C. & Parkin, D.E. (1999) A randomised trial comparing microwave endometrial ablation with transcervical resection of the endometrium for the treatment of women with heavy menstrual loss. *The Lancet*, **354**, 1859–1863.

27 Thijssen, R.F.A. (1997) Radiofrequency induced endometrial ablation: an update. *British Journal of Obstetrics and Gynaecology*, **104**, 608–613.

28 Overton, C., Hargreaves, J. & Maresh, M. (1997) A national survey of the complications of endometrial destruction for menstrual disorders: the MISTLETOE Study. *British Journal of Obstetrics and Gynaecology*, **104**, 1351–1359.

7

8 The Menopause and Hormone Replacement Therapy

THE MENOPAUSE

The menopause is the permanent cessation of menstruation due to failure of ovarian follicular development in the presence of adequate gonadotrophin stimulation. It is diagnosed retrospectively after 12 months of amenorrhoea. Age at menopause varies between individuals with a mean of about 50 years worldwide.

The climacteric

The Climacteric is the physiological period in a woman's life during which ovarian function regresses. In the perimenopause follicle-stimulating hormone (FSH) levels increase, oestradiol levels decrease and luteinising hormone (LH) levels remain unchanged until after the menopause. Although many perimenopausal cycles are ovulatory, progesterone levels are often lower.

The end of the menses

- Natural menopause can only be established in retrospect after 12 consecutive months of amenorrhoea.
- The median age of the menopause is 51 years.
- Premature menopause occurs in 1 per cent of women before the age of 40 (premature ovarian failure, POF).
- The reason for the timing of the last menses is unresolved.
- There is no clear-cut hormonal marker of the final menses.
- It occurs at an average oestradiol concentration of 110 pmol/l.
- FSH levels are approximately 50 per cent of their postmenopausal maximum.
- The perimenopause is characterised by great variability in circulating levels of FSH and oestradiol, accounting for the variety of symptoms.

• In the climacteric, there is an increased frequency of low luteal progesterone levels.

Physiological mechanisms of the menopause

During the perimenopause (about 4 years before menopause), concentrations of FSH, LH, oestradiol and oestrone vary unpredictably. Menstrual cycles get longer, gradually increasing from 28 days (range 26–32 days) to 60 days (range 35 to >100 days). Menstrual cycles get longer due to inadequate folliculogenesis, resulting in impaired corpus luteum function and inadequate progesterone secretion. At the start of the menopause, about 60 per cent of the cycles are still ovulatory. In the last 6 months preceding menopause, ovulatory progesterone levels occur in about 5 per cent of cycles. Cycles are then characterised by follicular oestradiol secretion which is insufficient to induce a mid-cycle LH surge, but sufficient to stimulate endometrial growth. Lacking the modifying effect of the normal luteal progesterone, it disintegrates easily, giving the symptoms of irregular and/or heavy bleeding.

In postmenopausal women, 3000 µg of androstenedione is produced daily, 95 per cent by the adrenal glands and 5 per cent by the ovaries. Androstenedione is converted to oestrone in the peripheral body fat. Increased body fat produces a greater amount of oestrone. Postmenopausal women convert about 1.5 per cent of androstenedione to oestrone (40 µg of oestrone per day). Obese women convert as much as 7 per cent of androstenedione to oestrone (200 µg of oestrone per day). Obese women are therefore more at risk of endometrial hyperplasia and adenocarcinoma of the endometrium.

Symptoms of the menopause

Decreased oestrogen produces:
• Hot flushes, night sweats and sleep disturbance
• Urogenital discomfort – atrophic urethral epithelium leading to micturition disorders
• Atrophic vaginal irritation and dryness, dyspareunia
• May include anxiety, depression, irritability, mood swings, memory problems and fatigue
• Other symptoms are joint pain and clumsiness.

The main clinical goal of hormone replacement therapy (HRT) (oestrogen or oestrogen plus progestogen) is to alleviate the symptoms of the menopause. There is substantive evidence from observational and epidemiological studies as to the indications and benefits of HRT [1–5].

EFFECTS OF OESTROGEN DEFICIENCY

1 The hot flush

- The hot flush is the characteristic acute symptom of the climacteric (Table 8.1). It is experienced as an explosion of heat, lasting 3–4 minutes, followed by profuse sweating.
- 75 per cent of postmenopausal women and about 40 per cent of perimenopausal women develop hot flushes.
- The hot flush is the result of changes in the brain's thermoregulatory centre located in the hypothalamus, despite a normal core body temperature. At the beginning of a hot flush there is a sudden drop in the body's thermoregulatory set point. The skin flush is preceded by an increase in blood perfusion which is followed by increases in peripheral skin temperature and heart rate.

Treatment of hot flushes

Hormonal treatment for vasomotor complaints may be continued for 1–2 years.

8

Table 8.1 Incidence, duration and causes of the menopausal hot flush.

No flushes (%)	15–25
Daily flushes (%)	15–20
Average duration of flushing (years)	1–2
Duration ≥5 years (%)	25
Premenopausal flushes (%)	15–25

Causes other than menopause
Psychosomatic stress
Phaeochromocytoma
Carcinoid tumour
Leukaemia
Thyroid disease

- **Oestrogen** almost entirely eliminates hot flushes.

Alternatives to oestrogen are:

- **Medroxyprogesterone** acetate (10 mg/day).
- **Dydrogesterone** (20 mg/day).
- **Tibolone** (2.5 mg continuously).
- **Depot- medroxyprogesterone acetate** (150 mg intramuscularly every 3 months).
- **Clonidine** (0.05 mg twice daily orally or transdermally). Clonidine is an α-adrenergic blocker. Its use is limited by adverse effects such as dry mouth, constipation, local skin irritation and drowsiness.
- **Methyldopa** (250–500 mg/day) is also effective.
- **Megestrol acetate** (20 mg twice daily) reduces flushes by 70 per cent.
- **Bromocryptine** and **naloxone** may also be effective.

2 Skin collagen

In the first 5 years of the menopause, up to 30 per cent of skin collagen can be lost. Changes in skin collagen and skin thickness are in proportion to the duration of menopause. Oestrogen therapy ameliorates this.

3 Urogenital tract change

Decreased oestrogen production leads to atrophy of the vagina – atrophic vaginitis. Atrophic vaginitis can present as itching, burning, dyspareunia and vaginal bleeding due to a thin epithelium. The trigone of the bladder and urethra are embryologically derived from oestrogen-dependent tissue and oestrogen deficiency can result in atrophy of these tissues, producing symptoms of urinary urgency, incontinence, dysuria and urinary frequency.

4 Vaginal atrophy

Treatment can include vaginal moisturisers. Oestrogen improves the integrity of vaginal tissue with beneficial effects on sensation, vasocongestion and vaginal secretions leading to enhanced arousal.

5 Osteoporosis

Osteoporosis is a complex multifactorial skeletal disease leading to an increased fracture risk because of a low bone mass, microarchitectural deterioration of bone tissue leading to poor bone quality and reduced bone strength.

6 Cognitive functioning and Alzheimer's disease

Oestrogen may mediate its effect on the central nervous system (CNS) through the stimulation of neurotrophic factors that influence nerve cell growth. Alternatively improvements may also be due to improved blood flow secondary to the protective effect of oestrogen on the vascular system.

7 Cardiovascular disease

The age-adjusted risk for coronary heart disease among post-menopausal women, whether surgical or natural, is twice that for premenopausal women [6,7].

It is thought that oestrogens have a protective effect in premenopausal women against atherogenesis. Women have a 10-year delay in the onset of coronary disease compared with men and a 20-year delay in myocardial infarction and sudden death. Current use or past use of postmenopausal oestrogen replacement therapy significantly reduces the risk of cardiovascular disease which persists into the eighth decade of life.

8

HISTORY TAKING PRIOR TO COMMENCING HRT

- Medical history
- Gynaecological details
- Personal and familial breast disease
- Diabetes
- Venous and arterial thromboembolic disease
- Liver disease
- Gastrointestinal disease
- Family history of osteoporosis, ovarian cancer and colonic cancer.

Investigations

Measure height, weight, blood pressure; breast, abdominal, vaginal and pelvic examinations; cervical smear, mammography, a lipid profile. Investigate risk factors with a personal or family history (Tables 8.2 and 8.3) [8].

EFFECTS OF OESTROGENS

- Oestrogens primarily target epithelial cells lining the reproductive tract and the ductolobular structures of the breast.
- Oestrogens play a key role in the maintenance of the calcium content of the skeletal structure.

Table 8.2 Risk assessment for venous thromboembolism when prescribing HRT.

Age
Obesity
Family history of thrombotic events
Past history of thrombotic events
Immobilisation
Dehydration
Surgery

Table 8.3 Investigations for potential thrombophilia. (RCOG (1999) [8].)

Activated partial thromboplastic time and prothrombin time
Antithrombin activity
Protein C activity
Total and free protein S antigen
Modified activated protein C resistance
Lupus anticoagulant and anticardiolipin antibodies (IgG and IgM)

Factor V Leiden

Routine haematology and biochemistry
FBC including platelet count; exclude thrombocythaemia
U&Es
LFTs
Urinalysis for protein

FBC, full blood count; U&E, urea and electrolytes; LFT, liver function test.

- Oestrogens maintain secondary sex characteristics (voice, skin texture, brain function).
- Oestrogens regulate the function of the cardiovascular system.
- Oestrogens influence cell adhesion molecules and motility of some cell types and facilitate collateral vessel formation.
- They modulate smooth muscle reactivity and other non-endothelium-mediated vascular effects.
- They enhance endothelial function via effects on nitric oxide/calcium channels.
- They may have an antioxidant effect, e.g. in their direct action on synapses to suppress oxidative impairment of membrane transport systems (a possible mechanism for protection against Alzheimer's disease).
- The effects of oestrogens are modified by oestrogen receptors.
- Oestrogens modify lipid metabolism and transport. They decrease low density lipoproteins (LDLs) and lipoproteins by about 11 per cent and increase high density lipoproteins (HDLs) by 4–12 per cent, depending on the associated progestogen. There is, however, a detrimental effect with elevation of triglycerides. Elevated total cholesterol and LDL cholesterol is a major risk factor for coronary heart disease (CHD) [9]. Hence the recommendation in 1993 from the National Cholesterol Education Program Adult Treatment Panel that oestrogen therapy be considered as a pharmacological alternative to conventional lipid-lowering agents for the management of elevated LDL cholesterol in postmenopausal women (Tables 8.4 and 8.5) [10]. Subsequently the Heart and Estrogen/Progestin Replace-

8

Table 8.4 World Health Organisation (WHO) classification of hyperlipidaemia. (Beaumont et al. (1970) [9].)

WHO type	Total cholesterol	LDL cholesterol	Triglycerides	Lipoprotein abnormality
I	High	Low/normal	High	Chylomicrons
IIa	High/normal	High	Normal	LDL
IIb	High	High	High	LDL
III	High	Low/normal	High	VLDL remnants
IV	High/normal	Normal	High	VLDL
V	High	Normal	High	Chylomicrons + VLDL

VLDL, very low density lipoprotein.

Table 8.5 The European Atherosclerosis Society classification of hypertriglyceridaemia.

Mild	1.2–2.3 mmol/l (100–200 mg/dl)
Moderate	2.3–5.6 mmol/l (200–500 mg/dl)
Severe	>5.6 mmol/l (>500 mg/dl)

Table 8.6 Indications for HRT.

Very severe climacteric complaints
Severe climacteric sleep disturbances and anxiety
Severe atrophic and symptomatic urogenital changes
High risk for osteoporosis and cardiovascular disease
Hypercholesterolaemia and oestrogen deficiency

ment Study (HERS) has refuted this for secondary prevention of CHD. The 'beneficial' effect on lipids is maximal using unopposed oestrogens, but this is only possible in women who have had a hysterectomy. The effect on lipids is attenuated by the addition of progestogens, the magnitude depending on the choice of progestogen (less for micronised progesterone than for medroxyprogesterone acetate). Transdermal preparations have a significantly smaller effect on LDL cholesterol and no effect on HDL cholesterol levels or triglycerides. Careful consideration needs to be given to the use of statins for cholesterol lowering as indicated. Statins (HMG-CoA reductase inhibitors) cause a 37 per cent reduction in LDL, a 7 per cent rise in HDL and a 16 per cent fall in triglycerides in women over a 5-year period [11].

- The aim of postmenopausal oestrogen therapy is to deliver the lowest dose of oestrogen to relieve acute symptoms (vasomotor) and prevent vaginal–urethral mucosal atrophy, and for prophylactic use efficacious doses are needed to maintain skin collagen, reduce bone resorption and restore equilibrium, protect the cardiovascular system and maintain brain cognitive function (Table 8.6).

- In order to maximise compliance a hormonal regimen should be selected that produces the least amount of uterine bleeding. In women with a uterus the lowest effective dose of progestogen should be used (i.e. that which maintains endometrial stability).

▪ The superiority of one oestrogen over another has not been established. For 0.625 mg oestrogen, 5 mg medroxyprogesterone acetate is necessary or the equivalent progesterone. It is given for at least 10–14 days a month (sequential), to prevent endometrial hyperplasia and malignancy, or throughout the cycle (continuous) with the aim of amenorrhoea.

TYPES OF ORAL OESTROGEN

17β-oestradiol, oestrone and oestriol are naturally occurring human oestrogens. Conjugated equine oestrogens (CEE) (e.g. Premarin) are obtained from the urine of pregnant mares and comprise 50–60 per cent of oestrone sulphate together with equine oestrogen such as equalin and 17α-dihydroequalin. They are analogous to purely human oestrogens and therefore are considered 'natural'. CEE formulations are standardised, whereas the biological activity of an E_2 preparation depends on its formulation and on the delivery system. The following give approximate equal potencies:

CEE	0.625 mg
E_2-valerate	2 mg
Micronised E_2	1.6 mg (approximately)
Transdermal delivery systems	50 µg

The natural oestrogen produced by the ovary is 17β-oestradiol which is rapidly oxidised to oestrone before being excreted as the weak oestriol in urine. Use of 17β-oestradiol implants or oestradiol valerate (Progynova) produces high levels of circulating oestradiol, thus simulating normal ovarian oestrogen production. CEEs act in a similar manner to oestradiol, but are metabolised by different enzymes and therefore have more complex and sustained actions on hepatic proteins and enzymes.

There is often not a clear medical indication for one particular formulation or delivery system. The patient can often decide on a preference for which type of formulation and delivery system (tablets, patches, gels, sprays, implants).

Examples of types of HRT available are listed in Tables 8.7 and 8.8.

All the natural oestrogens other than CEE are derived from plants, cactus or soya bean. There is no evidence that one type of oestrogen is any more effective than others in relieving menopausal symptoms or in the prophylactic prevention of osteoporosis or cardiovascular

8

Table 8.7 Examples of combined sequential hormone replacement therapy.

Type	Brand	Oestrogen	Formulation	Progestogen
Monthly	Climagest	Oestradiol 1 mg, 2 mg	Tablets	Norethisterone 1 mg
	Cyclo-Progynova	Oestradiol 1 mg, 2 mg	Tablets	Levonorgestrel 0.25/0.5 mg
	Elleste Duet	Oestradiol 2 mg	Tablets	Norethisterone 1 mg
	Estracombi	Oestradiol 50 µg	Patches, combined patches	Norethisterone 250 µg
	Estrapak 50	Oestradiol 50 µg	Patches and tablets	Norethisterone 1 mg
	Evorel-Pak	Oestradiol 50 µg	Patches and tablets	Norethisterone 1 mg
	Evorel Sequi	Oestradiol 50 µg	Patches, combined patches	Norethisterone 170 µg
	Femapak	Oestradiol 40 µg, 80 µg	Patches and tablets	Dydrogesterone 10 mg
	Femoston	Oestradiol 1 mg, 2 mg	Tablets	Dydrogesterone 10, 20 mg
	Improvera	Oestrone 0.93 mg	Tablets	Medroxyprogesterone 10 mg
	Menophase	Mestranol 12.5–50 µg	Tablets	Norethisterone 0.75–1.5 mg
	Nuvelle	Oestradiol 2 mg	Tablets	Levonorgestrel 0.75 mg
	Nuvelle TS	Oestradiol 80 µg + 50 µg	Patches, combined patches	Levonorgestrel 20 µg
	Premique Cycle	Conj. oestrogens 0.625 mg	Tablets	Medroxyprogesterone 10 mg
	Prempak-C	Conj. oestrogens 0.625 mg, 1.25 mg	Tablets	Norgestrel 0.15 mg
	Trisequens	Oestradiol 1–2 mg ± oestriol 1 mg	Tablets	Norethisterone 1 mg
Quarterly	Tridestra	Oestradiol 2 mg	Tablets	Medroxyprogesterone 20 mg

British National Formulary

8

Table 8.8 Oestrogen preparations.

Brand	Oestrogen	Formulation	Dose of oestrogen
Climaval	Oestradiol	Tablets	1, 2 mg
Dermestril	Oestradiol	Patches	25, 50, 100 µg
Elleste-Solo	Oestradiol	Tablets	1, 2 mg
Estraderm TTS or MX	Oestradiol	Patches	25, 50, 100 µg
Evorel	Oestradiol	Patches	25, 50, 75, 100 µg
Fematrix	Oestradiol	Patches	40, 80 µg
FemSeven	Oestradiol	Patches	50 µg
Harmogen	Oestrone	Tablets	0.93 mg
Hormonin	Oestradiol ⎫		0.6 mg
	Oestrone ⎬	Tablets	1.4 mg
	Oestriol ⎭		0.27 mg
Menorest	Oestradiol	Patches	37.5, 50, 75 µg
Oestrogel	Oestradiol	Gel	1.5 mg
Premarin	Conj. oestrogens	Tablets	0.625, 1.25 mg
Progynova	Oestradiol	Tablets	50, 100 µg
Progynova TS	Oestradiol	Patches	50, 100 µg
Sandrena	Oestradiol	Gel	0.5, 1 mg
Zumenon	Oestradiol	Tablets	1, 2 mg
Oestradiol Implant	Oestradiol	Implant pellet	25, 50, 100 mg

British National Formulary

disease. After oral ingestion oestradiol undergoes metabolism in the small intestine. Only 10 per cent reaches the circulation as oestradiol. Metabolism in the liver converts a large proportion of the oestradiol to oestrone. Therefore measurement of the serum oestradiol level is not a true reflection of the oestrogen level.

Ethinyloestradiol and mestranol are semi-synthetic oestrogens. They are considered less suitable for HRT because of their more potent effect on hepatic cellular function. Ethinyloestradiol is more potent and is readily absorbed from the intestine and passes unchanged to the liver. Oestradiol, a natural oestrogen preparation, undergoes considerable metabolism in the intestine and liver and is partly changed to the less potent oestrone.

NON-ORAL ADMINISTRATION OF OESTROGEN

Non-oral administration of oestrogen avoids enterohepatic metabolism. It can be useful for women with significant liver function abnormalities or high triglycerides. Non-oral routes include intra-muscular injection, implantation, vaginal creams, skin creams or gels and patches. Intramuscular oestrogen by injection causes wide variation in concentrations and therefore is not a suitable route for administration.

Transdermal oestrogen

Absorption of oestrogen through the skin and subcutaneous fat, vaginal epithelium, nasal or sublingual mucosa has the advantage of avoiding metabolism in the intestine and liver. Pure oestradiol administered directly into the systemic circulation causes a rise in plasma oestradiol concentration, producing an oestradiol:oestrone ratio similar to that found in premenopausal women. Theoretically, transdermal oestrogen may be preferable to oral oestradiol but there is no clinical evidence for the effects of this. Transdermal oestradiol causes a reduction in serum triglycerides which may be a beneficial independent risk factor for cardiovascular disease. Transdermal oestrogen does not impair glucose or insulin metabolism, whereas oral therapy causes a deterioration in glucose tolerance. There is no change in coagulation or fibrinolytic factors or renin substrate with transdermal oestradiol, compared with CEEs, which do cause some changes in these factors.

Transdermal oestrogen may be preferable for women with a history of deep vein thrombosis who, after being fully informed of potential risks and screened for inherited coagulopathies, wish to take HRT. Transdermal oestrogen does not produce rises in factors VII and X and protein C nor the decrease in antithrombin-III and protein S found with oral HRT.

The first oestradiol skin patch (Estraderm TTS) contains a reser-voir of oestradiol. There is an alcohol solvent behind a rate-limiting membrane and an adhesive layer. Newer transdermal systems consist of a single transparent matrix with an adhesive layer that contains the oestradiol. The dose delivered is proportional to the surface area of the patch in contact with the skin (Table 8.7). The most commonly used patches are those delivering around 50µg oestradiol per 24 hours. This method of administration may be prob-lematic in tropical climates because of skin reactions. A gel might be more suitable.

Gel

Percutaneous gels or creams are convenient and well suited to women who live in tropical climates and want to use a transdermal route. High moisture in climates makes local skin irritation from patches troublesome.

Oestrogen gels and creams are limited by the variability of the amount applied. With patches, reactions can occur at the application site in about 5 per cent of women who use adhesive patches and 10 per cent with alcohol-based patches. Drying the alcohol off sometimes helps, and avoiding moisture and putting them on different sites minimises the skin reactions.

Gel is the most popular method of administration of HRT in France. It is a hydro-alcoholic substance containing 0.06% w/w 17β-oestradiol and in the UK is packaged as a non-pressurised canister as Oestrogel. A dose of 0.75 mg oestradiol is dispensed as a starting dose applied to the arms or legs. A similar gel containing 1 mg 17β-oestradiol per gram of gel is also available (Sandrena).

Implants

Oestradiol implants are crystalline 17β-oestradiol pellets that are inserted subcutaneously into the anterior abdominal wall or the buttocks.

- 50 mg 6-monthly is the most commonly used oestradiol dose, giving circulating levels of approximately 400 pmol/l at 1 year. Each pellet may continue to release oestradiol for 2 years or more, which can lead to supraphysiological blood levels if the implants are given too frequently (tachyphylaxis).
- Therefore after stopping implant therapy cyclical or continuous progestogen should be continued for at least 2 years.

Localised oestrogen may be given vaginally (Table 8.9).

Combined patches

These provide both oestrogen and the protective progesterone in a patch formulation, thus obviating the need for an oral form of progesterone taking with oestrogen-only patches.

8

Table 8.9 Vaginal oestrogen preparations. (Greendale *et al.* (1991) [1].)

Geneic (proprietary) name	Formulation	Regimen
Oestradiol tablet (Vagifem)	Each tablet contains 25 µg oestradiol	One tablet twice weekly
Oestradiol ring (Estring)	Silicone elastomer ring with core that contains 2 mg oestradiol (released as 7.5 µg/24 h)	Replace every 90 days
Oestriol cream	1 mg/g	0.5 mg oestriol twice weekly

- Estracombi
- Levonorgestrel (Nouvelle TS)
- Norethisterone (Evorelsequi) for 14 days.

Tibolone (Livial) has oestrogenic and progestogenic and androgenic activity. The incidence of bleeding is 10–15 per cent during the initial months and about 4 per cent after 6 months.

PROGESTOGENS

Originally progestogens were developed in the early 1950s when the methyl group was removed at C_{19} to produce norethisterone – the best potent progestogen at the time (Fig. 8.1). The 17α-hydroxyprogestogens became available in the early 1960s with attempts of pharmaceutical companies competing for the oral contraceptive market. These are characterised by an acetate group at C_{17} and a 17-hydroxy derivative where the 17 OH group has been acetylated. A methyl group occurs at C_6 (e.g. Provera).

Types of progestogens

Natural progesterone

Natural progesterone (derived from plant sources including the yam) given orally has unpredictable absorption, and metabolism will influence final blood levels. Relatively high doses are required for an adequate endometrial response. Therefore, a variety of synthetic progestogens have been developed from various companies.

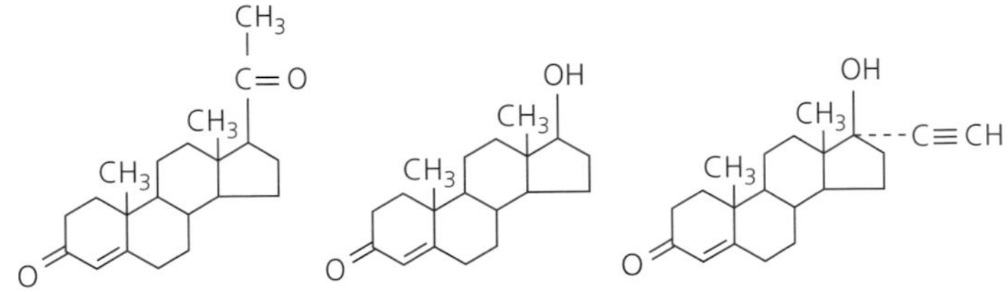

PROGESTERONE
4 pregnene –3, 20 dione

TESTOSTERONE

ETHISTERONE
17α ethinyl testosterone

Fig. 8.1 Types of progesterones.

19-nortestosterone derivatives

First to third generation oral sequential preparations contain C_{19} progestogens:

- Norethisterone
- Norgestrel
- Levonorgestrel
- Gestodene
- Desogestrel.

17α-hydroxyprogesterone derivatives – antiandrogen

- Medroxyprogesterone acetate
- Dydrogesterone.

These are less androgenic and allow greater flexibility in prescribing, especially in those women with premenstrual symptoms such as bloating, depression and headaches during the progestogen phase of treatment.

Table 8.10 shows empirical dosages of different progestogens commonly used to avoid endometrial hyperplasia and subsequent carcinoma which have metamorphosised onto the market.

Effects of progestogens, including side effects

- Induce a secretory change in the endometrium and breast alveolar cells.
- Inhibit breast and endometrial cell mitosis.

Table 8.10 Empirical doses of progestogens to avoid endometrial hyperplasia and subsequent carcinoma.

	mg/day
Progesterone (micronised)	200–300
Medroxyprogesterone acetate (MPA)	10
Norethisterone acetate (NETA)	1–2.5
DL-norgestrel (NORG)	0.15
Levonorgestrel (LNG)	0.075–0.15
Dydrogesterone	10–20
Cyproterone acetate	1–10
Desogestrel	0.15
Transdermal	
Norethisterone acetate (NETA)	0.25

- Produce slowing of smooth muscle cell activity which leads to bowel stasis, increasing flatus, weight gain and bloating.
- Premenstrual syndrome (PMS)-type syndrome.
- Depression, anxiety and irritability.
- Mastalgia.

HRT and progestogen intolerance

Progestogens may have androgenic and/or oestrogenic or antiandrogenic and/or antioestrogenic effects. Progestogens may also have mineralocorticoid and glucocorticoid-type effects.

The C_{19} nortestosterone derivatives (e.g. norgestrel and norethisterone) may have a higher risk of adverse effects than the less androgenic C_{21} derivatives (medroxyprogesterone and dydrogesterone). Effects such as acne and darkening of the facial hair tend to occur mainly with the 19-nortestosterone derivatives which can have androgenic effects due to their relatively strong binding affinity for the androgen receptor. Progesterone and dydrogesterone have no androgenic effects.

C_{21} progestogens, particularly medroxyprogesterone, have mild androgenic effects as their binding to the androgenic receptors is a little higher than that of progesterone. In addition, dosage has an effect.

Progestogens vary and therefore higher doses are required in some women compared to others. For example, MPA is absorbed well from the gut and achieves good blood levels but is not as potent as norethisterone. Therefore, higher oral doses of MPA must be given for an adequate endometrial response, and more unwanted progestogenic side effects can arise in women taking MPA compared to those taking lower doses of norethisterone. Some women may alleviate the adverse side effects by taking the progestogen in divided daily doses or at bedtime.

Mineralocorticoid activity

Most of the adverse physical symptoms associated with progestogen intolerance such as oedema, weight gain, bloating and migraine are attributed to the effect of progestogen on the renin–aldosterone system. This leads to retention of sodium and fluid gain.

OESTROGEN AND PROGESTOGEN REGIMENS

Types of regimen

- Cyclic
- Sequential
- Long cycle
- Continuous combined
- Gonadomimetic.

Cyclic HRT

The oestrogen is administered unopposed for 3 weeks out of every 4. The progestogen is added for 10–14 days each cycle, where a regular withdrawal bleed occurs. However, it is thought preferable that postmenopausal women have therapies that minimise or avoid bleeding.

Continuous combined therapy

Continuous combined therapy uses a progesterone every day to prevent the proliferative effect of oestrogen and to maintain an atrophic endometrium to prevent bleeding. The incidence of breakthrough bleeding may be as high as 80 per cent in the first 3 months. Continuous combined regimens cause amenorrhoea by inducing endometrial atrophy. However, the continuous progestogen can result in hypertrophy of the stroma which is highly vascular. Thirty to forty per cent of women experience erratic bleeding for up to 6 months and discontinue treatment during this time. Continuous combined regimens ought not to be administered unless the woman has had 12 months of amenorrhoea, because the endogenous ovarian activity gives rise to vaginal bleeding (Table 8.11).

Erratic vaginal bleeding is more frequent in women within 1 year of the menopause. The progesterone-only contraceptive pills provide a convenient low dose progestogen supplement if it is necessary to adjust the dose–response to bleeding or side effects.

Long cycle HRT

The regimen comprises oestradiol valerate (2 mg for 70 days) followed by medroxyprogesterone acetate (20 mg) in addition to the oestradiol for 14 days (days 71–84). Each cycle is completed with seven placebo tablets on days 85–91, e.g. Tridestra. The rate of endometrial hyperplasia is 1.9 per cent for the first 12 months and 0.5 per cent between 12 and 24 months.

Daily administration of oestrogen avoids breakthrough bleeding. Progestogens can be prescribed on a monthly (days 1–12 each month) cycle continuously or four times per year (quarterly regimen).

Progestogen protects the endometrium against the development of hyperplasia and neoplasia (Table 8.12). Progestogens may be administered sequentially for 10–12 days each 28-day treatment cycle. About 85 per cent of women on a sequential regimen have a withdrawal bleed either towards the end or immediately after the progestogen phase. To prevent cyclical bleeding on sequential regimens, progestogens are increasingly being given continuously – every day – in combination with oestrogen. Eventually it is hoped the endometrium becomes atrophic and therefore the woman becomes amenorrhoeic.

In general, CEE (0.625 mg) is combined with norethisterone (0.7–1 mg) for cyclic therapy, 0.35–0.5 mg for continuous, or with MPA – continuous 2.5–5 mg each day, or cyclic 5–10 mg for 12 days. MPA results in a low rate of endometrial hyperplasia (less than 1 per cent per year). The main reason to use 5 mg daily is to stop withdrawal bleeding. With continuous progestogen regimens bleeding is light to moderate but its timing is erratic and unpredictable. After 12

8

Table 8.11 Period-free hormone replacement therapy.

Type	Brand	Oestrogen	Formulation	Progestogen
Continuous	Climesse	Oestradiol 2 mg	Tablets	Norethisterone 0.7 mg
Combined therapy	Kliofem	Oestradiol 2 mg	Tablets	Norethisterone 1 mg
	Premique	Conj. oestrogens 0.625 mg	Tablets	Medroxyprogesterone 5 mg
	Kliovance	Oestradiol 1 mg	Tablets	Norethisterone 0.5 mg
	Evorel Conti	Oestradiol 50 µg	Patches	Norethisterone 170 µg
Gonadomimetic	Livial		Tablets	

8

Table 8.12 Progestogens used for prevention of endometrial hyperplasia in combination hormone replacement therapy.

Generic (proprietary) name	Cyclical dose (duration 12 days) (mg)	Continuous daily dose (mg)
Medroxyprogesterone acetate (Provera)	5–10	2.5–5
Dydrogesterone (Duphaston)	10–20[1]	Unknown
Micronised progesterone	200	100[2]
Norethisterone (Micronor; Primolut N)	0.7–1.0	0.35–0.5[1]

[1] Degree of hyperplasia protection achieved varies by dose.
[2] Limited data.

months of continuous combined hormone therapy, bleeding stops in about 90 per cent of women.

A sequential/cyclical regimen combines an oestrogen for 21 days (e.g. Trisequens, Estrapak, Nuvelle, Prempak-C) or a tailored regimen of Progynova (2 mg daily for 21 days; or e.g. Premarin 0.625 mg, Estraderm 50) each month together with a progestogen such as Provera (10 mg for 10–14 days).

Continuous combined HRT has the advantage of a lower dosage of progestogen with fewer side effects such as mastalgia, and has a decreased incidence of bleeding. Examples of such regimens are: oestrogen (e.g. Progynova 2 mg, Premarin 0.625 mg, Climaral 2 mg, Estraderm 50 or their equivalents) combined with a progestogen (e.g. Provera 2.5–5.0 mg, Primolut **N** 0.25–1.25 mg daily). Combined preparations include oestradiol 2 mg plus norethisterone acetate 1 mg, and 0.625 mg conjugated oestrogens plus 5 mg medroxyprogesterone acetate. Continuous combined HRT is most suitable for women who are at least 1 year post-menopausal. Light bleeding or spotting occurs in 40–60 per cent of women in the first 6 months of treatment, which decreases to approximately 10 per cent after 1 year of use.

If bleeding persists after the first 6 months, endometrial biopsy and hysteroscopy are indicated to exclude endometrial pathology. Although residual endogenous endometrial activity can cause irregular bleeding in those perimenopause, HRT should be changed to sequential for at least 1 year before restarting the continuous combined HRT.

For persistent breakthrough bleeding in postmenopausal women a sequential regimen may be preferable to have regular bleeding rather than 'nuisance' bleeding that is irregular.

SIDE EFFECTS OF HRT

Bleeding

- The longer a progestogen is administered, the less the endometrium proliferates with less of a risk of a withdrawal bleed.
- Continuous HRT may be associated with breakthrough bleeding that is due to atrophic endometrium with exposed fine capillaries and arterioles.
- The breakthrough bleeding can be arrested by discontinuing the progestogen for 5–7 days, which allows the oestrogen to stimulate regeneration of vessels and growth of the endometrium, thus stabilising it.
- If heavy or prolonged bleeding occurs on sequential therapy and pathology has been excluded, use the progestogen for a longer duration or a more androgenic progestogen.

Oestrogen therapy and intrauterine disease and irregular bleeding

Uterine fibroids are monoclonal tumours derived from a single myometrial cell. Oestrogens promote fibroid growth. Progesterone may also have a myogenic and growth-stimulating effect on fibroids. Endometrial polyps are present in 3.5–33 per cent of postmenopausal women.

Abnormal bleeding with sequential HRT (Table 8.13)

- Heavy or prolonged bleeding at the appropriate time of the cycle, i.e. towards the end of or immediately after the progestogen phase
- Breakthrough bleeding occurring at any other time.

In theory bleeding should not occur during continuous combined therapy or with tibolone. However, in practice approximately 40 per cent of postmenopausal women starting continuous combined oestrogen/progestogen regimens will experience some bleeding during the first 4–6 months of treatment. This bleeding is usually light. The probability of achieving amenorrhoea is greater if treatment is not started at least 12 months since the menopause because of the diminished endogenous ovarian function.

8

Table 8.13 Questions to ask in the management of abnormal bleeding on HRT.

When did the bleeding occur in relation to the oestrogen and progestogen phase?
How long does the bleeding last and how heavy is it?
Did amenorrhoea occur before treatment was commenced?
Is there a problem that suggests poor compliance, e.g. progestogens causing premenstrual tension, incorrect administration of medication, poor patch adherence, concomitant drug therapies?

Livial (tibolone) does not appear to cause endometrial stimulation and the incidence of bleeding is no higher than that with the use of a placebo.

Postmenopausal bleeding

Approximately 10 per cent of women stop HRT after a year of therapy mostly due to irregular vaginal bleeding. Other side effects are those from the oestrogen component (breast tenderness, leg cramps, nausea and headaches) and from the progestogen component (premenstrual syndrome, dysmenorrhoea, acne and fluid retention), as well as fear of cancer and general anxieties about treatment.

Endometrial hyperplasia in premenopausal women is almost always associated with anovulation. Endometrial hyperplasia (occurs in 10 per cent) contains a spectrum of histological changes, ranging from simple exaggeration of the proliferative stage of intraepithelial neoplasia similar to adenocarcinoma, and may present as irregular vaginal bleeding. There is only a small risk of the progression of simple hyperplasia without atypia to endometrial carcinoma. Between 20 and 80 per cent of women with untreated endometrial glandular hyperplasia with cellular atypia will eventually develop adenocarcinoma.

Endometrial biopsy with bleeding on HRT is required if:

- Light bleeding continues after the first 6 months of treatment with a continuous regimen.
- Bleeding recurs after amenorrhoea has been established.
- There is no obvious explanation of the bleeding, such as poor compliance.

Other causes of bleeding with HRT

- Poor gastrointestinal absorption
- Gastroenteritis
- Malabsorption syndromes (coeliac disease, Whipple's disease, inflammatory bowel disease, e.g. ulcerative colitis, Crohn's disease) may all affect the absorption of oral oestrogen and progestogen that could lead to abnormal bleeding.

Endometrial biopsy and hysteroscopy indications

Endometrial biopsy with or without hysteroscopy should be considered for:

- Heavy withdrawal bleeding
- Prolonged withdrawal bleeding
- Breakthrough bleeding during two or more cycles.

Approximately 4 per cent of the endometrium is sampled by the pipelle biopsy. Ultrasound measures endometrial thickness. An endometrial thickness >5 mm or irregularities in endometrial morphology where one area is thicker than another suggest the need for endometrial biopsy and hysteroscopy. Hysteroscopy enables visualisation of the whole surface of the endometrium. In switching from a sequential combined HRT to continuous combined treatment, a 28-day break-off from all HRT (wash-out period) is recommended.

Poor gastrointestinal absorption

In women with chronic malabsorption syndromes, the transdermal or subcutaneous route of administration of oestrogen should be used to avoid erratic gastrointestinal absorption. Progestogens can be administered transdermally, rectally, vaginally or intrauterine in combination with a non-oral oestrogen.

8

Mastalgia

- Mastalgia occurs because oestrogen induces mitosis and proliferation of breast cells.
- Progestogen inhibits mitosis but induces alveolar cells to produce secretions.
- Mastalgia may occur for a few weeks with administering continuous progestogen but then it subsides and the breasts become smaller and softer.

- Mastalgia may be treated by stopping the progestogen or increasing it to inhibit breast cell activity.

Bloating

- Progestogens affect the motility of smooth muscle cells and therefore they may cause slowing of gut peristalsis, bladder detrusor relaxation and other hollow organ changes.
- Slowing of gut peristalsis leads to constipation, increased gas formation, bloating and weight gain. Gall bladder stasis may be increased.

Fluid retention

- Fluid retention occurs as a result of increased back pressure in afferent vessels and increased capillary permeability.
- Oestrogen improves arteriolar and capillary endothelial and smooth muscle cell function, and so oedema should be reduced by oestrogen.

Weight gain

- It is commonly thought that HRT causes weight gain. All long-term studies have shown that menopausal women taking HRT gain less weight than those not taking it.

Progestogen side effects

- 20 per cent of women will have significant progestogen intolerance. Many of these would resolve within 2–3 months.
- Side effects can sometimes be counteracted with a mild diuretic such as 25 mg of either spironolactone or hydroclorothiazide. The diuretic should be given in the last week of added progestogen.
- Other alternatives are oral dydrogesterone or progesterone suppositories (200 mg/day for 12 days).

ENDOGENOUS OVARIAN ACTIVITY AND EXOGENOUS HORMONE TREATMENT

Giving HRT in pre- and perimenopausal women needs to be synchronised with their natural cycle. In premenopausal women with a regular 28-day cycle, progestogens should be administered starting on day 17 of the cycle (day 1 being the first day of bleeding) to coincide with the endogenous progesterone production. If the cycle is short, i.e. 20 days) the progestogen is added from days 8 through to 19. With a 42-day cycle, give the progestogen from days 30 to 41. Failure to do so will result in patients bleeding twice during the month: one bleed will be due to endogenous ovarian function and the second to exogenous hormone administration. In general, androgenic progestogens such as norethisterone and norgestrel appear to give better cycle control than those derived from a natural steroid progesterone.

Some patients will continue to bleed erratically because their own ovarian function is intermittent and unpredictable and all forms of sequential oestrogen/progestogen HRT are associated with irregular bleeding. In such patients the combined oestrogen/progestogen oral contraceptive pill can be used if there are no contraindications. The combined pill provides oestrogen and therefore relieves oestrogen deficiency symptoms. Unlike HRT the combined oral contraceptive pill suppresses ovarian function and thus gives good cycle control in perimenopausal women with previously erratic periods.

Perimenopausal women who take continuous combined therapies or tibolone will bleed erratically because of the endogenous ovarian function. Therefore continuous HRT therapy should not be given to pre- and perimenopausal women. It is ideally suited to women who have had 12 months of amenorrhoea in the menopausal age group.

Sequential therapies

With sequential therapies women who experience bleeding too early during the phase of progestogen addition may benefit from an increase in progestogen dose. Erratic bleeding suggests the presence of a submucous fibroid, endometrial polyp or carcinoma. Postcoital bleeding suggests the presence of cervical pathology. A speculum examination ought to be done together with a cervical smear.

The progesterone-releasing intrauterine device

The progestogen levonorgestrel-containing intrauterine device (LNG-IUS) (Mirena) releases 20 μg progestogen daily and will produce an atrophic endometrium. It is unlicensed for use in HRT but provides satisfactory antagonism to oestrogen and is particularly suitable for the woman who has side effects from any other type of progestogen.

THE THEORETICAL BENEFITS OF HRT

These are summarised in Table 8.14 [12]. After 60 years of age, 50–60 per cent of women are likely to suffer an osteoporotic fracture during

Table 8.14 Decision analysis to assess the value of oestrogen replacement therapy for 25 years in a hypothetical cohort of 10 000 women, assumed to be aged 50 years, extrapolated to age 75. (Gorsky *et al.* (1994) [12].)

Prevent	574 deaths
Decrease in fatal coronary heart disease events	48% (567 cases)
Decrease in deaths from hip fracture	49% (75)
Increase in deaths from breast cancer	21% (39)
Increase in deaths from endometrial cancer	207% (29)
Gain	3951 quality-adjusted life years compared with women not using oestrogen

25 years of oestrogen use prevents 38% (574) of total deaths from these four conditions

Decrease in non-fatal coronary heart disease	49% (889)
Decrease in hip fractures	67% (312)
Increase in breast cancer incidence	22% (136)
Increase in endometrial cancer	206% (206)
Decrease in adverse health events among those treated	28.5% (859)

Use of oestrogens for 5 years

Prevents non-fatal coronary heart disease events	6% (106)
Prevents hip fractures	1.5% (7)
Breast cancer increase	0.5% (3)
Endometrial cancer increase	31% (31)

Use of oestrogens for 10 years

Decrease in non-fatal coronary heart disease events	14% (263)
Decrease in hip fractures	6% (28)

their remaining lifetime. Hip fractures account for 10 per cent of total fractures in the 60–80 age group, increasing to 40 per cent in those over 80.

OSTEOPOROSIS

HRT is effective for the prevention and treatment of postmenopausal osteoporosis (Table 8.15) [13]. Oestrogen replacement therapy reduces the incidence of fractures of the distal radius and spine. The expected annual bone loss for premenopausal women aged 23–44 years is under 0.5 per cent. After a natural menopause bone loss averages 2 per cent per year. Every 10 per cent reduction in bone mineral density is linked with a two to three times increased fracture risk (Table 8.16).

The HRT-effected increase in bone mineral density, decrease in bone turnover and reduction in the risk of fractures decline rapidly after treatment is discontinued. Therefore treatment should be continued for women into their 60s and 70s. Women at high risk of fracture (Table 8.17) are likely to benefit most and should be identified

Table 8.15 Dose of oestrogen necessary to reduce the risk of osteoporosis in postmenopausal women.

0.625 mg per day conjugated oestrogen (for 21–25 days per month)

0.5 mg per day of micronised oestradiol or 0.05 mg of transdermal oestrogen patch

1500 mg per day of calcium in women greater than 65 years helps lessen bone loss

Adequate calcium intake minimises the amount of oestrogen necessary to prevent bone loss

Conjugated oestrogen may be reduced to 0.3 mg per day with an exogenous intake of 1500 mg calcium

Table 8.16 Lifetime risk of fracture for 50-year-old women.

Risk of hip fracture	16%
Risk of wrist fracture	15%
Risk of vertebral fracture	32%

Table 8.17 Risk factors for osteoporosis.

Personal history of a fracture, especially if not much force occurred
Family history of an osteoporotic fracture
Premature menopause or bilateral oophorectomy
Smoking
Low body weight
Decreased calcium intake
Decreased physical activity
Increased alcohol consumption

and treated with either HRT or another effective therapy. A 10 per cent loss of bone mass in general causes a doubling in the risk of fracture. Current use of HRT, especially in long-term users, is associated with a 30–50 per cent reduction in hip, spine and wrist fractures. It is likely that HRT must be given for at least 10 years to reduce significantly fractures that occur 10–30 years after the menopause [14].

Osteoporosis is characterised by a low bone mass and microarchitectural deterioration of bone tissue, leading to increased bone fragility and to susceptibility to fracture. Low bone mineral density is associated with an increased risk of fracture and women in the lowest quartile of bone mineral density have a 12-fold lifetime increased risk of hip fracture. The lifetime risk of fragility fractures in a 50-year-old woman is 30–40 per cent in white women. Most osteoporotic fractures occur after the age of 65. Doses of 0.625 mg conjugated oestrogens, 1–2 mg 17β-oestradiol and 50–100 mg transdermal 17β-oestradiol are effective, with less than 10 per cent of women showing bone loss.

Effects of the menopause on bone

A reduction in the bone mass or density accompanied by microarchitectural deterioration of the skeleton results in an increase in the risk of fracture. The loss of bone mass that occurs after the menopause disproportionately affects cancellous bone (the spongy bone present largely in vertebral bodies and within the ends of long bones). There is a decline in bone mass and alteration in the architecture of the bone. Trabeculae are responsible for giving bones their horizontal and vertical 'struts', and therefore bone becomes

markedly weakened by small changes in mass of cancellous bone. Fractures particularly predisposed to by osteoporosis are fractures of:
- Vertebral bodies (crush fracture)
- Fractures of the distal forearm (Colles' fracture)
- Fractures of the hip.

Techniques for detection of osteoporosis

- Single and dual X-ray absorptiometry (SXA, DXA or DEXA). DXA can be used to measure the lumbar spine, hip or wrist. DXA is the most accurate and precise technique currently available.
- Quantitative computerised tomography (QCT).
- X-ray absorptiometry.
- Ultrasound.

Osteoporosis has been defined by the World Health Organisation as a greater than 2.5 standard deviation (SD) in bone mass below the normal range for young adults. Bone density measurements are expressed in units which relate to the distribution of bone density relative to the mean for young adults. These numbers represent standard deviations from the mean and when related to the distribution of bone mass in the young population are usually referred to as the 'T score'. When related to an age-matched population they are called the 'Z score'. By the WHO definition an individual who has osteoporosis will have a T score of <−2.5. If the Z score is also low (e.g. −2 or below), that individual has substantially more bone loss than would be expected for her age and therefore there should be a greater index of suspicion as to a secondary cause of the bone loss. Thus a bone density down to a T score of −1 is normal, −1 to −2.5 is osteopenia and lower than −2.5 is osteoporosis.

There are several reliable methods for accurate and precise measurements of bone mass (Table 8.18). Results are expressed as bone mineral density either in absolute terms (g/cm^2), SD units from peak adult bone mineral density (T score), or SD units from bone mineral density adjusted for age (Z score). Both T and Z scores are adjusted for ethnicity and sex. The Z score is used in determining which patient might require additional investigation, because it is of value for indicating a loss of bone mineral density that can be reasonably accounted for solely on the basis of age, sex and menopausal status. Any patient in whom the Z score is lower than −2 should be evaluated for secondary causes of low bone mineral density (Table 8.19).

8

Table 8.18 Methods for measurement of bone mass.

Method	Measurement site
Dual X-ray absorptiometry	Forearm (proximal and distal radius)
	Lumbar spine (anteroposterior and lateral projections)
	Proximal femur
	Total body
Quantitative computed tomography	Lumbar spine (cancellous bone only or combined cancellous and cortical bone)
Single X-ray absorptiometry	Calcaneus
Radiographic absorptiometry	Phalanges (hand)
Ultrasonography	Calcaneus
	Patella

Table 8.19 Investigations for women with low bone mass.

Laboratory investigations	Potential diagnosis
Hypercalcaemia/hypophosphataemia	Primary hyperparathyroidism
Elevated blood urea nitrogen/creatinine	Renal failure/secondary hyperparathyroidism
Hypoalbuminaemia/hypoproteinaemia	Malnutrition/malabsorption
Hyperglobulinaemia	Multiple myeloma
Hyperbilirubinaemia/elevated hepatic enzymes	Chronic liver disease
Full blood count	
Anaemia	Malnutrition/malabsorption
	Multiple myeloma
Thyroid-stimulating hormone	Hyperthyroidism
24-hour urine	
Calcium <50 mg/volume	Malnutrition/malabsorption (consider measurement of 25-hydroxyvitamin D)
Calcium >250 mg/volume	Hypercalciuria
Free cortisol	Cushing's disease

8

Bone mineral density measurement is useful if after full counselling a woman is not keen on taking HRT. If a woman does not wish to take HRT, bone density may be measured by DXA to spine and hip. If it is low, the woman may be more amenable to recognising the benefits of HRT. Treatment should be recommended if bone mineral density at the hip or spine is < −2.5 T score. In the presence of one or more risk factors, raise the treatment threshold by 0.5 (i.e. to < −2). It is not necessary to measure bone density if the patient wishes to take HRT for other reasons. For the patient with a prior peripheral fracture (e.g. Colles'), treat when the T score is −1.5 or lower, and if other risk factors are present treat at −1 or lower. If bone mineral density measurement has been an integral part of the initial decision not to begin HRT (and bone density measurement is not low), a follow-up measurement after an interval of not less than 2 years may be appropriate.

If the Z score is −2 the following investigations should be done: routine biochemical profile, including calcium, full blood count, erythrocyte sedimentation rate (ESR) and thyroid-stimulating hormone (TSH) test will detect most secondary causes of accelerated bone loss, if not due to illness or drug therapy (e.g. prednisone). A vitamin D level may be appropriate if nutritional or gastrointestinal problems are possible.

Differential diagnosis

- Primary hyperparathyroidism (hypercalcaemia, hypophosphataemia)
- Renal failure (increased creatinine)
- Malabsorption, malnutrition (hypoalbuminaemia, hypoproteinaemia)
- Multiple myeloma (monoclonal hyperglobulinaemia)
- Chronic liver disease (hyperbilirubinaemia, elevated hepatic enzymes), thyrotoxicosis (suppressed TSH).

HRT and prevention of osteoporosis

Oestrogen stops and may partly reverse the effects of menopause on bone and retards bone loss. Long-term controlled clinical trial data have shown that oestrogen use stabilises bone mass in the forearm and spine for at least 10 years. Progesterone, particularly if it is an androgenic progesterone, may have an additive effect. HRT reduces the risk of fracture by up to 50 per cent (Table 8.20). Oestrogen acts directly on bone cells through high affinity receptors and prevents the early phases of bone loss. Over time it may increase bone density

Table 8.20 Incidence of fractures after 5 years of oestrogen use.

35 per cent of hip fractures compared with non-users
Oestrogen use for less than 5 years reduces the incidence of hip fractures by 50
  per cent in women who had a premenopausal oophorectomy
Greater than 5 years of use gives a 90 per cent reduced incidence of fracture
  compared with non-users

in both cortical and trabecular bone, but complete reversal of substantial loss is not possible.

Non-hormonal treatment for osteoporosis – alternatives to HRT

Bisphosphonates

- Bisphosphonates are synthetic analogues of inorganic pyrophosphate, an endogenous regulator of bone turnover.
- Bisphosphonates bind avidly to hydroxyapatite, inhibit osteoclastic bone resorption and are then buried within the skeleton where they remain with a half-life of 10–12 years or more.
- Bisphosphonates inhibit mineralisation of bone in a dose-dependent manner. It is the ratio of the dose that inhibits resorption to the dose that inhibits mineralisation that makes one bisphosphonate more acceptable in clinical use rather than another (e.g. sodium clodronate, disodium etidronate, disodium pamidronate and tiludronic acid). Examples are:
- **Alendronic acid** (Fosamax) is a third generation aminobisphosphonate.

Alendronic acid (10 mg/day) is taken in the morning with 200 ml water at least 30 minutes before breakfast or other beverage. After taking it, the patient should remain upright to reduce the incidence of oesophagitis. Long-term treatment reduces new vertebral fractures by up to 50 per cent and loss of height by 35 per cent. Concomitant use of the bisphosphonate disodium etidronate and HRT (plus calcium, 1000 mg daily) increases the bone mass density by more than either HRT or the bisphosphonate alone. Oestrogen plus androgen therapy also prevents osteoporosis. Androgens influence bone resorption directly and indirectly through conversion of testosterone to oestrogen by aromatase. Androgens stimulate bone formation and androgen blockade or deficiency results in bone loss.

• **Disodium etidronate** (400 mg daily) (Didronel) is used for 2 weeks and then **calcium** (1000 mg equivalent daily) for the remainder of the 3 months, then the cycle is repeated. It is taken fasting with water, avoiding food or other drugs for at least 2 hours (bisphosphonates are poorly absorbed).

Calcitriol

Calcitriol (1,25-dihydroxyvitamin D_3, Rocaltrol) is given at a dose of 0.25–0.5 μg/day. Blood calcium levels should be monitored at 2, 6, 12 and 24 weeks because of the risk of hypercalcaemia and hypercalciuria.

Selective oestrogen receptor modulators (SERMs)

SERMs (e.g. raloxifene 60 mg daily) do not treat symptoms of the menopause. SERMs selectively deliver oestrogen where required in bone and antagonise oestrogen's effects on the breast and endometrium. Raloxifene is licensed for the prevention of non-traumatic vertebral fractures in postmenopausal women at increased risk of osteoporosis.

Tibolone

This synthetic C_{19} steroid with weak oestrogenic, progestational and androgenic properties is an alternative to standard HRT. The dose is 2.5 mg/day. It is effective for treating postmenopausal osteoporosis.

Calcitonin

A polypeptide hormone produced by the parafollicular C cells of the normal human thyroid, calcitonin inhibits bone resorption in pharmacological doses. It may be administered as an intranasal calcitonin spray.

Summary: prophylactic and treatment options for osteoporosis

• HRT.
• Bisphosphonates.
• Selective oestrogen receptor modulators.
• Calcitriol.

- Calcitonin.
- Weight-bearing exercise together with adequate oestrogen and calcium intake (1500 mg daily = three portions of dairy food or calcium-enriched soy products) is also useful but not sufficient on its own.
- Regular weight-bearing exercise (half an hour of walking every day) also helps.
- Vitamin D (800 U) is useful as is sun exposure for half an hour a day, because vitamin D decreases with age.

CARDIOVASCULAR DISEASE AND OESTROGEN REPLACEMENT THERAPY: MECHANISMS OF PROTECTION

General factors that reduce the risk of cardiovascular disease should be encouraged (Table 8.21).

There are two possible mechanisms for the cardioprotective effect of oestrogens.

- They may protect the arteries by an indirect action through a change in the lipid profile or by a direct action at the arterial wall. Altered lipid profile accounts for about 20–30 per cent of the reduction of the cardiovascular risk [15].
- The direct oestrogenic effect at the arterial wall might be responsible for 70–80 per cent of the cardioprotection of HRT. Experimentally in the monkey, it has been shown that oestrogens delay the progression of a coronary atherosclerosis and increase the endothelium-dependent relaxation at normal cholesterol levels as well as with pre-existing atherosclerosis. In addition, there are sig-

Table 8.21 Factors that reduce the risk of cardiovascular disease.

Maintain ideal body weight – 35–55 per cent compared with those 20 per cent above ideal body weight
Stopping smoking reduces the risk of myocardial infarction by 50–75 per cent
Decrease in total cholesterol by 1 per cent decreases the risk by 2–3 per cent
Regular exercise reduces the risk by 45 per cent
There is a 2–3 per cent reduction in relative risk for every 1 mmHg decrease in diastolic blood pressure
Retaining ovaries through early menopause reduces the risk of a cardiovascular disease by at least two- to three-fold

nificant numbers of oestrogen and progesterone receptors in the endothelium and smooth muscle cells of human arterial vessels. These receptors appear to be involved in processes that modify platelet aggregation, cholesterol deposition, synthesis of endothelial-derived relaxing factor (EDRF), smooth muscle cell proliferation and prostaglandin changes. After 3 months of use of oestrogen replacement therapy in healthy postmenopausal women, the ejection fraction peak velocity of flow over the aortic valve, and blood flow increases.

In the 1980s theoretical and observational evidence suggested that HRT provided a protective effect of up to 50 per cent in preventing death from coronary heart disease, but these were not prospective randomised trials. CHD is the commonest cause of death and a leading cause of morbidity in postmenopausal women [16]. An overview of HRT and CHD in 25 studies reported by mid-1997 gave a relative risk of CHD for women ever using HRT compared to never users of 0.70 (confidence interval of 0.65–0.75) [17]. A cause and effect relationship is not proven. The evidence that HRT lowers the risk of coronary heart disease in women without a history of this disease is sufficiently strong to consider this potential benefit when deciding whether to use HRT [18].

The difficulties with the evidence as to the cardiovascular benefits of HRT, including that of the Nurses' Health Study, is the probable selection of relatively healthy and health-conscious women as users of HRT. There was probably an avoidance of HRT in women at risk of thrombotic events, thus excluding those at risk of CHD. HRT was used in women of higher socioeconomic groups, giving a more favourable mortality and morbidity.

The Postmenopausal Estrogen/Progestin Interventions (PEPI) Trial suggested that MPA may have reduced the oestrogen-associated rise in HDL cholesterol compared with other regimens.

The results from two large primary prevention trials, that are randomised placebo controlled trials of HRT including the Women's Health Initiative and the Women's International Study of Long-Duration Oestrogen After Menopause (WISDOM), which are currently recruiting from 12 countries a projected total of 34 000 postmenopausal women without heart disease, are awaited. WISDOM, a 10-year study, will randomise women into a placebo group and a group to receive conjugated equine oestrogen (0.625 mg) with or without medroxyprogesterone (2.5 mg daily) (depending on the presence or absence of a uterus), and will examine the rate of

Table 8.22 The HERS study: results.

Event	Treatment group	Placebo group	Relative hazard	95 per cent confidence interval	p value
Non-fatal MI or CHD death	179	18	0.99	0.81–1.22	0.91
Thromboembolic events	34	12	2.89	1.50–5.58	0.002
Coronary heart disease (fourth	57	38	1.52	1.01–2.29	
and fifth years)	33	49	0.67	0.43–1.04	
Number of events					

serious cardiovascular events during the trial and results should be available in 2005.

The HERS study

The Heart and Estrogen/Progestin Replacement Study (HERS) was the first randomised, double blind, placebo-controlled study to evaluate the outcome of HRT on subsequent cardiac events in postmenopausal women with established coronary heart disease, published in 1998 (Table 8.22) [19].

Of the 2763 women enrolled, 1380 were randomised to receive 0.625 mg conjugated equine oestrogens plus 2.5 mg medroxyprogesterone daily, and 1383 were randomised to receive a placebo. The mean age at enrolment was 66.7 years (SD 6.7 years). Follow-up was for an average of 4.1 years. The primary outcomes were non-fatal myocardial infarction (MI), CHD and death. The secondary outcomes included coronary revascularisation, unstable angina, congestive heart failure, resuscitated cardiac arrest, stroke or transient ischaemic attack and peripheral arterial disease. Over a mean of 4.1 years' follow-up, the trial reported no effect of HRT on recurrence of CHD, but there was a significant trend for decreasing risk with longer duration. Risk of CHD was unexpectedly substantially increased in the first 4 months in the HRT group, followed by a decline to a relative risk of 0.67 in the final 2 years. The same pattern of an early increase in risk followed by a late decrease was found of secondary prevention in the Nurses' Health Study cohort. These findings raise concern about prescribing hormones to those with prior myocardial infarction but do suggest long-term benefit. Because there are no published observational studies compared to HERS, the HERS study cannot appropriately be interpreted as refuting the findings for primary prevention from observational study.

Results of the HERS randomised study

This data concluded that starting HRT for secondary prevention of coronary heart disease was not recommended, but given the favourable pattern of coronary heart disease events after several years of treatment it could be appropriate to continue treatment in women already taking HRT. The early increase in CHD observed in the HERS data may be explained by a prothrombotic effect of HRT. The HERS study did not address the cardiovascular effect of HRT in women without established coronary artery disease. There are numerous observational studies and meta-analyses that strongly suggest that postmenopausal oestrogen replacement therapy or combined oestrogen/progestogen replacement therapy reduces the risk of symptomatic atherosclerotic coronary heart disease in both primary and secondary prevention settings. Questions related to the safety of HRT in women with possible subclinical CHD are unanswered at this time.

HRT AND THE RISK OF BREAST CANCER [Table 8.23]

8

Across all studies the risk of breast cancer increases 3.1 per cent for each year of oestrogen replacement therapy [20–22]. A real aetiological relationship between the use of oestrogen replacement therapy and breast cancer risk has not been established. Women with breast cancer with previous oestrogen replacement therapy use have higher survival rates than non-users with breast cancer.

Based on reanalysis of data on 51 000 women with breast cancer and 108 000 controls (from 51 worldwide studies), the Collaborative Group of Hormonal Factors in Breast Cancer reported that ever use of HRT was associated with an overall 14 per cent increase in the

Table 8.23 HRT and numbers of women per 1000 developing breast cancer. (Collaborative Group on Hormonal Factors in Breast Cancer (1997) [23].)

	Per 1000 women aged 50–70 years[1]
Non-users	45
Use of HRT for 5 years	47
Use of HRT for 10 years	51

[1] 51 epidemiological studies.
52 705 women with breast cancer.
108 411 women without the disease.

relative risk of breast cancer [23]. The relative risk was largely confined to current and recent users in whom the relative risk increased by 2.3 per cent for each year of use. This effect wears off within 5 years of stopping use. Among 1000 women who use HRT continuously for 10 years starting at the age of 50, it is estimated there will be an additional six breast cancers, raising the incidence from a background of 45 cases to 51 cases. Breast and endometrial cancers that are diagnosed in HRT users are less aggressive clinically than those in never-users. At 5 years the excess incidence of breast cancer is 2 cases for every 1000 women using HRT.

Recently it has been suggested that oestrogen/progestogen regimens increase the breast cancer risk beyond that associated with oestrogen alone [24].

Developing breast cancer

In the Colditz study, increase in death from breast cancer in HRT users may be attributed in part to the effects of prevalence bias [20,21]. By reducing cardiovascular morbidity and mortality HRT users live longer and succumb to illnesses which become more prevalent with ageing, breast cancer being one of them. Tamoxifen can produce severe and disabling vasomotor symptoms. However, it has been shown to reduce the incidence of contralateral breast carcinomas by approximately 40 per cent and in postmenopausal women has additional benefits in the prevention of cardiovascular disease and osteoporosis.

Conclusions

There is a small excess of risk with HRT use of 2.3 per cent per year of use. Most HRT-related cancers are localised to the breast.

HRT AND THOSE WITH ESTABLISHED BREAST CANCER

HRT has been thought to be relatively contraindicated in those with a history of previous breast cancer. This is based on:

- Epidemiological studies that have demonstrated an increased risk of developing breast cancer with prolonged ovarian function.
- It is a disease that has been shown to respond to hormone manipulation.
- Some premenopausal women with advanced breast cancer achieve benefit from surgical oophorectomy. Therefore exogenous oestrogens have been thought not to be indicated because of the risk of exposing patients to the risk of promoting the growth or dissemination of occult malignant cells.

Up to two thirds of breast cancer patients may develop a premature menopause or experience severe vasomotor symptoms as a result of adjuvant therapies, e.g. the use of the anti-oestrogen tamoxifen, ovarian ablation or chemotherapy-induced ovarian failure.

Recently the reported increase in risk of breast cancer with current or recent HRT use decreases to the population risk with time from stopping HRT. This supports the hypothesis that HRT is acting as a promoting rather than an inducing agent. Therefore HRT would have no effect on the lifetime risk of cancer. Although the breast cancer risk does not change with <5 years of oestrogen therapy, a population of women using oestrogen would live longer and thus have greater opportunities for some adverse health events to occur, such as breast cancer.

OESTROGEN REPLACEMENT THERAPY AND VENOUS THROMBOEMBOLISM

It is established that combined oral contraceptive (COC) use is associated with an increased risk of venous thromboembolism (VTE). This is thought to be due to oestrogen and is thought to be dose

Table 8.24 Venous thromboembolism.

	Per 10 000 women years
Idiopathic non-fatal thromboembolism in postmenopausal women	1
Premenopausal women	0.4
Mortality	1 per 100 000 aged 45
	1 per 10 000 aged 60
HRT and venous thromboembolism among postmenopausal women	3[1]

[1] Highest in women using HRT for <1 year who have not been exposed to exogenous oestrogens before.

Table 8.25 The HERS study and relative risk of venous thromboembolism.

Event	Relative risk	95% confidence interval
Aspirin	0.5	0.2–0.9
Lower leg fracture	18.1	5.4–60.4
Hip fracture	6	–
Hospitalisation for surgery	4.9	2.4–9.8
Other causes	5.7	3.0–10.8
Myocardial infarction	5.9	2.3–15.3

related. The biological potency of the oestrogens used in post-menopausal hormone therapy is about one quarter to one fifth that of oestrogens in the COC. Recent observational studies have suggested that postmenopausal hormone therapy causes a two- to four-fold increase in risk of VTE (Table 8.24).

Cohort and case-controlled studies have shown that the risk of idiopathic venous thromboembolic events (deep vein thrombosis or pulmonary embolus (VTE)) is low at 27–32 per 100 000 women years for HRT users, compared with 9–11 per 100 000 for non-users, so HRT increases the incidence of VTE three-fold. The incidence is greatest in the first year of use [25]. The HERS study identified that the risks were greater, perhaps due to the low risk selection bias of the former studies (Table 8.25) [26,27]. Twenty-three per cent of women on HRT with a lower leg fracture experienced a VTE in the first 3 months following a fracture. Hip fracture increased the risk of VTE six-fold. Increased risk persisted for 30 days after stopping HRT and for 90 days following lower limb fracture, hospitalisation or acute myocardial infarction. Therefore, from this study, consideration should be given to stopping HRT 30 days before until 90 days after surgery. All women on HRT undergoing surgery should have routine thromboprophylaxis – TED stockings and either heparin or low molecular weight heparin perioperatively.

OESTROGEN REPLACEMENT THERAPY AND FATAL COLORECTAL CANCER

Oestrogen replacement therapy protects against colorectal cancer, reducing the risk by approximately 50 per cent. This may be partly due to decreased bile synthesis and secretion associated with oestrogen replacement therapy [28].

DEMENTIA

Although animal studies on individual hormones and epidemiological findings on different HRT preparations have suggested a protective role in cognitive function and in Alzheimer's disease, there are insufficient data to draw conclusions [29]. It is therefore not appropriate to start HRT solely for the prevention or treatment of dementia and cognitive function. However, the strongest evidence for a beneficial effect of HRT in dementia comes from cell and animal studies.

Oestrogens may affect the pathological processes of Alzheimer's disease by:
- Affecting β-amyloid metabolism
- Promoting the activity of the cholinergic system
- Decreasing oxidative stress
- Inhibiting neuronal apoptosis
- Promoting synaptogenesis and synaptic plasticity, reducing the incidence of vascular dementia.

HRT and Alzheimer's disease

Oestrogen interacts with growth and neurotrophic factors. It can potentiate the extension of neuronal processes, promote the formation of synapses between nerve cells and alter the composition of neuronal circuits. It influences a number of neurological systems – cholinergic, noradrenergic and dopaminergic. They may moderate deleterious affects of stress on cognitive function. Other oestrogen effects could also enhance general brain function. Oestrogen increases cerebral blood flow. It augments the cerebral uptake and widespread utilisation of glucose, the primary energy substrate of the brain. Oestrogen replacement may result in up to a 50 per cent reduction in the risk for Alzheimer's disease. The potential of oestrogen replacement to protect against cognitive decline may be influenced by a woman's genes.

ANDROGEN REPLACEMENT

After the menopause the circulating level of androstenedione is half that prior to the menopause because of the reduction in ovarian secretion. The remaining active stromal tissue in the ovary is stimulated to an increased production of testosterone compared to premenopausal levels because of the elevated gonadotrophin. However, the total amount of testosterone produced postmenopausally is slightly decreased because the primary source is the peripheral conversion of androstenedione, which is reduced. The potential benefits of androgen treatment include improvement in psychological well being and an increase in sexually motivated behaviour.

Side effects include hirsutism and a negative impact on the cholesterol–lipoprotein profile. It may be given as an implant or as 1.25–2.5 mg methyltestosterone.

OTHER EFFECTS OF OESTROGEN

Oestrogen therapy improves visual acuity. It may protect against lens opacities and give symptomatic relief from keratoconjunctivitis sicca (dry eyes). Postmenopausal women (60–80 years) who have lower than average femoral neck bone mass have an increased risk of developing hearing loss. Oestrogen therapy may to some degree prevent a sensory neural hearing loss.

OESTROGENS AND DIET

Dietary interactions with oestrogen may produce a clinical impact. Oestrogens undergo extensive first pass metabolism both in the gastrointestinal tract and in the liver. Metabolism consists chiefly of sulphation and hydroxylation. The cytochrome P450 system catalyses the hydroxylation of oestrogen. Antioxidants can inhibit this action. Antioxidants such as flavanoids are present in high concentrations in fruit and vegetables, and grapefruit juice inhibits oestrogen metabolism producing an increase in bioavailability that is consistent with an inhibition of hydroxylation.

HRT AND DIABETES

Menopause is associated with the emergence of two of the principal features of diabetes:
(1) A deficient pancreatic insulin response to glucose
(2) Insulin resistance.

The menopause is associated with the development of an adverse lipid and lipoprotein coronary heart disease risk factor profile comprising:
- Raised total and LDL cholesterol
- Raised triglycerides
- Reduced HDL cholesterol, particularly the important HDL_2 subfraction.

Oestrogen replacement can reverse many of the adverse changes in carbohydrate and lipid metabolism associated with menopause in healthy women and these beneficial changes may extend to women with diabetes.

Administration of 17β-oestradiol (50 μg/day) transdermal patches results in a decrease in insulin resistance, an increase in pancreatic insulin response to glucose and improved insulin elimination.

Progesterone causes insulin resistance. Norethisterone acetate in combination with 17β-oestradiol does not appear to affect glucose or insulin levels.

8

HYPERLIPIDAEMIA

Women with elevated fasting serum triglyceride levels are at a higher risk of developing coronary heart disease than those with low or normal levels, and this relationship is stronger than the link with LDL (but weaker than that with HDL). Fasting serum triglyceride levels are an independent risk factor for coronary heart disease and ought to be taken account of. An increase of 1 mmol/l triglyceride level is associated with up to a 40 per cent increase in the risk of coronary heart disease in women. The prescriber should be aware of the influence of different HRT preparations on serum triglyceride levels.

Influence of HRT on triglyceride levels

Oestrogens lower serum total cholesterol levels. Different HRT regimens have diverse effects on fasting triglyceride levels, depending on factors such as their chemical structure and route of administration. Oral oestrogens increase fasting serum triglyceride levels in a dose-dependent manner by stimulating hepatic synthesis of a specific protein as part of a hepatic first pass response. However, the large VLDL particles are rapidly cleared. This is why elevated serum triglyceride levels (20–25 per cent) with oral oestrogens are not thought to be of concern. 17β-oestradiol has less effect. Transdermal oestradiol reduces triglyceride levels by up to 15–20 per cent. Androgens and progestogens with androgenic activities reduce fasting serum triglyceride levels, as does norethindrone. In women with severely elevated triglycerides (>5.6 mmol/l; >500 mg/dl), oral oestrogen should be avoided because of the risk of inducing gross hypertriglyceridaemia with abdominal pain and severe pancreatitis. Those with moderate elevation (1.2–5.6 mmol/l; 100–500 mg/dl) should have transdermal oestradiol.

HRT AND ENDOMETRIAL CANCER

Endometrial cancer occurs in about 0.3 per cent risk for 50-year-old women over the rest of their lives. The use of unopposed oestrogen results in a 2.3 increase in the relative risk of endometrial cancer. If it is short term (1–5 years) the relative risk is 3. The risk for oestrogen and progestogen is 0.8 [30]. Therefore unopposed oestrogen HRT with a uterus is contraindicated.

HRT following endometrial cancer of FIGO stages I and II does not have an adverse effect on outcome and therefore it is justifiable in women with severe symptoms and problems related to oestrogen deficiency. With more advanced endometrial cancer (stages III and IV), high doses of progestogens are often given. Such high doses of progestogens may mitigate vasomotor symptoms. However, they do not improve atrophic urogenital changes or prevent osteoporosis and cardiovascular disease as oestrogens do. In stage III and IV disease for lower genital tract symptoms oestrogen could be applied locally. Oestriol may be used because it does not stimulate endometrial tissue. It would relieve symptoms and improve the quality of life.

SUMMARY OF USE OF HRT [31]

The use of HRT has to be tailored to the needs and desires of the individual. Although there is considerable evidence about the health effects of long-term use of HRT, on average the balance between the risks and the benefits is not overwhelming in either direction. The effects of HRT are both short term and long term. The objective for starting HRT should be clearly identified to the patient. HRT may, for example, be recommended on a short-term basis for alleviation of symptoms, or long term for the prevention of osteoporosis.

REFERENCES

1 Greendale, G.A., Lee, N.P. & Arriola, E.R. (1999) The menopause. *The Lancet*, **353**, 571–580.

2 Grady, D., Ruben, S.M., Petitti, D.B. *et al.* (1992) Hormone therapy to prevent disease and prolong life in postmenopausal women. *Annals of Internal Medicine*, **117**, 1016–1037.

3 Harlap, S. (1992) The benefits and risks of hormone replacement therapy: an epidemiologic overview. *American Journal of Obstetrics and Gynecology*, **166**, 1986–1992.

4 Hunt, K., Vessey, M. & McPherson, K. (1990) Mortality in a cohort of long-term users of hormone replacement therapy: an updated analysis. *British Journal of Obstetrics and Gynaecology*, **97**, 1080–1086.

5 Lobo, R.A. (1995) Benefits and risks of oestrogen replacement therapy. *American Journal of Obstetrics and Gynecology*, **173** (Suppl 3), 982–989.

6 Kannel, W.B., Hjortland, M.C., McNamara, P.M. & Gordon, T. (1976) Menopause and risk of cardiovascular disease: the Framingham Study. *Annals of Internal Medicine*, **85**, 447–452.

7 Lerner, D.J. & Kannel, W.B. (1986) Patterns of coronary heart disease morbidity and mortality in the sexes: a 26-year follow-up of the Framingham population. *American Heart Journal*, **111**, 383–390.

8 Royal College of Obstetricians and Gynaecologists (1999) *Hormone replacement therapy and venous thromboembolism*. RCOG Guideline No. 19. RCOG, London.

9 Beaumont, J.L., Carlson, L.A., Cooper, G.R., Fejar, Z., Fredrickson, D.S. & Strassar, T. (1970) Classification of hyperlipidaemia and hypoproteinaemia. *Bulletin of the World Health Organisation*, **43**, 891–908.

8

10 NCEP Expert Panel on Detection, Evaluation and Treatment of High Blood Cholesterol in Adults (1993) Summary of the second report of the National Cholesterol Education Program (NCEP) Expert Panel on Detection, Evaluation and Treatment of High Blood Cholesterol in Adults (Adult Treatment Panel II). *Journal of the American Medical Association*, **269**, 3015–3023.

11 Miettinen, T.A., Pyorala, K., Olsson, A.G. *et al.* for the Scandinavian Simvastatin Study Group (1997) Cholesterol-lowering therapy in women and elderly patients with myocardial infarction or angina pectoris. Findings from the Scandinavian Simvastatin Survival Study (4S). *Circulation*, **96**, 4211–4218.

12 Gorsky, R.D., Koplan, J.P., Peterson, H.B. & Thacker, S.B. (1994) Relative risks and benefits of long-term oestrogen replacement therapy: a decision analysis. *Obstetrics and Gynecology*, **83**, 161–166.

13 World Health Organisation (1994) *Assessment of fracture risk and its application to screening for postmenopausal osteoporosis.* Technical Report Series. WHO, Geneva.

14 Naessen, T., Persson, I., Adami, H.O., Bergstrom, R. & Bergkvist, L. (1990) Hormone replacement therapy and the risk for first hip fracture. *Annals of Internal Medicine*, **113**, 95–103.

15 Writing Group for the PEPI Trial (1995) Effects of oestrogen on oestrogen/progestogen regimens on heart disease risk factors in postmenopausal women. Postmenopausal Estrogen/Progestogen Intervention (PEPI) Trial. *Journal of the American Medical Association*, **273**, 199–208.

16 Epstein, F.H. (1999) The protective effects of estrogen on the cardiovascular system. *New England Journal of Medicine*, **23**, 1801–1811.

17 Barrett-Connor, E. & Grady, D. (1998) Hormone replacement therapy, heart disease and other considerations. *Annual Review of Public Health*, **19**, 55–72.

18 Mendelsohn, M.E. & Karas, R.H. (1999) The protective effects of oestrogen on the cardiovascular system. *New England Journal of Medicine*, **340**, 1801–1811.

19 Hulley, S., Grady, D., Bush, T. *et al.* (1998) Randomized trial of estrogen plus progestin for secondary prevention of coronary heart disease in postmenopausal women: Heart and Estrogen/Progestin Replacement Study (HERS) research group. *Journal of the American Medical Association*, **280**, 605–613.

20 Colditz, G.A., Egan, K.M. & Stampfer, M.J. (1993) Hormone replacement therapy and risk of breast cancer: results from epidemiologic studies. *American Journal of Obstetrics and Gynecology*, **168**, 1473–1478.

21 Colditz, G.A., Hankinson, S.E., Hunter, D.J. *et al.* (1995) The use of oestrogens and progestins and the risk of breast cancer in postmenopausal women. *New England Journal of Medicine*, **332**, 1589–1593.

22 Nachtigall, M.J., Smilen, S.W., Nachtigall, R.D., Nachtigall, R.H. & Nachtigall, L.E. (1992) Incidence of breast cancer in a 23-year study of

8

women receiving estrogen-progestin replacement therapy. *Obstetrics and Gynecology*, **80**, 827–830.

23 Collaborative Group on Hormonal Factors in Breast Cancer (1997) Breast cancer and hormone replacement therapy: collaborative reanalysis of data from 51 epidemiological studies of 52 705 women with breast cancer and 108 411 women without breast cancer. *The Lancet*, **350**, 1047–1059.

24 Schairer, C., Lubin, J., Troisi, R., Sturgeon, S., Brinton, L. & Hoover, R. (2000) Menopausal estrogen and estrogen-progestin replacement therapy and breast cancer risk. *Journal of the American Medical Association*, **283**, 485–491.

25 Daly, E., Vessey, M.P., Hawkins, M.M., Carson, J.L., Gough, P. & Marsh S. (1996) Risk of venous thromboembolism in users of hormone replacement. *The Lancet*, **348**, 977–980.

26 Grady, D., Wenger, N.K., Herrington, D. *et al.* for the Heart and Estrogen/Progestin Replacement Study research group (2000) Postmenopausal hormone therapy increases risk for venous thromboembolic disease. *Annals of Internal Medicine*, **132**, 689–696.

27 Hoibraaten, E., Qvigstad, E., Arnesen, H., Larsen, S., Wickstrom, E., & Sandset, P.M. (2000) Increased risk of venous thromboembolism (VTE) during hormone replacement therapy (HRT): results of the randomised, double-blind, placebo-controlled Estrogen in Venous Thromboembolism trial (EVTET). *Thrombosis and Haemostasis*, **84**, 961–967.

28 Chute, C.G., Willett, W.C., Colditz, G.A., Stampfer, M.J., Rosner, B. & Speizer, F.E. (1991) A prospective study of reproductive history and exogenous estrogens on the risk of colorectal cancer in women. *Epidemiology*, **2**, 201–207.

29 Yaffe, K., Lui, L-Y., Grady, D., Cauley, J., Kramer, J. & Cummings, S.R. (2000) Cognitive decline in women in relation to non-protein-bound oestradiol concentrations. *The Lancet*, **356**, 708–712.

30 Grady, D., Gebretsadik, T., Kerlikwske, K., Ernster, V. & Petitti, D. (1995) Hormone replacement therapy and endometrial cancer risk: a meta-analysis. *Obstetrics and Gynecology*, **85**, 304–313.

31 Clinical Synthesis Panel on HRT (1999) Hormone replacement therapy. *The Lancet*, **354**, 152–155.

8

9 Urogynaecology

Rose Elder and Cornelius Kelleher

URINARY INCONTINENCE

Introduction

Urinary incontinence is an enormous health and social problem in both the developed and developing worlds. It is often considered a natural consequence of ageing and childbirth, and misguidedly many women tolerate and cope with their symptoms in the belief that little can be done to improve them. Urinary incontinence is the end result of many different disease processes which must be investigated to make an accurate diagnosis and enable effective treatment.

Definition

Urinary incontinence (UI) is defined by the International Continence Society as an involuntary loss of urine, which is a social or hygienic problem and is objectively demonstrable. Conversely continence is the ability to hold urine within the bladder at all times other than during micturition.

Prevalence

The prevalence of UI varies depending on the study population, the method of survey and the definition of urinary incontinence used. A UK MORI poll published in 1991 [1] showed that at least 3.5 million women (approximately 10 per cent) suffer from urinary incontinence, and a report published by the Royal College of Physicians of London (1995) showed that between 8 and 20 per cent of women over 45 years old have this complaint. The prevalence amongst elderly institutionalised women may be as high as 90 per cent. The costs of UI both in terms of morbidity and financial expenditure to individuals and society are enormous.

Control of micturition – anatomy and physiology

The lower urinary tract (bladder and urethra) converts the continuous involuntary production of urine by the kidneys into consciously controlled and appropriate voiding. This process requires the bladder to serve a dual role, that of maintaining low pressure storage and, when appropriate, contraction and expulsion of urine.

The detrusor muscle consists of smooth muscle fibres, which from a functional point of view are arranged to contract as a single syncitial mass. Three distinct muscle layers have been described histologically (outer and inner longitudinal fibres and middle circular), although there is known to be significant interchange between layers. The smooth muscle of the trigonal region is arranged differently and may be important in the control of the ureterovesical junction during voiding, preventing ureteric reflux.

The female urethra is a fibromuscular tube 3–5 cm in length attached to the posterior aspect of the pubic symphysis by the pubourethral ligament. It consists of an outer sleeve of striated muscle thickest mid-urethra (external urethral sphincter) and inner smooth muscle fibres. The smooth muscle is arranged as a thick inner longitudinal layer and a thin outer circular layer. The submucosa of the urethra has a rich vascular plexus, and the inner urethral epithelial surface is highly folded to allow complete apposition of the mucosa.

Paraurethral tissues interdigitate with those of the vaginal wall, and with the medial portion of the levator ani, and hence the pelvic side wall. Each of these intrinsic and extrinsic urethral factors contributes to the urethral continence mechanism.

The lower urinary tract is innervated by three sets of peripheral nerves:
(1) Pelvic parasympathetic nerves, which arise at the sacral level of the spinal cord, stimulate the detrusor and relax the internal sphincter.
(2) Lumbar sympathetic nerves, which inhibit the detrusor, modulate transmission in bladder parasympathetic ganglia and stimulate the bladder base and internal urethral sphincter.
(3) Pudendal nerves, which stimulate the external urethral sphincter.

The accommodation of the bladder to increasing volumes of urine is largely a passive phenomenon dependent on the quiescence of the parasympathetic efferent pathway. Micturition is dependent on parasympathetic activity, and inhibition of sympathetic outflow and external sphincter activity.

9

Table 9.1 Risk factors for urinary incontinence.

Pregnancy and childbirth
Age and the menopause
Race
Obesity
Hysterectomy
Genital prolapse
Functional impairment
Constipation
Diuretics and other prescribed medications
Pelvic radiation therapy

Classification

The epidemiology of urinary incontinence is complex, and many different independent aetiological factors are thought to be important. Risk factors of urinary incontinence are given in Table 9.1.

An accurate diagnosis of the cause of urinary symptoms requires urodynamic investigations. In questionnaire- or interview-based surveys only symptoms can be registered. For the purpose of prevalence data the relative proportions of stress, urge and mixed symptoms are usually reported. Approximately 50 per cent of all incontinent women are classified as stress incontinent although this percentage is lower amongst older women. The prevalence of urge incontinence is 20–30 per cent and increases with advancing age. Mixed urinary symptoms, 20–30 per cent, are very common and require appropriate urodynamic investigations to determine their cause (see Fig. 9.1).

Pregnancy and childbirth

Due to both hormonal and pressure effects, symptoms of both stress and urge incontinence are more common in pregnancy and are usually self-limiting [2]. Prevalence rates of 30–60 per cent of all pregnant women are reported. For a number of reasons women may develop urinary incontinence postpartum. Childbirth may result in stretching and weakening of the pelvic muscles and connective tissues. Nerve damage and direct trauma to the genital tract may also cause pelvic floor damage. There is a definite link between increasing parity and urinary incontinence. Elective Caesarean

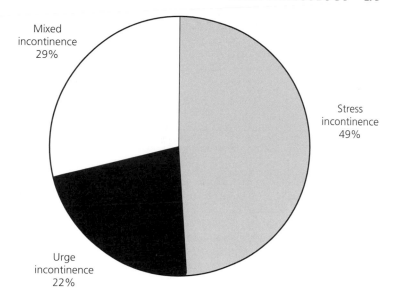

Fig. 9.1 Prevalence of different types of unrinary incontinence.

section may prevent pelvic floor damage and urinary incontinence, although this is not fully evaluated. Electromyography of the pelvic floor has shown denervation postpartum. The only factor in labour that was associated with severe damage was a long active (pushing) second stage [3].

Age and the menopause

Despite the fact that oestrogen receptors have been found within all parts of the lower urinary tract, the role of oestrogen therapy in the treatment or prevention of urinary incontinence has not been proven [4]. Hormone replacement therapy has been shown to prevent and reverse urogenital atrophic change, and improve irritative bladder symptoms. It has also been shown to reduce the frequency of post-menopausal urinary tract infections [5]. At present there is insufficient evidence that oestrogen therapy alone prevents or cures urinary incontinence, although it is a useful adjunct to other proven forms of treatment.

Table 9.2 The classification of urinary incontinence.

Genuine stress incontinence
Detrusor instability
Retention with overflow
Detrusor hyperreflaxia
Fistulae
Temporary, e.g. urinary tract infection, medications
Functional, e.g. immobility

Race

Racial differences in both UI and genital prolapse are difficult to fully quantify, but the incidence of urinary incontinence and prolapse appears to be similar in the black and white populations. Studies may be confounded by cultural factors affecting perception and presentation of urinary symptoms [6].

Obesity

Increased body mass index (BMI) has an association with both stress incontinence and detrusor instability. The prevalence of daily incontinence increases by an odds ratio of 1.6 per 5 BMI units [7]. Weight loss in the morbidly obese has been shown to improve continence after weight reduction operations. Urinary incontinence is reported by obese women to decrease with weight loss.

Hysterectomy

Hysterectomy has a controversial role in the aetiology of UI and needs to be studied further. It is important when hysterectomy is considered to enquire about urinary symptoms and, if present, to investigate and treat at the same time.

Functional impairment

Mobility impairment is associated with urinary incontinence. This could mean that the bathroom is difficult to reach as it is upstairs, or that clothing is difficult to remove.

Cognitive impairment

Demented patients more commonly experience UI compared with the non-demented. This association suggests a link between cognitive impairment and urinary incontinence. It may be due to the simple lack of awareness of the need to toilet or a manifestation of some neurological deficit resulting in cognitive disability.

Other factors

Constipation, diuretics, other drugs, pelvic irradiation, exercise, prolapse, childhood enuresis and smoking are all associated with urinary incontinence.

HISTORY

Urinary symptoms are a poor predictor of the cause of urinary incontinence. Diagnosing the cause of urinary symptoms requires urodynamic investigations. On the basis of an accurate history and physical examination, conservative therapy for UI can often be commenced providing there are no major contraindications to doing so.

The following information should be obtained from the patient and can often be collected with the use of standardised urinary symptom questionnaires [8].

- Onset and duration of urinary symptoms
- Frequency of incontinent episodes
- Frequency (the number of voids per day, i.e. greater than seven is abnormal)
- Nocturia (the number of voids per night – greater than one per night is abnormal in those aged less than 70 years)
- Urgency (a difficult-to-control desire to pass urine)
- Urge incontinence (leakage with urgency)
- Stress incontinence (leakage with an increase in intra-abdominal pressure)
- Voiding difficulties (poor stream, difficulty voiding, hesitancy, post-micturition dribble)
- Urinary tract infection (cystitis/dysuria)
- Haematuria
- Nocturnal enuresis (bed wetting)
- Incontinence coping strategies (e.g. use of pads).

General

- Fluid intake
- Caffeine/alcohol intake
- Menopausal status.

9

Past obstetric history

- Parity
- Symptoms during and after pregnancy
- Vaginal deliveries
- Weight of babies
- Difficulties during delivery (obstetric intervention, prolonged second stage).

Past gynaecological history

- Prolapse
- Malignancy/irradiation – the degree of damage is dose dependent. Acute symptoms are irritative, while chronic symptoms are related to decreased bladder compliance and decreased bladder capacity
- Pelvic pathology (e.g. fibroids)
- Previous pelvic/vaginal surgery.

Medical

- Cardiovascular – heart failure
- Respiratory – chronic cough, smoking
- Renal – renal problems
- Gastrointestinal – chronic constipation, faecal incontinence
- Endocrine – diabetes mellitus
- Ophthalmology – glaucoma
- Neurological – multiple sclerosis, spinal trauma, cerebrovascular accident, disc lesion
- Psychiatric – mental state, dementia.

Medication

- Diuretics (frusemide) cause diuresis.
- α-adrenergic blocking agents (terazocin) relax the bladder sphincter.
- β-adrenergic blockers (atenolol) may cause heart failure and deteriorate glucose tolerance in diabetics.
- Tranquillisers (diazapam) may sedate the patient and make getting to the toilet in time difficult.
- Tricyclic antidepressants (amitriptyline) may cause urine retention.

QUALITY OF LIFE

An important part of the assessment of urinary incontinence is the impact of urinary symptoms both on women's lifestyle and their quality of life (QoL). This can be measured with standardised validated QoL questionnaires (e.g. King's Health Questionnaire) [8]. Questionnaires focus both on the impact of individual urinary symptoms, and also on the more general aspects of QoL impairment.

- Physical function (activities of daily living)
- Psychological function (emotional and mental well being)
- Social functioning (relationships)
- Life satisfaction
- Perception of health status
- Pain
- Impact on life.

Simple measures to improve urinary incontinence

Urinary symptoms can often be improved by simple measures and these should be explained and or available to all patients (Table 9.3).

EXAMINATION

The initial overall appearance of the woman provides important information as to potential contributing factors to her incontinence. Poor mobility and dexterity can prevent her from getting to the toilet and undressing herself in time to pass urine. Reduction in weight or

Table 9.3 Simple measures to improve urinary incontinence.

Avoid excessive fluid intake during the day and last thing at night
Avoid the intake of bladder irritants, e.g. caffeine
Avoid excessive alcohol consumption (alcohol is a diuretic)
Void prior to intercourse if intercourse incontinence is a problem
Take a fluid load prior to and void after intercourse if experiencing intercourse-
    related urinary tract infections
Avoid constipation
Stop smoking
Lose weight if obese (BMI >30)

altering the medication for heart failure may improve her urinary incontinence.

General appearance

- Patient mobility
- Cognitive status
- Height and weight
- BMI (weight (kg)/height (m)^2) >25.

Abdominal examination

- Note scars, hernias and masses.
- Palpation of the bladder post-micturition is indicative of voiding difficulties and/or overflow incontinence.
- Ultrasound or catheterisation is more accurate for the assessment of post-micturition residual urine volume.

Neurological examination

Strength, sensation and reflexes of lower limbs and dermatomes S2–4.

Pelvic examination

- Genitalia for oestrogen status, previous scarring
- Prolapse (rectocele, enterocele and cystocele)
- Size of uterus and ovaries, pelvic masses
- Urethral mobility
- Rectal – sphincter tone, faecal impaction, rectal mass
- Residual urine.

The Q-tip test involves using a lubricated cotton bud inserted into the urethra. While the patient lies flat on the bed the Q-tip will be at an angle of about 30°, with the Valsalva manoeuvre this will increase in angle and display the hypermobility of the pelvic floor.

The inspection of the external genitalia may reveal atrophy secondary to oestrogen deficiency or excoriation from chronic exposure to urine. Attempts to demonstrate incontinence with the Valsalva manoeuvre should be attempted supine, but also when the patient is standing.

Vaginal examination may reveal anterolateral protrusion into the vagina and may represent detachment of the pubocervical fascia from the attachment to the arcus tendinous fascia on the pelvic side wall. Central protrusions of the anterior vaginal wall may represent defects in the supports to the base of the bladder. Cervical or vaginal apex descent below the level of the ischial spines is evidence of defective vaginal suspension.

Posterior vaginal wall descent at the vaginal vault may involve the protrusion of the small bowel (enterocele) and/or the rectum (rectocele). At rest there may be a loss of the transverse crease at the junction of the lower third and middle third of the vagina. A hypermobile urethrovesical junction may be noted when getting the woman to perform the Valsalva and seeing the bladder neck descend.

Neurological examination may uncover conditions such as multiple sclerosis. Tone, power, sensation and reflexes need to be assessed in the lower limbs. For continence the dermatomes of S2–4 are especially important as this is where the innervation of the bladder arises.

Children should be examined for evidence of spina bifida occulta.

Sacral nerve reflexes are tested with the bulbocavernous reflex. This involves gently touching the clitoris, which should cause a contraction of the external anal sphincter (absence may indicate a lower motor neurone defect of the sacral nerve). Anal tone and sensation are also important to record.

INVESTIGATIONS

Simple investigations and basic urodynamics are widely available. Specialised investigations may only be available in secondary or tertiary referral centres.

Simple (suitable for the general practice setting)

- Urinalysis/mid-stream urine culture and sensitivities
- Voiding diaries/frequency volume chart
- Pad test.

Basic urodynamics (available in all units routinely investigating UI)

- Uroflowmetry
- Subtracted cystometry

- Videocystourethrography
- Cystourethroscopy
- Intravenous pyelogram (IVP).

Specialised (often only available in tertiary referral units)

- Urethral pressure profilometry
- Bladder and urethral ultrasound
- Cystourethrography
- Electromyography
- Ambulatory urodynamics.

Mid-stream urine

Uncomplicated urinary tract infections are a cause of incontinence that is easily diagnosed and treated. Urine infections will also aggravate any symptoms that the patient already has and complicate any other investigations that are done.

Frequency volume charts

These are objective assessments of women's fluid intake and output, frequency and nocturia. They also confirm the timing and frequency of incontinent episodes. They are useful to document inappropriately large volumes of fluid intake. These charts are also helpful when teaching bladder drill.

Pad testing

This test involves the wearing of preweighed perineal pads to assess the volume of urine lost. Urine loss is documented by measuring the increase in pad weight. The period of testing can be over a short time (usually 2 hours), with a known amount of fluid (250 ml) instilled into the bladder or more commonly performed after ingestion of 1 l of fluid, or over a longer time (24–48 hours) with physiological bladder filling and a series of exercises being performed. The short test usually involves a series of standard exercises to provoke urine loss.

Uroflowmetry

This is a non-invasive investigation, which requires passing urine onto a flowmeter. The flowmeter calculates the rate of urine flow,

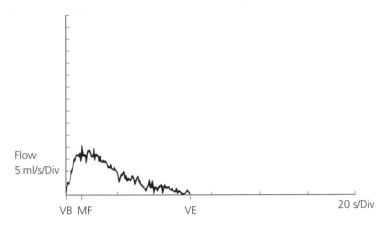

RESULTS

Max Flow Rate	20.2	ml/s
Average Flow Rate	7.9	ml/s
Voided Volume	391	ml
Delay Time	0	s
Voiding Time	51	s
Flow Time	49	s
Time to Max Flow	6	s
Residual Volume	30	ml

Fig. 9.2 An example of normal uroflowmetry.

the volume voided and produces a graphical representation of the flow of urine over time.

Important information gained from this are voided volume, maximum and average flow rate, flow time and time to maximum flow (Fig. 9.2).

Subtracted cystometry

Cystometry is a method by which the pressure/volume relationship of the bladder is measured and it is an important evaluation of both physiological and pathological detrusor activity. It is also used to assess bladder sensation, capacity and compliance. The most commonly used technique is the retrograde filling of the bladder with fluid via a urinary catheter. The intravesical pressure and volume are used to generate a pressure–volume curve with the results. Normal saline is used to fill the bladder. Radiopaque contrast medium is used if radiological imaging of the bladder is to be performed. Simultaneous measurement of both intravesical and intra-abdominal (rectal) pressure allows calculation of subtracted detrusor pressure (intravesical pressure minus abdominal pressure).

Cystometry has two main phases:

(1) **Filling.** The bladder is filled at a rate of 50–100 ml/min. Recordings are made at the first desire to void (>100 ml) and bladder capacity (≥400 ml). Compliance during filling and the presence or absence of detrusor contractions are recorded. Asking the patient to cough during examination may demonstrate urinary incontinence or provoke detrusor activity. If incontinence occurs in the absence of a detrusor contraction then the urine loss is due to a weakness in the urethral closure mechanism, and a diagnosis of genuine stress incontinence can be made.

(2) **Voiding.** If the patient is asked to void after filling, the voiding detrusor pressure can be recorded.

Videocystourethrography

Using a radiopaque contrast medium to fill the bladder allows the bladder to be visualised using an image intensifier. Bladder anatomy and function can be assessed while standing, straining and voiding. Trabeculation, fistulae, vesicoureteric reflux and diverticulae may be seen.

Cystourethroscopy

Examination of the bladder and urethra with a cystoscope is important when there is a history of haematuria, urgency and marked frequency. Bladder stones, mucosal appearance and focal lesions can be evaluated and bladder biopsies taken.

Intravenous pyelogram

To perform an intravenous pyelogram requires adequate renal function. Renal dysfunction, obstruction, congenital abnormalities, fistulae, stones and tumours may be detected.

Urethral pressure profilometry

This is a specialised investigation in which a microtip transducer catheter is placed in the bladder and withdrawn at a constant rate. A graphical pressure curve is created demonstrating the measured closure pressure of the urethra. This investigation is used to document outflow obstruction or sphincter failure.

Bladder and urethral ultrasound

Ultrasound is an especially attractive investigation as it is non-invasive and independent of renal function. It can assess post-void urine residual, bladder morphology and wall thickness, presence of renal stones and large tumours, ureteric dilatation and renal morphology.

Ambulatory urodynamics

This investigation utilises microchip transducer technology and portable cystometry apparatus to allow prolonged cystometry to diagnose the cause of urinary symptoms. It is more physiological than conventional laboratory urodynamic investigations. It is usually performed when a diagnosis of the cause of urinary symptoms is important and cystometry has failed to identify one.

GENUINE STRESS INCONTINENCE

Genuine stress incontinence (GSI) is defined as the involuntary loss of urine when the intravesical pressure exceeds the maximum urethral closure pressure in the absence of detrusor activity. Women usually complain of symptoms of stress incontinence but may also complain of other urinary symptoms. Cystometry is required to establish the diagnosis and exclude other causes of urinary incontinence.

The management of GSI is either conservative or surgical.

Conservative

- Pelvic floor exercises
- Weighted cones
- Electrical stimulation

- Devices, e.g. tampon, urethral insert (Reliance)
- Medication, e.g. α-adrenergic agents, hormone replacement therapy (HRT).

Surgical

- Abdominal bladder neck suspension, e.g. colposuspension, Marshall Marchetti Krantz (MMK)
- Slings, e.g. tension-free vaginal tape (TVT), Aldridge sling
- Periurethral injectables
- Endoscopic bladder neck suspension
- Anterior repair
- Artificial urinary sphincter.

Conservative therapy

Conservative therapy is used when:
- The patient refuses or is undecided about surgery
- The patient is medically unfit for surgery
- Childbearing is incomplete
- There is uncontrolled detrusor instability or voiding difficulty.

Pelvic floor exercises

Regular strength training exercises increase the number of activated motor units, frequency of excitation and muscle volume [9]. Various protocols for teaching pelvic floor exercises have been reported. A protocol should probably include three sets of 8–12 slow velocity maximal contractions sustained for 6–8 seconds each, performed three to four times a week and continued for 15–20 weeks [10]. Exercises should be taught properly and women assessed to determine their understanding of the exercises and their ability to perform them to achieve a good result. Recently published data demonstrate that properly taught pelvic floor exercises are more effective than either electrical stimulation or vaginal cones for the treatment of GSI [11].

Vaginal cones

Graded weight vaginal cones can be used to strengthen the pelvic floor muscles. The weighted cone is held in the vagina for 15 minutes four times a day, increasing the weight of the cone as the pelvic floor strength improves (Fig. 9.3).

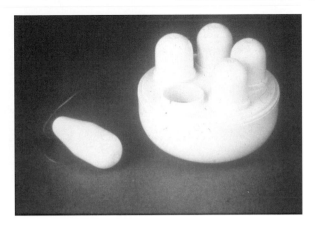

Fig. 9.3 Vaginal cones are used to aid pelvic floor strength.

Electrical stimulation

Utilises either intravaginal, extravaginal or anal plug electrodes to stimulate contraction of the pelvic floor muscles.

Devices

A variety of devices are available for the relief of GSI and are most applicable for women who have leakage at specific times only, e.g. sporting activities. Devices are either designed to elevate and compress the urethra and anterior vaginal wall (e.g. Conveen Contiguard) or to occlude the urethra (e.g. Reliance insert) (see Fig. 9.4).

Surgical management

The first procedure is the most likely to cure GSI and therefore should be carefully planned and executed.

Colposuspension

This is currently the most widely advocated surgical procedure for the correction of GSI. Meta-analysis from retrospective and prospective studies shows an objective cure rate of 89.8 per cent following a colposuspension in the absence of previous surgery [12]. The randomised trials which compare colposuspension with either bladder buttress, long needle suspension or MMK suggest a consistent cure

9

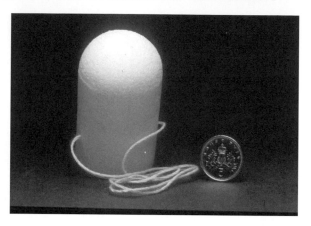

Fig. 9.4 Devices can be used to occlude the urethra.

rate of 85–90 per cent [13–15]. Trials are currently ongoing to evaluate the outcome of colposuspension performed laparoscopically.

Burch colposuspension

Procedure
A low transverse suprapubic incision is made to open the space retropubically and the bladder neck is mobilised bilaterally off the underlying fascia by blunt dissection against two fingers placed in the vagina. Two to four long-term absorbable or non-absorbable sutures are tied between the paravaginal fascia and the ipsilateral ileopectineal ligament.

Complications

These include blood loss, detrusor instability (17 per cent), voiding difficulties (mean of 10.3 per cent, range 2–27 per cent), failure (19 per cent), vaginal wall prolapse 13 per cent) and urinary tract damage (Fig. 9.5) [16].

Laparoscopic Burch colposuspension

Procedure
The laparoscopic Burch colposuspension is not widely used and is presently undergoing randomised controlled trials. It is the same

9

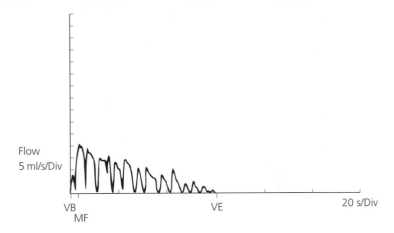

RESULTS

Max Flow Rate	21.1	ml/s
Average Flow Rate	8.0	ml/s
Voided Volume	413	ml
Delay Time	0	s
Voiding Time	60	s
Flow Time	51	s
Time to Max Flow	4	s
Residual Volume	40	ml

Fig. 9.5 Disordered voiding showing intermittent urinary flow is often due to hypocontractile detrusor function and straining to void.

technique as the open Burch procedure but via a laparoscopic approach. An umbilical 10 mm or 5 mm port is introduced for the camera. Two lateral 5 mm ports are inserted midway between the umbilicus and pubic bone. The retropubic space may be insufflated directly, or the abdominal cavity can be insufflated and a transperitoneal approach to the retropubic space is used. A pledget is attached to a grasping forcep and used to expose the fascia adjacent to the bladder neck, stripping the bladder and the surrounding fatty tissue medially. The lateral vaginal wall is elevated with a finger in the vagina and the tissue grasped with grasping forceps. An Ethibond suture is inserted and two bites of the vagina are taken prior to placing the suture through the iliopectineal ligament (Cooper's

9

ligament). The suture is tied using an extra- or intracorporeal knot. Usually two or more sutures are placed on each side of the bladder neck. A redivac drain is placed in the retropubic space. A urinary catheter is left in place for 24 hours prior to catheter clamping to ensure adequate voiding when it may be removed.

Complications
Complications are similar for Burch colposuspension.

Marshall Marchetti Krantz

Procedure
The Marshall Marchetti Krantz procedure is performed using the same abdominal incision as the Burch colposuspension. Sutures are placed between the paravaginal fascia on either side of the bladder neck and the periosteum of the pubis.

Complications
These are similar to the Burch colposuspension, but the procedure does not cure cystocele to the same degree as colposuspension and 5 per cent of patients suffer osteitis pubis [15].

Slings

Traditionally sling procedures are performed as secondary operations when the vagina is scarred and narrowed, and when intrinsic sphincter deficiency is present. This usually requires both an abdominal and vaginal incision. Slings are constructed from either organic (e.g. rectus sheath) or inorganic (e.g. non-absorbable polypropylene – PTFE, Marlex, Prolene) material. The cure rate is similar to that of retropubic bladder neck suspension, although the complications are greater.

Procedure
A strip of material is tunnelled underneath the bladder neck and/or proximal urethra and then attached to the rectus muscle or the abdominal wall.

Complications
These include detrusor instability (16 per cent), postoperative voiding disorder (10 per cent) and bladder laceration.

Table 9.4 Dosages of antimuscarinic drugs.

Oxybutynin 5 mg b.i.d. – normally t.d.s., maximum q.i.d. In the elderly 2.5–3 mg
  b.i.d. initially, increased to 5 mg b.i.d. according to response and tolerance
Tolterodene 2 mg twice daily
Propiverine 15 mg b.i.d. – t.d.s. increased to maximum of 15 mg q.i.d. In the
  elderly initially 15 mg b.i.d. increased if necessary to 15 mg t.d.s.

Tension-free vaginal tape

A new procedure, the tension-free vaginal tape (TVT), is currently gaining popularity and undergoing multicentre randomised controlled trials. The procedure is performed under sedation and local anaesthesia. Following a mid-urethral anterior vaginal wall incision and dissection, a sleeved abrasive prolene tape is inserted as a tension-free sling using a needle introducer and catheter retractor. The tape is inserted through a vaginal incision on either side of the urethra and withdrawn through two small 1 cm incisions each made 4 cm from the midline, 1 cm above the pubic bone. Following adjustment of tension on the tape to prevent urinary leakage when the patient coughs, and cystoscopy to ensure correct placement of the tape, the plastic sleeve is removed. The abrasive nature of the tape maintains its position, and all that is necessary to complete the procedure is to trim the tape and close the incisions. Although currently still under formal evaluation, the limited morbidity of this procedure would confer significant benefit to patients if its long-term efficacy is established [17].

Anterior repair

This is not the operation of first choice for surgical treatment of genuine stress incontinence. The objective cure rates do not compare well with other operations. Studies report a wide range of success rates. The major advantage of the buttress procedure is the lack of complications including the relative lack of voiding difficulties postoperatively and a shorter hospital stay.

Procedure

An anterior longitudinal incision is made in the vaginal wall. The bladder neck is mobilised and elevated using 'Kelly' or 'Pacey' sutures. The pubovesical fascia is approximated and the vagina

9

closed. This operation can be done in conjunction with a vaginal hysterectomy.

Complications
There is an increased risk of failure.

Long needle suspension

Initially described by Pereyra and later modified by Stamey, these procedures are rarely used as their long-term efficacy is less than other operations.

Procedure
A long needle is used to thread sutures on either side of the bladder neck between the anterior abdominal fascia and the vaginal wall. Stamey used cystoscopy to judge placement of sutures and to ensure there were no sutures in the bladder.

Periurethral injectable (bulking agents)

A variety of different substances are available for injection into the proximal urethra to act as a cushion of tissue that enhances the urethral closure mechanism. This procedure is usually used when previous surgery has failed, and the urethra is relatively fixed and immobile. The procedure is associated with minimal morbidity. The substances most widely used are collagen and microparticulate silicone. The subjective cure rate at 2 years is 70–80 per cent, although objective cure is somewhat less at 48 per cent [18].

Procedure
Injections are performed either peri- or transurethrally under local, regional or general anaesthetic. A cystoscope is used to guide the paraurethral or transurethral injection of the chosen substance. A new injection device has recently been introduced for microparticulate silicone injections which allows accurate transurethral injection without the need for cystoscopic guidance. This procedure has a quick recovery time and low morbidity and so is ideal for the patient who is unfit for surgery.

Complications
It is generally considered to be relatively free of side effects, although there have been some reports of urgency, haematuria and short-term urinary retention.

DETRUSOR INSTABILITY

Definition

Detrusor instability (DI) is defined by the International Continence Society as a condition in which the detrusor is shown objectively to contract either spontaneously or on provocation, while the subject is attempting to inhibit micturition. In the presence of demonstrable neurological pathology, e.g. multiple sclerosis, the term 'detrusor hyperreflexia' is used.

DI is usually managed conservatively, although in severe intractable cases surgery may be helpful. The pathophysiology of DI is poorly understood and consequently many different treatments are available, none of which are perfect. The mainstay of conservative therapy is a combination of drug treatment and bladder drill.

History will often include:

- Frequency (more than seven voids per day)
- Nocturia (more than one void at night)
- Urgency
- Urge incontinence
- Nocturnal enuresis.

It is increasingly recognised that many women with overactive bladder symptoms can be managed without the need for initial urodynamic investigations, and that not all women with detrusor instability suffer from urge incontinence. The term overactive bladder (OAB) has been introduced to include all those patients with symptoms suggestive of bladder overactvity, irrespective of whether their symptoms result in urge incontinence.

A list of the common treatments for DI is shown below:

- Drug therapy
- Behavioural therapy (bladder drill biofeedback, hypnotherapy)
- Electrical stimulation
- Acupuncture
- Augmentation cystoplasty
- Cystodistension
- Phenol injections.

Drug therapy

Most drug therapies work via antimuscarinic effects on the parasympathetic cholinergic nerves supplying the detrusor muscle, e.g. oxybutynin, tolterodine, propiverine and imipramine. Antimuscarinic drugs treat urinary frequency, urgency and incontinence by increasing the bladder capacity and by diminishing unstable detrusor contractions. A major disadvantage of antimuscarinics is the occurrence of side effects, e.g. dry mouth, blurring of vision, constipation and reflux. They may precipitate glaucoma.

Oxybutynin has additional smooth muscle relaxant effects unrelated to its antimuscarinic effect.

Tolterodine has greater specificity for M3 muscarinic receptors and therefore has a more direct effect on the detrusor muscle with less systemic side effects.

The tricyclic antidepressants imipramine, amitriptyline and nortriptyline are sometimes effective in the management of the unstable bladder because of their antimuscarinic properties. Imipramine has both an effect on α receptors in the urethra, and central effects, both of which also contribute to its mode of action.

Practical prescribing
(1) Start off at a low dose to minimise initial side effects.
(2) Encourage fluid restriction and bladder drill.
(3) 'When required' (p.r.n.) use of these drugs should be tried if patients are unable to take them continuously.
(4) Follow-up is essential as many women discontinue treatment in the first few weeks following commencement of therapy.

Which drug for which patient
Oxybutynin, tolterodine and propiverine are useful for treatment of frequency, urgency and urge incontinence. A new slow-release oxybutynin preparation has recently been introduced which allows once daily dosing and may improve treatment compliance.

Imipramine is most often used for nocturia and nocturnal enuresis, but can be used during the day and prior to intercourse for coital incontinence.

DDAVP (1-desamino-8-D-arginine vasopressin) is a long-acting analogue of vasopressin used for the treatment of nocturia and nocturnal enuresis. It is given intranasally or orally and is effective for 12 hours. It is effective at reducing diuresis during sleep and therefore should be avoided in women with heart failure who diurese to a greater extent at night.

Behavioural therapy

Bladder drill, first described as 'bladder discipline', involves a regimen of timed voiding. With a normal daily intake of fluid (approximately 1.5l) women are gradually taught to increase the interval between voids. Bladder retraining programmes vary but need to include some key elements: patient education on the mechanisms of continence and incontinence; a scheduled voiding regimen with gradually progressive voiding intervals; urgency control strategies including distraction and relaxation techniques; self-monitored voiding behaviour; and positive reinforcement from trained staff. The initial voiding interval is 30 minutes greater than that documented on frequency volume charting. The interval is increased by 30 minutes as the target interval is achieved. This requires personal discipline and motivation and can be made easier with the use of a voiding diary. The goal is to achieve voiding at 3-hourly intervals.

Electrical stimulation

Inhibition of detrusor contractions following vaginal or anal electrical stimulation has been shown to be effective for the treatment of DI. It is believed to occur by inhibition of the detrusor via pudendal nerve reflexes.

Acupuncture

Acupuncture employing both traditional, e.g. spleen and stomach, sites and segmental lumber and sacral needling has been shown to improve the symptoms of DI. A similar effect has been demonstrated with electro-acupuncture and transcutaneous electrical nerve stimulation (TENS).

If the above measures fail to improve the symptoms of DI it is important to review the patient's symptoms and perform additional investigations, e.g. cystourethroscopy, bladder biopsy and further neurological assessment. For patients with intractable symptoms surgery may be appropriate but is not without complications.

9

Augmentation cystoplasty

This operation involves augmenting the transected bladder using either a tubularised or detubularised portion of bowel. This is a major surgical procedure. The aim of surgery is to increase the bladder capacity and reduce unstable bladder contractions. Complications include voiding difficulties, mucus in the urine, urinary tract infections and, in the long term, risks of neoplastic changes within the bowel segment. Patients are usually taught to clean intermittently and self-catheterise prior to surgery. Despite the complications this is the most successful operation to date for severe intractable DI.

Cystodistension

Overdistension of the bladder at the time of cystoscopy was first popularised by Helmstein in 1966. Studies have shown limited long-term efficacy and short-term complications including bladder rupture.

Phenol injections to the nerve plexuses of the bladder are no longer in common practice.

Detrusor hyperreflexia

Treatment is generally similar to that of idiopathic DI. Due to associated detrusor sphincter dyssynergia, women often require a method for overcoming voiding difficulties and urinary retention following treatment, particularly if commenced on anticholinergic therapy. This usually involves the use of intermittent self-catheterisation by the patient or her carer. If this is difficult due to a lack of manual dexterity, other means of bladder drainage may be used.

Hyperreflexia can also be managed with the intravesical instillation of anticholinergic drugs at the time of intermittent catheterisation. This minimises the systemic side effects of these drugs experienced when they are taken orally.

Capsaicin, a neurotoxin, has been used with some success for the treatment of intractable pain and overactivity of the detrusor amongst patients with neurological pathology following intravesical administration.

OVERFLOW INCONTINENCE/DIFFICULTY VOIDING

Overflow incontinence is a condition in which the bladder exceeds its capacity to hold urine and leakage occurs. This can either be when the bladder is grossly enlarged and flaccid or occasionally with a small trabeculated bladder. Long-term back pressure and vesico-ureteric reflux can cause secondary kidney damage resulting in hydronephrosis and deteriorating renal function.

Aetiology

Detrusor hypotonia

This most commonly occurs secondary to bladder overdistension occurring after childbirth or surgery.

Neuropathology causing bladder atony includes lumbosacral nerve disease resulting from disc compression, spinal tumours, myelomen-ingocele or multiple sclerosis. Neuropathy secondary to diabetes can also result in detrusor hypotonia.

Outflow obstruction

This is an uncommon cause of voiding difficulty in women and is most commonly seen in the presence of severe genital prolapse. It is also seen after surgery to the urethra, employed either to correct urethral abnormalities (e.g. diverticulae) or to correct urethral sphincter incompetence.

Symptoms

Women with overflow incontinence may complain of mixed urinary symptoms including frequency, nocturia, urgency and stress and urge incontinence. In addition they usually complain of voiding dif-ficulties, and recurrent urinary tract infections.

Investigations

Physical examination may demonstrate a palpable bladder, and ultra-sound or catheterisation will show a large post-void urinary residual (>100 ml).

Uroflowmetry will show poor maximum flow rate (>15 ml/ second), a prolonged flow time, a reduced mean flow rate, and an intermittent or prolonged flow curve.

Cystometry will demonstrate either a low flow/high pressure pattern of voiding seen in outflow obstruction, or a low pressure/low flow pattern seen in detrusor hypotonia (See Fig. 9.5).

9

Urethral pressure profilometry will demonstrate a high urethral closure pressure in the presence of urethral obstruction.

Treatment

The aim of treatment is to facilitate bladder emptying either by improving detrusor function, relieving outflow obstruction or providing a form of bladder drainage if these are not possible to achieve.

Improving detrusor function

Drugs

Bethanechol (10–25 mg t.i.d.) is a parasympathomimetic that causes parasympathomimetic nerve stimulation. It possesses the muscarinic rather than nicotinic effects of acetylocholine. Voiding difficulty is improved by it increasing detrusor muscle contraction.

Side effects, particularly in the elderly, include generalised parasympathomimetic side effects such as sweating, bradycardia and intestinal colic, vomiting and blurred vision.

Contraindications include intestinal or urinary obstruction or the increased muscular activity of the urinary or gastrointestinal tract is harmful in e.g. asthma, bradycardia, hypothyroidism, recent myocardial infarction, epilepsy, hypertension, pulmonary vagotomi and peptic ulceration.

Neural stimulation

This comprises neurosurgically implanted devices.

Decreasing outflow obstruction

- Repairing prolapse
- Urethral dilatation
- Urethrotomy (if proven stricture).

Bladder drainage

- Intermittent self-catheterisation
- Indwelling catheterisation
- Urethral pump devices
- Urinary diversion (if associated severe incontinence).

CONCLUSION

The appropriate investigation and management of urinary incontinence will improve the quality of life of women with lower urinary tract symptoms. Although a cure is not always achievable, all patients can expect significant symptomatic improvement.

REFERENCES

1 Brocklehurst, J.C. (1993) Urinary in continence in the community – analysis of the MOR1 poll. *British Medical Journal*, **306**, 832–834.

2 Cutner, A. (1997) The urinary tract in pregnancy. In: *Urogynecology* (ed. L.D. Cardozo), pp. 417–443. Churchill Livingston, New York.

3 DeLancy, J.O.L., Fowler, C.J., Keane, D. *et al*, (1998) Pregnancy, childbirth and the pelvic floor. In: *Incontinence. International Consultation on Incontinence* (eds P. Abrams, S. Khoury & A. Wein), pp. 287–294. Health Publications.

4 Fantl, J.A., Cardozo, L.D. & Ekberg, J. (1994) Oestrogen therapy in the management of urinary incontinence in the postmenopausal woman and meta-analysis. HUT committee report. *Obstetrics and Gynecology*, **8**, 12–18.

5 Raz, R. & Stamm, W.E. (1993) A controlled trial of intravaginal oestriol in postmenopausal women with recurrent urinary tract infection. *New England Journal of Medicine*, **329**, 753–756.

6 Bump, R.C. & Norton, P.A. (1988) Epidemiology and natural history of the pelvic floor dysfunction. *Obstetrics and Gynecology Clinics of North America*, **25**, 723–746.

7 Brown, J.S., Seeley, D.G., Fong, J., Black, D.M., Ensrud, K.E. & Grady, D. (1996) Urinary incontinence in the older woman: who is at risk? *Obstetrics and Gynecology*, **87**, 715–721.

8 Kelleher, C., Cardozo, L.D. & Khullar, V. (1997) A new questionnaire to assess quality of life of urinary incontinent women. *British Journal of Obstetrics and Gynaecology*, **104**, 1374–1379.

9 Dinubile, N.A. (1991) Strength training. *Clinics in Sports Medicine*, **10**, 33–62.

10 Wilson, P.D., Bo, K., Bourcler, A. *et al.* (1999) Conservative management in women. In: *Incontinence* (eds P. Abrams, S. Khoury & A. Wein), pp. 579–636. Health Publication.

11 Bo, K., Talseth, T. & Holme, I. (1999) Single blind randomised controlled trial of pelvic floor exercises, electrical stimulation, vaginal cones and no treatment in management of genuine stress incontinence in women. *British Journal of Medicine*, **318** (7182), 487–93.

12 Jarvis, G.J. (1994) Surgery for genuine stress incontinence. *British Journal of Obstetrics and Gynaecology*, **101**, 371–374.

9

13　Bergman, A., Ballard, C.A. & Koonings, P.P. (1989) Comparison of three different surgical procedures for genuine stress incontinence – prospective randomised study. *American Journal of Obstetrics and Gynecology*, **160**, 1102–1106.

14　Bergman, A., Koonings, P.P. & Ballard, C.A. (1989) Primary stress urinary incontinence and pelvic relaxation – prospective randomised comparison of three different operations. *American Journal of Obstetrics and Gynecology*, **161**, 97–100.

15　Bergman, A. & Elia, G. (1995) Three surgical procedures for genuine stress incontinence – 5-year follow-up of a prospective randomised trial. *American Journal Obstetrics and Gynecology*, **173**, 66–71.

16　Jarvis, G.J. (1998) Surgical treatment for incontinence in adult women. In: *Incontinence. International Consultation on Incontinence*, pp. 637–668. Health Publications.

17　Nilsson, C.G. (1998) The tension-free vaginal tape procedure for treatment of female urinary incontinence. A minimally invasive surgical procedure. *Acta Obstetrica et Gynecologica Scandinavia*, **168** (Suppl), 34–37.

18　Monga, A.K., Robinson, D. & Stanton, S.L. (1995) Periurethral collagen injections for genuine stress incontinence: a 2-year follow-up. *British Journal of Urology*, **76**, 156–160.

9

10 Sexual Health and Disease

Janet Say

SEXUAL HEALTH

Sexual health is the integration of the physical, emotional, intellectual and social aspects of sexual being, in ways that are positively enriching. Today, the speciality of sexual health may encompass sexually transmitted infections and their management, genital dermatology, reproductive health, sexual abuse and psychosexual medicine.

Sexual health history taking

- The taking of a sexual health history should not be daunting, and neither the clinician nor patient should be embarrassed.
- Direct questions regarding sexual activity at the end of the routine gynaecological history are probably indicated in most situations.
- The patient may be asymptomatic but admit to a partner having symptoms.
- Specific questions about vaginal discharge, dysuria, pelvic pain and dyspareunia should be asked. There may be a history of a rash, irritation, soreness, lumps or ulcers.
- It is important to define the onset of the symptoms and their relationship to sexual intercourse, urination and menstruation.
- Has the patient had similar symptoms before?
- A history of previous sexually transmitted infections should be taken.
- A risk history will indicate the chances of finding an asymptomatic disease, i.e. practising unprotected sexual intercourse.
- Ask when sexual intercourse last took place, and how long the patient has been with their present partner(s). Document events over the last 3 months.
- What is the gender of their present partner(s)?
- Has the sexual activity occurred with a regular or casual partner or occurred overseas?

- What was the type of sexual intercourse – vaginal? oral? anal?
- Is there a risk for human immunodeficiency virus (HIV)? The history includes questions about sexual intercourse overseas, with a foreigner, with an intravenous drug user or intravenous drug use itself and/or the sharing of needles.
- Is there a hepatitis B and C risk? Ask specific questions about vaccination for hepatitis B and the use of recreational drugs, needle using and sharing.
- Where there are facilities and protocols for onward referral, a history regarding previous sexual assault can be taken, i.e. 'Have you had any sex you did not want, that was forced on you, as an adult or as a child?'

Sexual health examination

- Complete visualisation of the external genitalia can only be made in the lithotomy position using a good light.
- Examine the pubic area for dermatoses, pubic lice.
- Inspect the external genital area, introitus, vestibular area, urethra and around the upper thighs.
- Palpate the inguinal nodes. Are they tender? If so, the genital area should be touched carefully, particularly on inserting a speculum.
- Internal examinations – choose a speculum suitable for the patient. Use warm water as a lubricant (KY and other lubricants often contain antibacterial disinfectants). Include a bimanual examination.
- Some extremely painful conditions may preclude a speculum examination, e.g. trichomoniasis and genital herpes.

Routine screening swabs to exclude disease (in order of being taken)

- Swab the posterior fornix, particularly for *Trichomonas* and the lateral vaginal wall for *Candida*.
- Cervical swab for gonorrhoea taken in Amies transport media.
- A cervical smear (Papanicolaou, if indicated) is taken next.
- *Chlamydia* swab from the cervical os.
- Urethral swab in transport media for gonorrhoea and urethral swab for *Chlamydia* (enzyme immunoassay); both cervical and urethral swabs may be placed in the same container.
- If activity includes oral or anal sites, swabs for gonorrhoea in Amies transport media and *Chlamydia* cultures are taken in specific

Chlamydia transport medium. A proctoscopy may be indicated if there are symptoms.
- Routine blood tests to be taken and repeated, if necessary, at 3 months post-risk activity include syphilis, hepatitis B, hepatitis C and HIV. This will depend on the type of risk. Pretest counselling must be provided.

Normal flora of the female genital tract and associated infections [1]

- At birth, maternal flora, *Trichomonas* and *Candida*, may be vertically transmitted. *Trichomonas* survives for 1–2 weeks only, as oestrogenisation wears off.
- From 2 months to puberty there is colonisation by skin flora. The cuboidal epithelium is susceptible to *Neisseria gonorrhoea* and *Chlamydia trachomatis*.
- Post-puberty the stratified squamous epithelium, pH 4.5, is colonised by lactobacilli at a concentration of 10^8–10^9 (bacterial vaginosis (BV) = 10^{11}). Anaerobes are small and constant in numbers. Colonisation with gut flora occurs, e.g. ureaplasma with penetration of the hymenal barrier.
- Introduced *Staphylococcus saprophyticus* and Gram-negative rods are associated with uroepithelial colonisation and increased risk of honeymoon cystitis (enhanced by a diaphragm).
- Strains of *Staphylococcus aureus* and tampons can be associated with toxic shock syndrome.
- In postmenopausal women, atrophic changes occur and there is a rise in pH, with a fall in numbers of lactobacilli related to the fall in oestrogen levels.

Lactobacilli

At puberty the cyclical influence of oestrogen encourages increased glycogen in the epithelial cells so that Gram-positive rods, lactobacilli, proliferate and predominate.

Hydrogen peroxide (H_2O_2)-producing lactobacilli, e.g. *Lactobacillus crispatus*, maintain the vaginal flora milieu. As well as providing the acid pH (4.5), by producing lactic acid from glucose, the H_2O_2 destroys implanted exogenous bacteria. Lack of these types of lactobacilli is positively associated with an increased incidence of BV and this has been associated with an increased prevalence of HIV.

10

The normal discharge from the vagina – child-bearing age group

- Normally there is a non-odorous white to grey floccular discharge that varies throughout the cycle.
- This includes the loss of the cervical mucous plug at ovulation and a fall in oestrogen, premenstrually, leads to exfoliation and watery granular discharge with a lower pH.
- *Cytology*: cells are polygonal, flat squamous, a few polymorphs, more premenstrually.
- Round to oval parabasal cells are indicative of lowered oestrogen, common in desquamative vaginitis and perimenopausally.

SEXUALLY TRANSMITTED INFECTIONS

Vaginitis – abnormal vaginal discharge

- This may include discharge from the upper genital tract, e.g. cervicitis, salpingitis.
- Therefore, take swabs from the vagina *and* cervix for possible pathogens, e.g. *Chlamydia*, gonorrhoea and herpes simplex (where indicated).
- Organisms that cause vaginal discharge can occur as an overgrowth, e.g. *Candida* and bacterial vaginosis.
- *Trichomonas* is always sexually transmitted (except in the neonate, where vertical transmission occurs).
- Discharges may be caused by mixed pathogens, with mixed symptoms and clinical signs; requiring laboratory elucidation (Table 10.1).

Bacterial vaginosis – odorous discharge

- The commonest cause of vaginal discharge is an overgrowth of mixed organisms, mostly gut anaerobes, *Gardnerella*, *Mobiluncus* spp. in high numbers.
- There is a lack of lactobacilli and a rise in pH of the secretion from 5.0 to 7.0.
- It is not sexually transmitted, but has been associated with increased sexual activity, lesbian partners, douching and increased risk ($\times$2) with intrauterine device (IUD) insertion.
- The cause is unknown, but it is presumably associated with the overwhelming of normal vaginal lactobacilli by exogenous organisms and their products.

10

Table 10.1 Vaginitis: clinical diagnosis – symptoms, signs and treatment.

	Candida	Trichomonas vaginalis	Bacterial vaginosis
Aetiology	Yeast, invasive pseudomycelium	Motile flagellated protozoan	Overgrowth, anaerobes, streptococci, Ureaplasma Prevotella, Gardnerella, Mobiluncus, group B streptococci
Incubation period	1–2 days to 1 week	2–28 days	5–14 days
Discharge	White curdy	Green frothy	Grey homogenous
Examination	Plaques Vaginal wall mucosa red, swollen, superficial ulceration	Red strawberry mucosa (2%) discharge watery, posterior fornix	Flourpaste discharge Coating on vaginal wall
pH	<4.0	6–7.0	5–6.0 + Whiff test +
Diagnosis	Microscopically 40–60% positive for yeasts and hyphae Wet prep. Gram Potassium hydroxide 10% (70% positive)	Wet prep. Acridine orange stain Cervical smear polymorphs +++	Clue cells present No lactobacilli Curved Gram-negative rods Mixed organisms
Culture medium	Sabourauds Dextrose agar	Trichomonas broth Culture media	
Treatment	Imidazole creams for 3–6 days Pessaries – stat Oral agents in chronic disease for 6 months (Table 10.4)	Nitromidazoles Metronidazole 400 mg b.i.d. for 5–7 days 2 g metronidazole stat doses	Metronidazole 400 mg b.i.d. for 5–7 days Metronidazole vaginal gel 0.75% nocte for 5 days or clindamycin vaginal cream 2% nocte for 7 days
Partners treated	Not indicated	Indicated Metronidazole 400 mg b.i.d. for 5-7 days (not stat doses)	Not indicated

10

Clinical signs, symptoms and management
  See Table 10.1.

Diagnosis of BV (Amsel's criteria)
  Three of the four criteria:
  - Grey homogenous flour-paste-coating discharge
  - pH >4.5
  - Clue cells (lack of lactobacilli) on microscopy. Clue cells are polygonal epithelial cells smothered in Gram-negative coccobaccilli (*Gardnerella vaginalis*)
  - Fishy (amine) odour when 10 per cent potassium hydroxide added to the vaginal discharge.
  - A laboratory diagnosis involving grading criteria of the Gram stain (Nugent) may recognise an intermediate group, e.g. post-antibiotics.

Upper genital tract associations with BV
  - Ascending infection has been associated with gynaecological procedures, e.g. termination of pregnancy (TOP), hysterectomy, IUD insertion.
  - BV organisms are part of the polymicrobial aetiology of pelvic inflammatory disease (PID). Whether they are just a secondary invader or a primary cause is not yet known.
  - In pregnancy BV is associated with preterm delivery, postpartum endometritis, fever and earlier miscarriage [2].
  - Early studies of the use of prophylactic antimicrobial therapy, in the months pre-delivery, have not been shown so far to successfully prevent these complications.

Treatment (Table 10.1)
  - Not indicated in asymptomatic women
  - Not indicated for sexual partners
  - Indicated before certain surgical procedures (e.g. TOP [3])
  - The role of therapy in pregnancy to prevent preterm labour is still under investigation (local clindamycin may have an adverse effect).
  - Recurrent BV, anecdotally, has been associated with altered anatomy, abnormal pooling of secretions, following vaginal hysterectomy.

10

Candidiasis (thrush) – itchy discharge

- *Candida albicans*, a yeast, is causative in 90 per cent of cases and can produce pseudomycelium.
- *Candida glabrata* and *Saccharomyces cerevisiae* (Baker's yeast) are uncommon and more resistant to imidazoles. Antifungal sensitivities may be helpful.
- The majority of women acquire *Candida* at some stage with up to 20 per cent of women being asymptomatic carriers of *Candida* spp.
- *Candida* infection may result from the use of broad-spectrum antibiotics and may be worse in pregnancy because of the oestrogen levels and immunosuppression.

Clinical diagnosis – symptoms, signs and treatment
See Table 10.1.

Recurrent cyclical candidiasis (four or more attacks per year)
- This may be a familial variety (non-secretors' Lewis blood group).
- It may be a marker for severe underlying disease, e.g. malignancy, diabetes or thyroid disease.
- It is common with immunodeficiency, ongoing steroid or antibiotic therapy.
- Often an invasive pseudomycelium switch occurs and may be related to increased prostaglandin E_2 (PGE_2) encouraged by mucosal immunoglobulin E (IgE) [4].

Management of Candida infection
- All local imidazole vaginal treatment preparations are equal in efficacy (cure rate 80 per cent), and their use depends on preference of the patient and prescriber.
- Some local preparations are more hypersensitising, e.g. tioconazole.
- It is essential to ensure vulval care, avoiding the use of coloured, perfumed products such as soaps, toilet paper, pads, sprays, additives to bath water, on mucous membranes.
- Ensure local skin diseases are managed, e.g. eczema, psoriasis, lichen sclerosis.
- Treatment of the male partner is only indicated if he is symptomatic (penile itch, rash, swelling).
- Advise the woman that adequate healing time is necessary ('rest the injured limb'), i.e. delay normal sexual function up to 2 weeks, or exacerbations can occur.

10

Treatment of candidiasis (Tables 10.2 and 10.3) [5]

- A variety of topical and oral azole therapies give an 80–95 per cent clinical and microbiological cure rate in acute vulval vaginal candidiasis in non-pregnant women
- Pregnancy – colonisation rates that are asymptomatic are as high as 30–40 per cent of women. Topical azoles may be used. Oral therapies are contraindicated.
- There is no evidence that treating asymptomatic male sexual partners benefits the woman partner. Occasionally the male partner can present with symptoms postcoitally that are due to *Candida* and the

Table 10.2 Topical therapies for the treatment of candidiasis. (With permission from Clinical Effectiveness Group (1999) [5].)

Drug	Formulation	Dosage regimen
Clotrimazole[1]	Pessary	500 mg immediately
Clotrimazole[1]	Pessary	200 mg × 3 nights
Clotrimazole[1]	Pessary	100 mg × 6 nights
Clotrimazole[1]	Vaginal cream (10%)	5 g immediately
Econazole[2]	Pessary (Ecostatin 1)	150 mg immediately
Econazole[2]	Pessary	150 mg × 3 nights
Fenticonazole[2]	Pessary	600 mg immediately
Fenticonazole[2]	Pessary	200 mg × 3 nights
Isoconazole[1]	Vaginal tablet	300 mg × 2 immediately
Miconazole[2]	Ovule	1.2 g immediately
Miconazole[2]	Pessary	100 mg × 14 nights
Nystatin	Vaginal cream (100 000 units)	4 g × 14 nights
Nystatin	Pessary (100 000 units)	1–2 × 14 nights

[1] Effect on latex condoms and diaphragms not known.
[2] Product damages latex condoms and diaphragms.

Table 10.3 Oral therapies for the treatment of *Candida* infection. (With permission from Clinical Effectiveness Group (1999) [5].)

Drug[1]	Formulation	Dosage regimen
Fluconazole	Capsule	150 mg immediately
Itraconazole	Capsule	200 mg twice daily for 1 day

[1] Avoid in pregnancy/risk of pregnancy and breastfeeding.

woman partner may be colonised but asymptomatic. Treating the woman may resolve the male symptoms.
- Follow-up swabs (post-treatment) are unnecessary.

Chronic cyclical candidiasis (Table 10.4)
This occurs in less than 5 per cent of women.
- Six-month courses of pulse therapy with oral antifungals may be necessary but this is not recommended in pregnancy.
- Liver function and white blood cells (WBC) need monitoring.
- Relapse rates may be as high as 50 per cent of women treated.

Trichomoniasis (Trichomonas vaginalis) – sore discharge

- This is a motile protozoan sexually transmitted infection (STI), involving the urethra and vagina.
- Classic symptoms are a florid watery, green, frothy, malodorous discharge. Two per cent will have a 'strawberry cervix' with petechial haemorrhages.
- Fifty per cent of women may be asymptomatic. Trichomonas is commonly associated with other STIs. The incidence increases with age in many countries.
- The incubation period is up to 28 days, so it may present post-treatment for gonorrhoea.
- Occasionally there is a spontaneous cure, but low grade symptomatic and asymptomatic infection may be present for many years.
- In pregnancy trichomoniasis is associated with amnionitis and increased risk of prematurity.
- There is growing evidence of an increased risk of acquisition of HIV in adults.

Table 10.4 Regimens for the treatment of chronic candidiasis. (With permission from Clinical Effectiveness Group (1999) [5].)

Fluconazole 100 mg weekly (p.o.) × 6 months
Clotrimazole pessary 500 mg weekly × 6 months
Itraconazole 400 mg monthly (p.o.) × 6 months
Ketoconazole 100 mg daily (p.o) × 6 months

NB: Low risk of idiosyncratic drug-induced hepatitis. Monitor liver function tests monthly.

10

Clinical disease – symptoms signs and treatment
See Table 10.1.

Management of **Trichomonas vaginalis**
- Ensure concomitant full course of treatment of male partner(s).
- Ensure screening is done for other STIs, gonorrhoea and *Chlamydia*.
- Follow-up testing of cure, particularly in pregnant patients, is indicated.
- Nitroimadazole – full and partial resistance is rare.

Desquamative vaginitis

This is a rare condition of unknown aetiology, associated with a very profuse yellow discharge (often requiring the use of pads) and marked superficial dyspareunia [6].
- On examination there is often redness around the inner aspects of the vulva and introitus.
- The profuse discharge usually has a raised pH.
- The mucous membranes of the vagina and cervix in severe cases may have a typical erythematous appearance with a cobblestone-like pattern, more obvious on colposcopy.
- On microscopy there are many round or oval parabasal cells and a profuse numbers of polymorphs. β-haemolytic streptococci are often isolated in culture.
- When other pathogens are excluded the optimum treatment appears to be clindamycin cream (2 per cent) inserted vaginally at night each night for 2 weeks. Some perimenopausal patients require oestriol (Ovestin) cream as a course for some months to ensure there is no relapse.

LOWER GENITAL TRACT BACTERIAL INFECTIONS

Chlamydia trachomatis (strains D–K) [7]

- This is the commonest sexually transmitted bacterial infection of the genital tract.
- It is an intracellular energy parasite (using the host's cells for adenosine triphosphate (ATP)) which has a complex life cycle, but is sensitive to antibiotics.

10

- The peak incidence in women is 19 years, with a history of recent change in sexual partners.
- It causes cervicitis (probably associated with an increased ectopy, area of glandular epithelial cells, which are target cells), urethritis, vaginitis (prepubertal) and proctitis.
- There is an increased incidence in pill users.
- There is an increased incidence in those practising unprotected sex.

Clinical signs and symptoms of Chlamydia

- Up to 90 per cent of women are asymptomatic (may present because the male partner is symptomatic).
- There is an incubation period of 2–4 weeks.
- Early mild dysuria may occur with a change in vaginal discharge, central lower abdominal pain (endometritis) and menstrual disorders, but these are uncommon symptoms.
- Commonly there is no evidence of cervicitis.
- Cervicitis may show as yellowish cervical discharge on a cotton tip swab, and/or friability and bleeding on contact.

Complications of Chlamydia

- Upper genital infection includes ascending endometritis, salpingitis in up to 20 per cent.
- Re-exposure to *Chlamydia* is associated with an increased incidence of chronic tubal disease that is immune mediated.
- With two attacks of chlamydia with or without gonorrhoea PID, there is a 30–50 per cent incidence of tubal factor infertility, a 15 per cent incidence of ectopic pregnancy, and a 25 per cent incidence of chronic pelvic pain and adhesions.
- Fitz–Hugh–Curtis syndrome – perihepatitis – occasionally occurs as a complication of PID, with severe subcostal pain sometimes referred to the shoulder tip.
- Reiter's disease, a seronegative reactive arthritis affecting mostly lower limbs, is uncommon in women.
- Adult conjunctivitis is rare.
- Transmission to the neonate may cause conjunctivitis (50 per cent) on the sixth day post-delivery and pneumonitis (8 per cent) at 6 weeks to 3 months. Screen and treat parents.

10

Laboratory diagnosis of Chlamydia [8]

Swabs for enzyme immunoassay are taken from the cervix *and* urethra (low incidence groups). It has a sensitivity of up to 80 per cent, specificity 92–100 per cent. Laboratory confirmatory tests, particularly with enzyme immunoassay, are essential.

- Cellular material must be obtained on the swabs.
- Swabs from throat and rectal areas require culture (medicoforensic). Specificity is 100 per cent.
- Urine tests in females have a lower sensitivity.
- The molecular techniques of ligase chain reaction (LCR) and polymerase chain reaction (PCR) are highly sensitive and specific. Self-applied swabs of the vagina and introitus may be important 'non-invasive' future screening methods.
- *Chlamydia* serology is mostly a research tool, e.g. retrospective diagnosis of the aetiology of tubal infertility.
- An IgM ≥16 microimmunofluorescent antibody level (MIF test) is diagnostic of neonatal pneumonia.

Treatment of uncomplicated Chlamydia *lower genital tract infections*

- Azithromycin, 1.0g orally stat, or
- Doxycycline, 100mg orally b.i.d. for 7 days (cheaper), or
- Erythromycin, 500mg q.i.d. for 7 days, in pregnancy and lactation.

Alternatively, in non-pregnant patients with hypersensitivy to the above antibiotics, give ofloxacin, 200mg b.i.d. for 7 days.

Important points on management

- *Chlamydia* is a 'ping-pong' infection – local immunity is inadequate and reinfection common – so that all partners must be treated synchronously to prevent this.
- Re-exposure to *Chlamydia* (i.e. untreated male partner) enhances the immune response leading to a higher risk of tubal infertility. Heat shock proteins have a probable role [9].
- Disease prevention includes condom use, compliance, partner notification and education on the disease, all of which are all essential in the index case.
- Follow-up to re-enforce the above is recommended. Tests of cure are unnecessary, but can be offered at 6 weeks (to expose an untreated third party?).

10

Neisseria gonorrhoeae

- *Neisseria gonorrhoeae* is a Gram-negative, bean-shaped diplococcus seen inside polymorphs.
- It causes urethritis, cervicitis, proctitis and rarely pharyngitis and vaginitis (prepubertal).
- The incidence of gonorrhoea in the UK is increasing along with resistance to antibiotic therapy, e.g. ciprofloxacin.
- Concomitant infections with *Chlamydia* and *Trichomonas* are common.
- Ascending infections (in 20 per cent) cause destruction of tubal ciliated epithelial cells and an acute inflammatory response, followed by resolution and fibrosis causing tubal damage.

Clinical signs and symptoms of Neisseria gonorrhoeae
- The majority are asymptomatic
- Symptoms can include a purulent vaginal discharge
- Lower abdominal pain from ascending infection (hitches ride on sperm)
- Urethritis or cystitis (sometimes haemorrhagic)
- Abnormal menstrual bleeding
- On examination purulent cervicitis, yellow or normal-looking vaginal discharge
- On bimanual examination, central and adenexal pain if ascending infection.

Complications of gonorrhoea
- PID, ectopic pregnancy, sub/infertility
- Pyosalpinx, adhesions, chronic pelvic pain, tubo-ovarian abscess
- Fitz–Hugh–Curtis syndrome
- Bartholinitis – purulent discharge from duct (but this is an uncommon cause)
- Adult conjunctivitis occasionally occurs
- Disseminated gonococcal infection (DGI) occurs in 1 per cent, manifested as a peripheral rash, flitting joint pains, arthritis and tenosynovitis, often of the upper limbs
- Transmission to the neonate may occur as a severe purulent conjunctivitis within 24–48 hours of delivery. The parents should be screened and treated.

10

Laboratory diagnosis of gonorrhoea

- Cervical, urethral Gram stain smears for initial diagnosis (approximately 50 per cent sensitivity)
- Culture swabs taken from the urethra, cervix, rectum and throat, depending on sexual activity
- Swabs directly plated on Thayer–Martin medium are optimum or can be transported to the laboratory immediately in Amies transport media
- Isolation of organism by culture is essential for sensitivity testing
- PCR is available and combined with *Chlamydia*, more expensive.

Antimicrobial treatment of gonorrhoea

- At present, treatment comprises ciprofloxacin, 500 mg stat orally
- If the organism is sensitive to penicillin, give ampicillin 3 g plus probenecid 1 g orally stat (safe in pregnancy)
- If there is ciprofloxacin resistance, give ceftriaxone, 250 mg i.m. stat (safe in pregnancy), or
- Ofloxacin 400 mg orally stat, or
- Spectinomycin 2 g i.m. stat (safe in pregnancy) (not effective in pharyngeal infection).

Special considerations regarding treatment

- All patients and present partner(s) should be offered concomitant antichlamydial therapy.
- All partners need synchronous treatment to stop the ping-pong effect.
- Give counselling education on compliance and condom use. Any partner(s) in the previous 60 days should be notified or advised to seek medical screening and therapy.
- Follow-up testing of cure is recommended, preferably in the first week, at least once.

Cystitis

Chlamydia, gonorrhoea and *Trichomonas* may cause symptoms suggestive of cystitis. In the sexually active woman where no definitive usual bacterial pathogen has been isolated on mid-stream urinalysis (MSU), an STI screen is indicated as part of 'honeymoon cystitis' work-up.

UPPER GENITAL TRACT BACTERIAL SEXUALLY TRANSMITTED INFECTIONS – PELVIC INFLAMMATORY DISEASE

PID may include cervicitis, endometritis, salpingitis, tubo-ovarian and pelvic abscess and peritonitis.

▪ PID can be from direct spread, i.e. appendicitis (1 per cent).

▪ Secondary PID occurs from ascending infection, 75 per cent of cases in women <25 years.

▪ *Chlamydia* and gonorrhoea are the commonest aetiology, also anaerobes, including those from BV. Twenty per cent may be from post-surgical procedures.

▪ Chronic PID may be caused by actinomycosis (IUD use) and tuberculosis.

▪ Ascending infections may follow gynaecological procedures including TOP.

▪ Long-term sequelae include ectopic pregnancy, chronic pelvic pain from adhesions and infertility, with an incidence of 13 per cent (one episode), 30 per cent (two episodes) and 60 per cent (three episodes).

▪ HIV-positive women tend to have more severe PID with complications, i.e. tubo-ovarian abscess and slow response to antimicrobial therapy.

▪ PID may be asymptomatic (only 30 per cent of post-*Chlamydia* tubal factor infertility women had pain).

Contraception and PID

▪ Barrier techniques, e.g. condoms, prevent acquisition of PID pathogens.

▪ The combined oral contraceptive pill (COC) may promote, indirectly, chlamydial cervical colonisation because of an increase in the size of an ectropion. However, it possibly strengthens the mucous plug, limiting ascending infection.

▪ IUDs are much improved but are still associated with a significant risk of ascending infection and are more ideally suited to the woman who has completed her family.

Clinical signs and symptoms of PID

▪ In general only 65 per cent of PID is confirmed at laparoscopy.

▪ Symptoms included lower abdominal pain. Central suprapubic pain may be endometritis and lateral pain typical of salpingitis. Deep

10

dyspareunia, pyrexia, abnormal vaginal bleeding or discharge may occur.

- *Chlamydia* is commonly associated with endometritis (central pain). Exclude cystitis.
- Cervical excitation occurs along with central and lateral pelvic pain (usually bilateral) as minimal criteria.
- If severe, signs of peritonitis and a mass in the fornices may be present.
- Fitz–Hugh–Curtis syndrome may be associated with PID and can be diagnosed, at laparoscopy, by seeing violin string adhesions between the liver capsule and diaphragm.

Other diagnostic criteria for PID – may increase specificity of diagnosis

- The Centers for Disease Control (CDC) recommend this could include a rise in temperature >38.3°C [10].
- Raised erythrocyte sedimentation rate (ESR) and/or WBC count – *Chlamydia* is rarely associated with leukocytosis.
- Isolation of *Chlamydia* or gonorrhoea from the cervix correlates with the pathogens in the upper genital tract in 80 per cent of cases.
- Endometrial biopsy, laparoscopy, fallopian tube sampling and pelvic ultrasound are other diagnostic aids.
- Inadequately treated disease may progress to tubo-ovarian abscess. This may respond to high dose systemic antimicrobial therapy. Rarely is drainage necessary.

Differential diagnosis of PID

- Ectopic pregnancy often presents as unilateral pain. The pregnancy test is positive. It occurs in 8 per cent of first pregnancies in patients with a history of PID. There is a 20 per cent risk in subsequent pregnancies.
- Acute abdomen, e.g. appendicitis, ruptured ovarian cyst, endometriosis, cystitis, bowel disease.

10

Management of PID

Outpatient

In mild disease, polymicrobial infection with polyantimicrobial therapy is indicated (see below) to cover *Chlamydia*, gonorrhoea and anaerobes.

Inpatient

Patients should be admitted if they are under 20 years of age, with severe disease, peritonitis, pregnancy, HIV positive, tubo-ovarian complications, no response to oral therapy, uncertain diagnosis, post-gynaecological procedures, ensuring intravenous therapy. All partners must be advised to be treated synchronously.

Outpatient therapy

There have been few double-blind placebo trials of oral therapy, but it can include ciprofloxacin (500 mg oral stat) plus doxycycline (100 mg b.i.d. for 14 days minimum) plus metronidazole (400 mg b.i.d. for up to 2 weeks) with or without augmentin (500 mg t.d.s. for 2 weeks).

Treatment of inpatients

- Cefoxitin (2 g t.d.s i.v.) plus doxycycline (100 mg b.i.d. i.v.) followed by oral doxycycline (100 mg b.i.d.) + oral metronidazole (400 mg b.i.d.) up to 14 days.
- Clindamycin (900 mg t.d.s i.v. daily) plus gentamicin (2 mg/kg i.v. loading dose followed by 1.5 mg/kg t.d.s.) followed by either clindamycin orally (450 mg q.d.s. daily) to complete 14 days or oral doxycycline (100 mg b.i.d.) plus oral metronidazole (400 mg b.i.d.) to complete 14 days.
- With hypersensitivity problems, ofloxacin (400 mg b.i.d. orally) plus metronidazole (400 mg b.i.d. orally) for 14 days.

Special considerations

- In pregnancy, PID has a greater risk of morbidity for the mother and fetus. Intravenous therapy is recommended, although specific regimens have not been trialled.
- If assessment at follow-up in 72 hours shows no improvement, further investigations are indicated, including possible surgical intervention.
- Further follow-up at 1 month should occur to assess compliance and resolution of symptoms, as well as partner notification and synchronous therapy.

10

STIS AND SEXUAL ASSAULT [11]

- The isolation of *Neisseria gonorrhoeae* in a *child* or *young person* may be the only marker.
- *Chlamydia trachomatis* after the age of 3–4 years may also be corroborative forensic evidence.
- *Trichomonas* infections in young people are also liable to be forensically relevant.
- PID should be considered as a differential diagnosis for pelvic pain in young adolescents. It may be from non-consenting sexual activity.
- These infections may also be acquired following *adult* sexual assault, although their role as forensic evidence is complex in women in consenting sexual relationships.
- All patients suspected of, or complaining of, recent non-consenting sex should be referred to the appropriate local agencies for management urgently. Medical forensic examination may be necessary.
- Laboratory specimens need to be processed as a 'chain of evidence' to be forensically viable.
- DNA-positive semen specimens may survive for only up to 7 days (cervix) post-assault.
- Post-assault pregnancy prophylaxis and antibiotics for STI prophylaxis [10], along with hepatitis B vaccination and anti-HIV prophylaxis, may be indicated.

SYPHILIS (*TREPONEMA PALLIDUM*)

- Any positive syphilis serology (Venereal Disease Reference Laboratory (VDRL) – non-specific treponemal test; rapid reagin (RPR) test – non-specific treponemal test; *Treponema pallidum* haemagglutination (TPHA) test; fluorescent treponemal antibody (absorbed) (FTA abs)) should be discussed immediately with an appropriate specialist (genitourinary medicine or infectious diseases physician).
- Urgent referral is required in pregnancy. A Jarisch–Herxheimer reaction following treatment may be a risk to the pregnancy.
- A recent pandemic affects Russia and some northern European countries.
- Immigrants and refugees from Asian, African and South American countries should be screened if they have not been already.
- Atypical genital ulcers require follow-up syphilis serology for up to 3 months to exclude a primary lesion.

10

Secondary syphilis

Secondary syphilis (6 weeks to 6 months after acquisition) has highly infectious mucous membrane lesions, i.e. oral cavity snail-tract ulcers, genital area, flat wart-like areas, condyloma lata. There may be a generalised maculopapular rash (including palms of hands and soles of feet), rubbery lymphadenopathy, etc. This continues for 2 years (15 per cent up to 4 years) if untreated.

Tertiary syphilis

This may manifest in 35 per cent of untreated patients after 5 years as cardiovascular disease, e.g. aortic aneurysm, neurological disease (tabes dorsalis).

GENITAL HERPES – HERPES SIMPLEX TYPES 1 AND 2

Herpes simplex viruses (HSV) are similar to other members of the herpes group in that they can be excreted over many years through mucous membranes, i.e. through oral and genital secretions. Although they are not always sexually transmitted (e.g. primary herpetic whitlow of finger), they are ubiquitous in the sexually active age group, e.g. approximately 10–25 per cent of women in antenatal clinics. Sixty to seventy per cent of patients are asymptomatic for the classical ulcers around the mouth or genital region, but can still intermittently excrete the virus and probably transmit it unknowingly. The latent infection resides in the sensory nerve ganglion and virus travels down the nerve to the endings in the skin. If local immunity is inadequate replication follows and a recurrence may occur. Genital HSV 1 is increasing in Europe (50 per cent) as people practice 'safer' oral sex.

Neonatal herpes has high morbidity and mortality. Ninety per cent of cases are presumed to be associated with primary disease of the mother's cervix at delivery. Less than 5 per cent of cases of neonatal herpes arise through contact with mothers suffering recurrent disease. Five per cent may be acquired postpartum.

Primary genital herpes infection

- Infection follows the first encounter with HSV 1 or 2, i.e. no protective antibody, severe infection with infectivity for several weeks.

- It has an incubation period of 3–20 days, maybe longer.
- It often presents with a flu-like illness, tiredness, and 5 per cent have severe headache (aseptic meningitis).
- Vulval swelling and itchiness may precede increasing numbers of small painful ulcers, which may coalesce.
- Severe external dysuria and tender inguinal lymphadenopathy are common symptoms.
- The effects on sympathetic bladder supply, atonic bladder with retention, and constipation (radiculopathy) should be assessed.
- Spinal and sciatic pain are occasionally part of aseptic meningitis.
- Proctitis, perianal pain and severe perineal nerve pain occur rarely.

Primary genital herpes – signs

At examination, severe pain, particularly in primary disease, can rightly preclude initial speculum examination.

- Examine the vulva for punched-out extensive or localised ulceration, secondary infection which occasionally occurs with skin pathogens, e.g. *Staphylococcus* or *Streptococcus*.
- Cervicitis can be an erosive, haemorrhagic, exfoliative cervicitis, with a profuse, watery, necrotic discharge (pH 7.0). Occasionally, a few developing, ulcerating vesicles may be present on the ectocervix or there may be no obvious signs. A positive cervical culture for herpes may be found in the majority of primary cases (90 per cent).
- Palpate for tender, swollen inguinal nodes draining from the site of infection.
- A few ulcers present at the anal margin may mark a profuse, haemorrhagic, ulcerating proctitis on proctoscopic examination.
- Retention of urine, bladder up to umbilicus, should be excluded in all cases.

Complications of genital herpes

- Urinary retention may not respond to aciclovir once established.
- Suprapubic catheterisation may be necessary with hospital admittance.
- Urinary tract infection from 'obstructive uropathy' may be a secondary infection.
- Secondary skin pathogen infections, i.e. spreading cellulitis.

- Adhesion of labia and lacunae formation may require plastic repair later.
- Severe pain may require non-steroidal anti-inflammatory drugs (NSAIDs) or morphine derivatives.

Genital herpes – diagnosis

- Viral culture swab taken from blister, ulcer or cervix
- Fluorescent antigen detection from ulcer swabs
- PCR (in-house, highly sensitive) viral swab
- Gull HSV 1 and HSV 2 commercial antibody has a window period up to 6 months from the primary infection. Western blot confirmatory testing is encouraged.

Primary genital herpes – management

- Specific antiviral therapy with aciclovir (200 mg five times a day for 5 days)
- Famciclovir (250 mg t.i.d. for 5 days)
- Valaciclovir (500 mg b.i.d. for 5 days)
- Salt water baths (a handful or two of ordinary salt in a bath); encourage micturition in bath and separating adhesing labial folds
- Local anaesthetic gel applied pre-micturition or pre-defecation
- Treatment of urinary tract infection (UTI) where indicated
- Educate the patient at the first visit regarding watching bladder function and to expect antiviral chemotherapy to provide symptomatic improvement in 48 hours
- On follow-up, counselling regarding risks to partner, risks in pregnancy, features of the disease and expectation of recurrences and suppressive therapy is necessary. Reassurance is a very important part of management.

Recurrent genital herpes

- Many infections may be subclinical, i.e. just slight tenderness, tingling, may be mild redness which presumably is an abortive attack.
- Up to 35 per cent of patients may expect frequent recurrences genitally after initial diagnosis.
- Recurrences are 80–90 per cent if HSV 2 is present, 50 per cent if HSV 1 is present (less infectious).

10

- The recurrent lesion lasts up to 6 days from the development of the blister through to ulcer, scabbing and healing.
- Viral cultures are generally only positive in the first 48 hours of the recurrent lesion.
- Patients should be encouraged to present early for confirmatory clinical diagnosis or to take their own swabs.
- Herpes causes up to 80 per cent of recurrent erythema multiforme and is also the cause of Mollaret's meningitis (recurrent aseptic meningitis).
- The majority of patients may see recurrences more frequently in the first few months after the primary infection.
- Increased stress (anxiety) has been associated with increased frequency of recurrence.
- Salt water baths, use of hair dryer to ulcers and local anaesthetic gels provide symptomatic relief.
- After 6 months of recurrences it may be appropriate to suggest oral therapy.

Recurrent genital herpes – management

Episodic antiviral treatment

- This is variable in its efficacy. Patients start therapy at the beginning of the prodromal symptoms.
- Treatment comprises aciclovir (200 mg five times a day), valaciclovir (500 mg b.i.d.) and famciclovir (125 mg b.i.d.), all for 5 days.

Suppressive therapy

- Patients should be advised about the suitability of suppressive therapy as it is a commitment for at least a year.
- Recurrent episodes every 4–6 weeks, or very severe local and systemic symptoms or interference with psychological well being and relationships may be indications.
- Therapy comprises aciclovir (400 mg b.i.d.) for a minimum of 9 months up to 15 months depending on circumstances.
- Alternatives include famciclovir (250 mg b.i.d.) or valaciclovir (500 mg/day).
- Patients should be warned after 1 year to cease therapy, to keep a diary and wait for at least two recurrences before recommencing suppressive therapy.

10

Herpes serology

- Serological tests for herpes have limited indications and protocols for these have not been internationally defined.
- Where the couple is discordant (e.g. if the male and not the female partner has a history of genital herpes), there may be an indication for the female partner to be checked in pregnancy, if she is worried about the risk of transmission of herpes to the baby at delivery.
- Occasionally herpes serology has been useful in medicolegal situations.
- Where there is an inability to diagnose recurrent or atypical lesions in the past, there may be corroborative evidence from serology (unusual).
- Pretest counselling is essential to explain all the different scenarios which may eventuate from the positive serology to HSV 1 or HSV 2. Is the patient personally prepared to deal with these positive results? Can the relationship stand it?

Differential diagnosis of genital ulcers

Mixed co-infections can occur.

- Atypical ulcers may be caused by syphilis – screen with dark-ground microscopy and serology. Tropical sexually transmitted infections, e.g. chancroid (*Haemophilus ducreyi*), require specific cultures. Donovanosis and lymphogranuloma venereum are very rare.
- Rarely bullous dermatological disorders, e.g. pemphigus, may mimic herpes. Immunological biopsy is diagnostic.
- Behçets disease – other systemic symptoms and manifestations should be searched for – often this is associated with mouth ulcers, joint pains, skin rashes, etc. Biopsy is non-specific.
- Ulceration may follow trauma, including dermatitis artefacta.
- Aphthous ulceration, with a history of mouth ulcers as well, is occasionally diagnosed.
- Genital ulceration, large painful lesions of the vulva, occurs rarely with early glandular fever, usually in younger age groups.

GENITAL WARTS – HUMAN PAPILLOMAVIRUS (HPV)

- Papillomaviruses are a heterogenous group of DNA viruses which occur predominantly in squamous epithelium, causing hyperplastic

10

papillomatous, verrucous squamous or subclinical epithelial lesions in humans.

- Over 150 different types have been identified (on the basis of nucleic acid homology).
- Over 24 are site specific for the genital region, HPV type 6/11 is benign, others including 16/18, 31 and 33 have been associated with premalignancy and dysplasia of the genital tract.
- Since the 1970s there has been a massive increase in the diagnosis of genital exophytic warts (type 6/11).
- There has also been an increase in the incidence of genital intraepithelial neoplasia in younger age groups, particularly vulval intraepithelial neoplasia (VIN).
- Transmission is through direct sexual contact [12]. There is a 10–15 per cent risk per change of partner in acquiring genital HPV types. Fomite transmission or autoinoculation probably occur but are difficult to prove.
- Vertical transmission occurs between mother and baby rarely leading to external HPV or laryngeal papillomatosis (type 6/11).
- Specific capsid antibody to the genital types takes an average of 8 months to develop [13].
- Cell-mediated immunity in the form of cytotoxic memory cells is essential in preventing further acquisition of the virus and development of the lesions.
- One hundred per cent of cervical cancers are associated with oncogenic types of HPV (see Chapter 14).
- Prevention of cervical cancer and early management of cervical intraepithelial neoplasia (CIN) are dependent on cervical screening programmes, through regular cervical smears picking up CIN changes on the cervix.

Natural history of HPV – genital exophytic warts (condyloma accuminata)

- Only 1–4 per cent of those infected with genital HPV types develop exophytic warts.
- The incubation period is earliest 2 months, average 8 months and up to 2 years or more.
- The virus gets implanted into the basal layer cells of the epidermis and stimulates proliferation of the keratinocytes [14].

- The virus replicates in the upper layer of the epidermis in cells that are becoming keratinised and dying.
- In this way the natural keratinocyte's differentiation cycle is used to excrete the virus outwards away from immune competent mechanisms in the subepidermis.
- There is a proliferation of virus for about 6 months leading to crops of exophytic condyloma accuminata in susceptible individuals.
- Thirty per cent or more may be removed by the normal immune mechanisms at this stage.
- Patients may require therapy for aesthetic reasons before then.
- Stimulation of interferons and other cytokines encourage the dendritic cells to leave the site and present antigen in the draining lymph nodes.
- T helper cells return to the wart site and cytotoxic T cells destroy the virus, some becoming memory cells.

Genital warts – clinical signs

- Lumps, commonly cauliflower-like, involve the vulva, introitus, vestibular and perianal area as well as on the cervix or inside the vagina.
- When they involve the mucous membrane, including the inner aspect of the labia, they may be hidden in the perihymenal folds – pink, soft warts with little keratinisation.
- They can be flat in a carpet, single or multiple.
- Occasionally they are associated with itching and concomitant candidiasis.
- If large or excoriated they can bleed.
- The only clue may be a partner who has been diagnosed with warts.
- In pregnancy the warts may reach a large size, very rarely are there complications with this. Regression occurs after delivery in many patients.

10

Management of genital warts

(Table 10.5) [15].

Table 10.5 Summary of treatment options for genital warts. (After New Zealand HPV Project (2001) [15].)

Forms of treatment	Usage	Response rate (%)	Recurrence rate (%)	Advantages and disadvantages	Use in pregnancy
Patient-applied					
Podophyllotoxin (0.5% solution, 0.15% cream)	External genital warts	37–95	0–35	Results are dependent on patient compliance. Not for large (>10cm²) wart areas	No
Imiquimod (5% cream)	External anogenital warts	37–85	13–19	Immune enhancer. Most effective on moist warts, introitus, perianal	No
Provider-administered					
Cryotherapy, liquid N₂ or cryoprobe	External anogenital, vaginal, cervical, urethral, anal or oral warts	60–97	20–79	Effective for moist and dry warts, pain can be reduced by use of Emla cream. Safety and efficacy are highly dependent on skill level, equipment and experience	Yes
Podophyllin (15–25%)	External anogenital, vaginal or urethral warts	19–80	23–70	Most effective on moist warts, wash off after 4 hours, unknown shelf life, may contain mutagens, variable concentration of active components. Avoid large wart areas and over-application	No

10

Trichloracetic acid (80–90%)	External anogenital, vaginal or anal warts	50–100	6–50	Inexpensive, effective for moist warts. Needs careful application because spreads easily and burns. Avoid large warts	Yes
Electrocautery or diathermy (bipolar or monopolar)	External anogenital or oral warts	35–94	22	Prompt wart-free state, results depend on skill level and training, requires equipment, longer clinic visit, local or general anaesthetic	Yes
Surgical excision	Extensive anogenital, oral or anal warts	93	8–35	Prompt wart-free state, results depend on skill level and training, requires equipment, longer clinic visit, local or general anaesthetic	Yes
Laser therapy (CO_2 laser)	Extensive anogenital warts	60–100	3–77	Prompt wart-free state, may require local or general anaesthesia, results and safety are dependent on skill level. Expensive	Yes

10

Genital warts – other considerations

- Other structures such as hymenal remnants, vestibular papillosis (hypertrophic papillary excrescences usually bilateral on inner labia minora), perianal skin tags and molluscum contagiosum lesions may be mistaken for warts.
- Always screen patient and partner for other STIs.
- Anti-*Candida* treatment is often necessary as well.
- Patients should be educated on the range of treatments available and be participants in the decision of treatment options.
- Patients should be encouraged to use salt water baths and Xylocaine gel pre-micturition as supportive measures during therapy.
- Counselling is important regarding transmission risks – this is not a ping-pong infection. Exacerbations are dependent on individual local immunity.
- Education is required on the difference between the oncogenic-associated types and ordinary genital warts.

HEPATITIDES

Hepatitis A, B, C and probably D can be transmitted through sexual activity. Preventative vaccination is available for hepatitis A and B.

HUMAN IMMUNODEFICIENCY VIRUS (HIV 1 AND 2)

Special considerations in HIV-positive women presenting to gynae-cology services include:

- Pelvic inflammatory disease (see above) may be more severe, run a more protracted course, be less responsive to antibiotics and may require drainage if abscess formation develops.
- Prophylactic antibiotics for gynaecological surgery and procedures, including TOP, may have to be prolonged.
- Recurrent and severe vaginal candidiasis is common and may require systemic antifungal therapy.
- Genital warts may have a poor response to the usual therapies and higher recurrence rates.

10

- Cervical dysplasia may be more advanced, with a greater recurrence rate despite ablation.
- The CDC have recommended cervical smear at diagnosis and a repeat 6 months later, then yearly smears [10]. Routine colposcopy has also been recommended.
- Screening for HIV in pregnancy is cost effective where new management regimens have limited transplacental transmission to less than 2 per cent.

OTHER CONDITIONS AFFECTING THE EXTERNAL GENITAL AREA

Conditions causing pruritis

Infectious conditions

- **Tinea cruris** may be caused by *Epidermophyton floccosum* or *Trichophyton rubrum var. interdigitalae* commonly. It is best to diagnose these lesions by taking a skin scraping from the well-defined edge of this erythematous rash. Treatment with local imidazole creams may take several weeks and the patient must be warned to continue the applications twice a day, even when the rash appears to have gone, for up to at least 2 weeks. Oral antifungals may be indicated.
- **Scabies** (*Sarcoptes scabiei* mite) tunnels into the epidermis and in the genital region often causes nodular lesions which are extremely itchy. It is important to examine other typical sites for this infestation. All sexual partners, and indeed household contacts, should be treated with permethrin (5 per cent cream) or malathion (0.5 per cent lotion) (not in pregnancy or young children). The patient should be warned that although there is a marked response in the severity of the itch, the immunological response to the infestation may be associated with pruritus that continues for up to a month after effectual mitocidal therapy.
- **Pubic lice** (*Phthirus pubis*) – the crab louse hangs on to pubic hairs upside down sucking blood from the skin and the resultant bite is, in most individuals, extremely itchy. Nits are often present on the pubic hairs. All sexual contacts should be treated with malathion (0.5 per cent) overnight or permethrin (1 per cent cream, which is safe in pregnancy and breastfeeding). All patients should be screened for other sexually transmitted infections.

10

Dermatological causes of pruritis in the genital region

- **Dermatitis** (chemical, allergic, contact) can arise from any coloured or perfumed agent in contact with mucous membranes and skin, e.g. soaps, toilet paper, bath additives. Removal of the allergenic agent and substitution to aqueous cream (soap alternative) for washing relieves symptoms. Disinfectants, preservatives and nickel are other allergens.

- **Atopic eczema**, **seborrhoeic dermatitis** and **intertrigo** can occur around the vulva, although the appearance may not be that typical of these conditions in other parts of the body. Often there is swelling, redness, sometimes folliculation and also scaling of the outer vulva. This can be secondarily infected with *Candida*, skin staphylococci or streptococci.

- Chronic excoriation may lead to thickening of the skin with changes of lichenification, increased skin markings, loss of hair and boggy thickening. Biopsy confirms **lichen simplex chronicus**. This intractable, insomnia-making itch-scratch-itch cycle can be stopped by using intensive medium dose steroids and antihistamines as sedatives at night over a period of several weeks.

- **Psoriasis**. Pruritis may occur in a minority of patients but many are colonised with candidiasis by the time they present. Clinically the classic, well-demarcated, silvery scaly, plaque-like lesions may not be obvious although there is usually a bright red edge to the lesions. Even biopsy may not be confirmatory. Most patients cannot tolerate tar preparations in this site, so that very judicious careful monitoring of low to medium dose steroid therapy is necessary under supervision. Sometimes only the genital area is involved, including the natal cleft and occasionally the umbilicus.

- **Lichen sclerosus**. This genital skin condition of unknown aetiology (occasional peripheral lesions) begins as thinning of the epidermis (retepegs flattening), telangectasia, bruising and fissuring of the skin. This can alternate with areas of firm and thickened white plaques which in themselves are itchy, but often secondarily infected with *Candida*. The architecture of the labia is altered. High potency steroids (clobetasol) over some weeks with a reducing interval of application ameliorates most symptoms dramatically. Follow-up must be yearly to exclude the small (less than 5 per cent) risk of squamous cell carcinoma. Dermatological referral may be indicated (see Chapter 11).

10

Conditions causing pain, including painful sex

- **Pyogenic abscess** involving mucous glands, simple and sebaceous gland cysts. Folliculitis, bartholinitis and hydradinitis may occur on the external genitalia, infected with skin or anaerobic flora, and there may be a tender draining inguinal lymphadenopathy.
- Soreness and pain from **infections** such as herpes, *Trichomonas* and *Candida* may preclude sexual activity.
- **Lichen planus**, the rare erosive type, particularly, may be intractably painful.

Dyspareunia – painful sex

Superficial dyspareunia

- A third of women may suffer this at some stage of their lives.
- **Primary superficial dyspareunia** (difficulties from first intercourse) may be associated with anatomical problems, e.g. thickened, banded hymen, or psychogenic problems, e.g. negative programming.
- **Acute secondary superficial dyspareunia** may be associated with many inflammatory or painful conditions of the vulva and vagina (see above).
- **Chronic superficial dyspareunia** can sometimes feel 'deep' to the patient but may be descriptive of pain around the perihymenal area, which occurs with sexual penetration or tampon insertion. This may be caused by ongoing inflammatory conditions or be part of vulvodynia.

Vulvodynia – painful vulva, vulvar dysethesia

- **Vulvar vestibulitis** occurs in young women under 30 years of age, usually under 25, who are in a non-problematic, long-term, established sexual relationship. A group of these follow chronic *Candida* infection which possibly could have led to inflammation and obstruction to the minute ducts of the minor vestibular glands that surround the perihymenal area. There may be a history of other inflammatory conditions – herpes, warts – but often there may be no clear background aetiology (spontaneous local).
- The diagnosis is made by using a cotton tip swab to touch around the hymenal area and elicit pinpoint exquisite tenderness, particularly between 4 and 8 o'clock.

10

- There may be localised redness of the mucous membranes and a typical vulvoscopy vascular pattern, although this is not always present and the subjectivity of these tests has recently been questioned.
- Continuing attempts to remain sexually functional are often complicated by the setting in of reflex vaginismus. This in itself may become a major problem with severe pelvic floor muscle spasm associated with pain, and may require electromyographic biofeedback of the pelvic floor muscles.
- Vulvar vestibulitis is symptomatically treated by using 2 per cent lignocaine gel pre-penetration (occasionally Emla cream) to allow penetrative sex and continued function.
- Vaginal dilator programmes, psychosexual counselling, deep pelvic floor relaxation exercises and physiotherapy of the pelvic floor may help through the months until the condition resolves of its own accord.
- This is an extremely testing time for relationships and both partners should be involved in the therapeutic management.
- Surgery is a last resort and must be extremely well considered.

Dysaesthetic vulvodynia (spontaneous generalised)
- This is a condition diagnosed by exclusion. It is usually found in women over 40 years of age complaining of burning or tingling or unpleasant sensations in the whole perivulval area and saddle region. On examination there is nothing specific to see. This condition is thought to be a dysaesthesia, possibly related to pudendal nerve entrapment, and in a small subset, historically related to a prolonged second stage of labour. It is treated as nerve pain by small doses (10–75 mg) of the tricyclics amitriptyline or imipramine at night for at least 3 months, ongoing. Surgery to free the pudendal nerve has been described.

Deep dyspareunia – pelvic pain with deep penetration
- This may be positional from hitting the ovary or other pelvic structures covered in peritoneum. Occasionally it is due to fixed retroversion of the uterus.
- Pain may be anterior at the base of the bladder and indicative of trigonitis or possibly interstitial cystitis.
- Chronic pain may be due to pelvic conditions such as endometriosis, ovarian mass, past PID or adhesions. Ultrasound imaging and

laparoscopy may be indicated. Large and small bowel disease may be causative.

▪ Pain without any obvious signs, which does not fit any real pattern, despite investigations, may be part of a somatisation problem following severe previous psychotrauma, particularly sexual.

REFERENCES

1 Holmes, K.K., Sparling, P.F., Mardh, P.-A., Lemon, S.M., Piot, P. & Wasserheit, J.N. (eds) (1999) *Sexually Transmitted Diseases*, 3rd edn. McGraw-Hill, New York.

2 Hillier, S.L., Nugent, R.P., Eschenbach, D.A. *et al.* (1995) Association between bacterial vaginosis and preterm delivery of low birth weight infants. The VIP study group. *New England Journal of Medicine*, **333**, 1373–1742.

3 Blackwell, A.L., Emery, S.J., Thomas, P.D. & Wareham, H. (1999) Universal prophylaxis for *Chlamydia trachomatis* and anaerobic vaginosis in women attending for suction termination: an audit of short-term health gains. *International Journal of Sexually Transmitted Disease and AIDS*, **10**, 508–513.

4 Rogers, C.A. & Beardall, A.J. (1999) Recurrent vulvovaginal candidiasis: why does it occur? *International Journal of Sexually Transmitted Diseases and AIDS*, **10**, 435–441.

5 Clinical Effectiveness Group (Association of Genitourinary Medicine and the Medical Society for the Study of Venereal Diseases) (1999) UK guidelines on sexually transmitted infections and closely related conditions. *Sexually Transmitted Infections*, **75** (Suppl 1), 519–522.

6 Sobel, J.D. (1994) Desquamative inflammatory vaginitis. A new subgroup of purulent vaginitis responsive to topical 2 per cent clindamycin therapy. *American Journal of Obstetrics and Gynecology*, **171**, 1215–1220.

7 Gilbert, G.L. (ed.) (1993) Infectious diseases: challenges for the 1990s. In: *Balliere's Clinical Obstetrics and Gynaecology, International Practice and Research*, **17 (1)**, pp. 159–193. Balliere Tindall, London.

8 World Health Organisation (1999) *Laboratory tests for the detection of reproductive infections*. WHO, Regional Office, Western Pacific.

9 La Verda, D., Kalagoglu, M.V. & Byrne, G.I. (1999) *Chlamydia* heat shock proteins and disease. New paradigms for old problems. *Infectious Diseases in Obstetrics and Gynaecology*, **7**, 64–71.

10 United States Department of Health and Human Sciences Centers for Disease Control and Prevention (1998) Guidelines for treatment of sexually transmitted diseases. *Centers for Disease Control Morbidity and Mortality Weekly Report*, **47**, RR-1.

10

11 Doctors for Sexual Abuse Care (2000) *The medical management of sexual abuse*, 5th edn. Doctors for Sexual Abuse Care, Auckland, New Zealand.

12 Koutsky, L. (1997) Epidemiology of genital human papillomavirus infection. *American Journal of Medicine*, **102**, 3–8.

13 Carter, J.J., Koutsky, L.A., Wipf, G.C. *et al.* (1996) The natural history of human papillomavirus type 16 capsid antibodies among a cohort of university women. *Journal of Infectious Diseases*, **174**, 927–936.

14 Stanley, M. (1999) Mechanism of action of imiquamod. Review. *Papillomavirus Report*, **10 (2)**, 23–29.

15 New Zealand HPV Project (1999) *Guidelines for the management of genital warts and/or genital HPV in New Zealand* (adapted). New Zealand HPV Project, Auckland, New Zealand.

10

11 Endometriosis and Chronic Pelvic Pain

Endometriosis is a pathological cause of pelvic pain that is part of the differential diagnosis of chronic pelvic pain, the aetiology of which is multifactorial.

Physical disorders include irritable bowel syndrome, adhesions, pelvic inflammatory disease, interstitial cystitis, musculoskeletal factors and nerve-related pain. As with all chronic pain, psychological factors modify it and it can cause varying degrees of dysfunction. Chronic pelvic pain (CPP) is pain in the lower abdomen or pelvis of at least 6 months' duration, occurring continuously or intermittently, not associated exclusively with menstruation or sexual intercourse and not relieved by analgesics and not associated with any precise physical cause. It results in significant altered physical activity and mood disturbance and ultimately results in a dysfunctional lifestyle.

History taking in relation to interpreting causation of chronic pelvic pain should include an acknowledgement from the physician of the reality of the patient's pain and identify factors which contribute to the pain. Definitive treatment may be multidisciplinary but the gynaecologist has a precise role in providing a laparoscopic diagnosis if indicated (40 per cent of diagnostic laparoscopies do not identify any pathological cause of CPP) and treatment of endometriosis. Morbidity from laparoscopy may be up to 0.6 per cent and can be serious.

DEFINITION OF ENDOMETRIOSIS

Endometriosis is an enigmatic disease. It is the presence of ectopic tissue with the histological structure and function of the uterine mucosa. Endometriosis is characterised by proliferation, differentiation and subsequent invasion into the underlying tissue. Histological confirmation must identify both endometrial glands and stroma. Haemosiderin-laden macrophages are identified in up to 80 per cent of endometriotic biopsies. It affects women in the reproductive age

11

group (2–5 per cent), with higher rates in those of low parity or in those who have not had ovulation switched off.

Proposed aetiological physiological mechanism

- Coelomic metaplasia. Under the influence of certain unspecified stimuli, mesothelial cells might undergo a metaplastic change to endometrium.
- Transplantation of exfoliated endometrium. Lymphatic, vascular and iatrogenic routes may disseminate endometriosis. Transtubal regurgitation is the most common route.
- Retrograde menstruation (Sampson's theory) occurs possibly as a result of a hypotonic uterotubal junction in women with endometriosis, allowing increased menstrual regurgitation.

Endometriosis at laparoscopy

Superficial peritoneal implants arise because of implantation but these are found in most women and often regress spontaneously. Cystic ovarian and deep infiltrating endometriosis is a disease state caused by both genetic factors in predisposed individuals exposed to environmental risk factors. Pain is caused by the release of inflammatory mediators of pain such as bradykinins and prostaglandins. Pain from endometriomas and nodular disease may be caused by traction on tissues or by infiltration or stretching of nerves themselves.

SYMPTOMS OF ENDOMETRIOSIS AND DIAGNOSIS

Dysmenorrhoea

Dysmenorrhoea varies in severity and duration and from cycle to cycle.

Symptoms are often initially mild. They encapsulate a chronic gnawing quality and finally cause dysfunction in life patterns. Endometriosis is an enigmatic disease. Women with only a few scattered implants of endometriosis may have the most severe complaints of pelvic pain compared with those with dense adhesions and large amounts of active disease, including endometriomas, who may

11

be totally asymptomatic, i.e. there is poor correlation between the extent of disease and the severity of the symptoms. Often the pain occurs before the onset of menstrual flow and worsens with flow. Peritoneal irritation and pain is caused through leaking implants and production of prostaglandins in the menstrual fluid.

Menstruation involves prostaglandin-induced arterial vasospasm and uterine contractions to raise intrauterine pressure and expel uterine contents. Dysmenorrhoea is the result of pressure developing within the endometrial cavity which depends on the magnitude of the contractions as well as the calibre of, and the pressure within, the exits of the uterine cavity – the cervical canal and the fallopian tube ostia.

Dyspareunia

Pain on deep penetration that is reproducible on pelvic examination is the only type of dyspareunia suggestive of endometriosis. It can often be well localised and is more severe at the end of the cycle with menstruation. Deeply invasive lesions (implants which invade 5 mm or more) are more strongly correlated with symptoms of pelvic pain and dyspareunia than superficial lesions. Deeply invasive endometriosis occurs almost entirely in the depth of the pelvis, 55 per cent in the pouch of Douglas, 35 per cent in the uterosacral ligaments and 11 per cent in the uterovaginal fold. Endometriotic deposits in the cul-de-sac are frequently surrounded by hard fibrotic material. This contains active endometriotic glandular tissue. Hard deposits are often very tender on vaginal examination [1].

Premenstrual spotting

This occurs in up to 35 per cent of patients with endometriosis and occurs several days before the onset of flow.

CLINICAL FINDINGS

Viable endometriotic implants may occur on the perineum and vaginal mucosae. The cervix may be deviated because of retraction of the ipsilateral uterosacral ligament. The uterus may be immobile and retroverted or fixed in the cul-de-sac by pelvic adhesions. The uterosacral ligaments should be palpated for the presence of nodules

11

which are often tender. Pain with vaginal examination is elicited better during menses because the implants are relative larger and more tender. The adnexal regions may have ovarian masses due to the presence of endometriomas.

Endometriosis can affect the urinary tract. The bladder is the most common site, followed by the ureter and kidney. When the bladder is affected symptoms include dysuria, urgency and frequency. Haematuria, flank and abdominal pain are more common with ureteral and/or kidney involvement. Ureteral endometriosis may result in loss of renal function due to hydronephrosis. Endometriosis may occur in other sites, including diaphragmatic, pleural and lungs.

Endometriosis affects up to 20 per cent of women (as seen at laparoscopy) and from 25 to 40 per cent of those with subfertility. The mode of inheritance is probably polygenic and multifactorial.

An altered cellular immune response to autologous antigens, together with possible alterations in cell-mediated immunity, predisposes some women to endometriosis.

INVESTIGATION

Endometriosis may be imaged by ultrasound scanning (see Chapter 6), particularly identifying endometriomas, but the substantive diagnosis is made at laparoscopy.

AIMS OF MANAGEMENT

- To relieve symptoms
- Make an accurate diagnosis
- To improve the quality of life.
  Treatment choices are dependent on
- Reproductive history and fertility plans
- Nature and severity of the symptoms
- Previous treatments and their success
- Location and severity of disease.

If immediate fertility is a major concern medical treatment is contraindicated. There is no fertility benefit from drugs used to suppress ovulation and thus induce amenorrhoea. The months of treatment merely deprive women of ovulatory cycles exposed to the possibility of conception and there is no improved subsequent fertility rate.

11

The approximate recurrence rate of endometriosis after medical therapy is 30–50 per cent, and about 20 per cent of patients have recurrence over 5 years after surgical excision of endometriosis.

VISUAL FEATURES OF ENDOMETRIOTIC LESIONS AT LAPAROSCOPY

Visual descriptions have included terms such as: red raspberries, purple raspberries, blueberries, blebs, peritoneal pockets, whitish scar tissue, stellate scar tissue, strawberry-coloured lesions, red vesicles, white vesicles, clear vesicles, powder burns, peritoneal windows, yellow-brown patches, brown-black patches, adhesions, clear polypoid lesions, red flame-like lesions, black puckered spots, white plaques with black puckers and chocolate cysts (Fig. 11.1).

Classification of different peritoneal endometriotic lesions

Superficial lesion can be:
- Red (red vesicular, flame-like or vascularised polypoidal)
- Black (classical black puckered)
- White (scar tissue with or without pigmentation).

Red lesions are proliferative lesions showing great similarity with the upper levels of the endometrium. Black and white lesions are less active or inactive and have decreased vascularisation and increased scarring. The chronic shedding seen in red lesions induces an inflammatory reaction, causing fibrosis and scarring and ultimately healing of the implant.

Typical or classically recognised lesions of endometriosis are black-brown 'powder burn', and black or puckered black stellate lesions.

Atypical lesions may be clear and vesicular (like sago) or white and opacified. They may appear as glandular excrescences or haemorrhagic vesicles. Defects in the pelvic peritoneum can also occur, characterised by scarring overlying endometriotic implants.

Laparoscopy

The pelvic cavity should be systematically inspected and should include all surfaces of the ovaries, the ovarian fossae, pelvic peritoneum (particularly the cul-de-sac, ureters, and bladder peritoneum), uterine ligaments, sigmoid colon, appendix, fallopian tubes

11

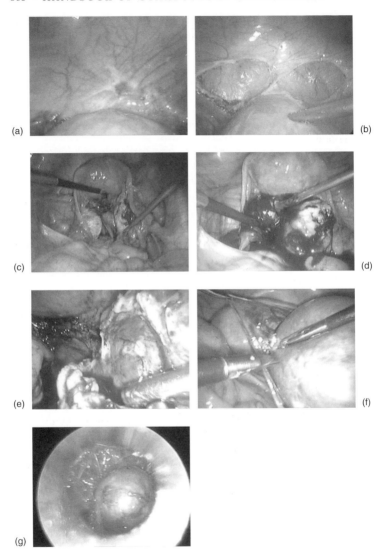

Fig. 11.1 (a) Classic powder burn endometriosis on the bladder dome.
(b) Pouch of Douglas endometriosis – scarred. (c) As after excision.
(d) Endometriotic chocolate cyst. (e) As after excision. (f) Endometrioma
being excised from the ovary. (g) As in a bag after excision intact.

11

and rectovaginal septum. Laparoscopy with its 8 times magnification can identify peritoneal lesions as small as 400 mm in diameter.

Endometriotic lesions may be identified as the most active implants which are aggressive and painful by filling the pelvis with irrigation fluid. Clear vesicles appear three-dimensional. The tissue balloons from the peritoneum.

Biopsy of lesions increases the diagnosis of endometriosis from 40 up to 80 per cent, since up to one third of women have atypical lesions.

Ovarian endometrioma

More than 90 per cent of endometriomas occur as an extraovarian pseudocyst. The pseudocyst wall is formed by the inverted cortex. The frontal or lateral surface of the ovary is the most frequent site of occurrence where the folding-in process of the cortex is shown.

Nodular endometriosis

Deep endometriosis is a nodular lesion histologically characterised by a dense structure which is composed of fibrous tissue and smooth muscle cells with islands or strands of glands and stroma (adenomyosis). The major component of the nodular lesion is not endometrial but fibromuscular tissue with sparse finger-like extensions of glandular and stromal tissue. The nodular lesion is characteristically located at pelvic supportive structures such as the uterosacral ligaments, the retrocervical fascia, the rectovaginal septum and the ovarian ligaments. It is a proliferative lesion and shows poor or absent secretory changes during the luteal phase of the menstrual cycle, and vasodilatation rather than necrosis and bleeding at the time of menstruation.

This myeloproliferative type of endometriosis is found in 25 per cent of lesions of the uterosacral ligament and in up to 90 per cent of lesions of the rectovaginal septum.

The normal laparoscopic view of the pelvis should show a hollow concave space between the rectum and the back of the uterus. Sponge-holding forceps ought to be inserted into the vagina to put up the posterior fornix. It is then easily seen if the cul-de-sac is normal between the rectum and the back of the uterus.

11

When isolated cul-de-sac obliteration occurs the rectum is pulled up and forwards and becomes attached to the back of the uterus. If the sponge holder is inserted into the posterior fornix the outline of the forceps will not be seen laparoscopically. The disease may extend posteriorly to involve the serous and muscularis layers of the rectum or sigmoid colon. This may extend to the lateral wall of the pelvis with involvement of the ureter and iliac vessels.

CLASSIFICATION OF ENDOMETRIOSIS (rAFS) [2]

Endometriosis has been reclassified by the American Fertility Society in an attempt to delineate the extent of ovarian involvement and adhesive disease in patients with endometriosis and provide for comparisons for the efficacy of medical and surgical treatment (Table 11.1) in trials. However, it is difficult to use and there is still a lack of worldwide consistency in classification of disease.

It is also important to record the depth of infiltration, size and distribution of lesions as there is some evidence that depth of invasion of lesions correlates with severity of pain.

TREATMENT

Medical treatments' including oral contraceptives, danazol, progestogens, gonadotrophin-releasing hormone (GnRH) agonists and gestrinone, produce temporary relief of symptoms. No drug eradicates endometriosis or produces long-term cure, particularly in those women with deeply invasive disease. Discontinuation of medication usually results in a recurrence of pain within 12 months.

Endometriosis and subfertility

Medical treatment does not enhance fertility because it interferes with the opportunity for pregnancy to occur by providing a contraceptive effect. Therefore long-term data show a decreased pregnancy rate. In contrast surgical treatment is effective in the treatment of infertility. Pregnancy rates are up to 40 per cent higher than with non-surgical treatment.

11

Table 11.1 Revised American Fertility Society (rAFS) classification of endometriosis. (With permission from Buttram (1985) [2].)

	Endometriosis		<1 cm	1–3 cm	>3 cm
Peritoneum		Superficial	1	2	4
		Deep	2	4	6
Ovary	R	Superficial	1	2	4
		Deep	4	16	20
	L	Superficial	1	2	4
		Deep	4	16	20

	Posterior culdesac obliteration	Partial	Complete
		4	40

	Adhesions		$<\frac{1}{3}$ enclosure	$\frac{1}{3}$–$\frac{2}{3}$ enclosure	$>\frac{2}{3}$ enclosure
Ovary	R	Filmy	1	2	4
		Dense	4	8	16
	L	Filmy	1	2	4
		Dense	4	8	16
Tube	R	Filmy	1	2	4
		Dense	4	8	16
	L	Filmy	1	2	4
		Dense	4	8	16

Stage I (minimal)	1–5
Stage II (mild)	6–15
Stage III (moderate)	16–40
Stage IV (severe)	>40

R, right; L, left.

MEDICAL THERAPY FOR ENDOMETRIOSIS
Analgesia

Symptoms may be managed effectively with general non-specific measures: analgesia combined with relaxation, exercise and psychological support. Dihydrocodeine may be effective, together with non-steroidal anti-inflammatories and paracetamol.

11

The combined oral contraceptive pill

This may be preferable because it has the least adverse side effects profile. A 'tri-cycle regimen' (3 weeks) continuously for 3 months followed by a week's break is most efficacious for the symptoms of endometriosis.

Progestogens

Dydrogesterone and medroxyprogesterone acetate are given continuously in moderately high doses and lead to inhibition of ovulation and lowered oestradiol levels. Their precise mode of action is unclear but they are likely to have a direct inhibitory effect on endometriotic tissue.

- The dose can be started at 20–30 mg/day and increased in subsequent cycles to 50–100 mg/day if necessary to achieve amenorrhoea.
- Side effects include nausea, breast tenderness, bloating, fluid retention, depression, weight gain, moodiness, acne and breast discomfort. Spotting or irregular heavy bleeding may be a problem but can be reversed by increasing the dose. Long-term oral progestogens may cause an increased risk of cardiovascular disease because of their increase in low density lipoproteins (LDL) and decrease in high density lipoprotein (HDL) levels.

Danazol (Table 11.2)

This is a synthetic derivative of 17α-ethinyltestosterone which causes
- Inhibition of ovulation
- Suppression of menses.

Dosage
The dosage is 200–800 mg daily in two to four divided doses, initially at a dose of 800 mg in four divided doses. The maintenance dose may be a reduced dose, and is given for up to 6 months at a time.

- Danazol induces a state of hypogonadism but women are not hypo-oestrogenic. It induces a state of oestrogenised anovulation with mild androgenisation.
- It causes regressive changes of the vaginal mucosa and marked atrophy of the endometrium.

11

Table 11.2 Side effects of danazol.

	Percentage
Weight gain	4
Seborrhoea	2
Mild hirsutism	5
Oedema	6
Hair loss	
Voice change	3
Menstrual disturbance – spotting, amenorrhoea, flushing	6
Vaginal dryness and irritation	4
Sweating	3
Hepatic dysfunction – rare hepatic effects are cholestatic jaundice, hepatic adenoma, rashes	3
Nausea	2
Vomiting, constipation, indigestion and gastroenteritis, muscle cramps, spasms or pains, arthralgia, headache, emotional lability, irritability, nervousness, anxiety, changes in appetite and depression	
Elevated blood pressure and exacerbation of existing hypertension, increased insulin requirements in diabetic patients	

- It gives relief of presenting symptoms of dysmenorrhoea, pelvic pain and dyspareunia.
- There is resolution of ectopic endometrial implants and induration of the cul-de-sac.
- It gives improvement in haemoglobin value.
- It alters the serum lipid concentrations and sex hormone-binding globulin but not to a clinically significant extent.
- It can cross the placenta and thus virilise the external genitalia of the female fetus. There is no effect on the male fetus.
- It produces a significant improvement in pain with the atrophy of the ectopic endometrium.
- Side effects include irregular vaginal bleeding. Features of androgenisation include a mild anabolic effect manifested by increased muscle mass resulting in an increase in the lean body mass–fat ratio. Muscle spasms or twitches occur because of a direct stimulatory effect on striated muscle.
- Side effects attributable to androgenic activity are acne, oily skin or hair, mild hirsutism, oedema, weight gain, deepening of

11

the voice, decrease in breast size, and occasionally clitoral hypertrophy.

▪ Other side effects are gastrointestinal disturbances, increased or decreased blood cell count, headache, backache, dizziness, tremor, depression, fatigue, sleep disorders, muscle spasm or cramp, alopecia, skin rash, hyperglucogenaemia, abnormal glucose tolerance, decreased serum HDL cholesterol, increased serum LDL cholesterol, occasionally elevation of liver function tests and cholestatic jaundice. Some patients may get tachycardia and intracranial hypertension and visual disturbances.

▪ Voice changes are not reversible. The adverse side effects have been widely publicised and consequently there is often widespread consumer resistance to this drug.

Precautions with the use of danazol

Although danazol inhibits ovulation pregnancies can occur and barrier contraception ought to be advised.

Thrombosis and thrombophlebitis have been reported, as have cholestatic jaundice, alteration of lipoproteins – decreased HDL and increased LDL – and decreased glucose tolerance.

Gestrinone (Dimetriose)

Gestrinone is a synthetic steroid hormone with an antiprogestin activity. It has a weak androgen and progestogen activity. Its main action is on the hypothalamic–pituitary axis where it inhibits gonadotrophin release with a weak inhibitory effect on synthesis. It also possesses anti-oestrogen activity. The suppression of the ovulatory gonadotrophin peak is seen after the first month of treatment. The resulting decrease in oestrogen ovarian secretion leads to endometrial atrophy. Gestrinone also has antiprogesterone activity on cell receptors in both the endometrium and the extrauterine ectopic implants.

Dosage

The dosage is one capsule (2.5 mg) twice a week. The first dose should be taken on the first day of the menstrual cycle and the second 3 days later and thereafter on the same 2 days of the week for the duration of treatment, which should be 6 months. If spotting occurs the dose can be increased to three capsules per week. Barrier contraception should be used because pregnancies can occur despite the inhibition of ovulation in many women.

Adverse reactions

These are usually related to the slight androgenic activity of gestrinone. Spotting, acne, seborrhoea, fluid retention, weight gain, hirsutism, hair loss, decrease in breast size, voice change and other androgen side effects may occur. Other undesirable effects include headaches, irritability, gastrointestinal disorders, changes in libido, hot flushes, cramps, arthralgia, increase in liver transaminase, and isolated cases of benign intracranial hypertension.

GnRH agonists (Fig. 11.2)

- GnRH agonists suppress pituitary follicle-stimulating hormone (FSH) and luteinising hormone (LH) secretion and this decreases ovarian oestrogen secretion dramatically [3].
- Thus they induce a state of hypogonadism or pseudomenopause. Use can only be for 6 months because of bone demineralisation. Hypo-oestrogenic side effects (atrophic vaginitis and vasomotor hot flushes) may be severe. The cost is high. They are indicated except in the most severely symptomatic patient recalcitrant to other treatments who requires only temporary treatment.
- Many different GnRH agonists are available [4]. There is no clear evidence that any one is superior in terms of pain relief or decrease in endometriotic deposits. They are rapidly degraded by the gastrointestinal tract.
- Administration is nasal, subcutaneous (daily) or as subcutaneous depo injections or intramuscular injections (monthly). The latter have the advantage of consistency of the endocrine response and greater compliance.
- GnRH agonists induce bone loss greater than after a natural menopause, averaging 1 per cent per month during a 6-month treatment period. There is a significant loss of bone mineral density at the lumbar spine of 1.5–12 per cent after 6 months of GnRH agonist treatment. Losses of 1–4 per cent for the femoral neck and 5 per cent for the distal radius have been reported. Recovery of bone mineral density does not appear to be universal, although some bone loss is reversible after cessation of GnRH agonist therapy. Some may be permanent.

11

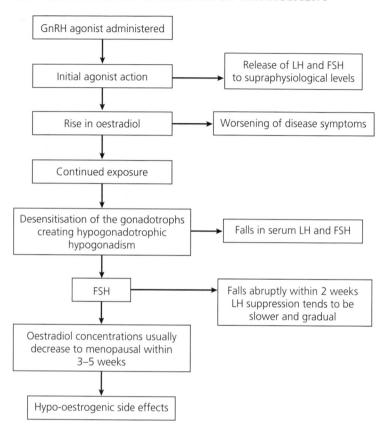

Fig. 11.2 Mechanism of action of GnRH agonists.

Systemic effects of GnRH agonists

Twelve to thirty per cent experience intermittent spotting or bleeding. One or two per cent may experience profuse vaginal bleeding. Menstruation returns 69–84 days after discontinuing GnRH agonists. Hot flushes can be reduced by the administration of combined HRT. Medroxyprogesterone acetate (15–100 mg/day) also has beneficial effects on hot flushes and sweating.

Tibolone (2.5 mg) and norethisterone (ranging from 1 to 10 mg daily) are also effective. The addition of norethisterone (5–10 mg) significantly improves vaginal dryness and dyspareunia compared with GnRH agonists only. Medroxyprogesterone acetate (15 mg) improves libido in 10 per cent of women. Oestrogens may also reduce memory deficits induced by GnRH agonist treatment alone.

Add-back therapy

- 'Add back' therapy (tibolone or a progesterone plus or minus an oestrogen) can be used with no loss of efficacy to relieve menopausal effects, prevent bone loss and allow therapy to continue beyond 6 months. Leuprolide acetate with add-back therapy has been used for over 12 months [5].
- Continuous combined therapy has benefits over cyclical therapy. In postmenopausal women with a history of endometriosis the continuous combined oestrogen–progestogen replacement regimen is preferred over cyclic regimens.
- Alternatively, the oestrogen component of add-back therapy should contain a minimum of 0.625 mg (or the equivalent, such as conjugated 2 mg oestradiol valerate or 0.05 mg transdermal oestradiol combined with medroxyprogesterone acetate). Medroxyprogesterone acetate is less androgenic. It abolishes FSH recovery, lowers sex hormone-binding globulin, thus increasing the levels of free oestradiol and testosterone. It is lipid neutral and protects against bone loss. Medroxyprogesterone acetate may be inferior to norethisterone in the treatment of endometriosis, but when combined with oestrogen its effects are similar. It is unclear whether 5 or 10 mg is the preferred dose.
- Treatment with GnRH agonists should include a mechanical form of contraception.
- In a randomised trial comparing danazol to GnRH agonists, 10–20 per cent required further treatment within a year. Discontinuation of danazol therapy is usually associated with a recurrence of pelvic pain within 12 months.
- Most women with endometriosis who subsequently become menopausal do not experience reactivation of endometriosis with the commencement of hormone replacement therapy (HRT). Adding back oestrogen after giving GnRH agonists does not stimulate the disease. It is thought that it is the cyclical nature of ovarian steroid release which is essential for the development and maintenance of fibroid and endometriotic growth. Low circulating oestradiol levels (110 pmol/l) are the minimal degree of hypo-oestrogenism that will

11

reliably produce atrophy of the endometriotic gland. Adding back small amounts of oestrogen increases circulating levels enough to maintain the integrity of tissues such as bone with relief of vasomotor symptoms. Fibroids and the degree of endometriosis stay static.

▪ GnRH agonists may be a useful primary therapeutic option in women with endometriosis in the American Fertility Society stages II–III, and as an adjuvant to surgery for stage IV disease. GnRH agonists significantly reduce painful symptoms of endometriosis and the extent of endometriotic implants. Symptomatic relief is achieved within a month of commencing therapy. This may continue for up to 6 months after cessation of treatment. Maximal reduction in this stage of disease may occur at 6 months. For endometriosis the addition of 100 mg medroxyprogesterone acetate or tibolone for add-back therapy reduces the undesired hypo-oestrogenic side effects of GnRH agonists.

Mifepristone

The antiprogesterone mifepristone (RU486) (100 mg daily for 3 months) results in improvement in pelvic pain for the first cycle of treatment. A further 50 mg daily for 6 months results in a 55 per cent reduction in the incidence of implants. Mifepristone suppresses ectopic endometrial bleeding.

SURGICAL TREATMENT

If patients have surgical treatment of their endometriosis at the time of their diagnostic laparoscopy, drugs are no longer the automatic first-line treatment. A specific trial of therapy is warranted for those with:

▪ Recurrent or persistent pain where there is no obvious residual endometriosis at repeat laparoscopy.

▪ Residual disease where there is a wish to avoid further surgery because of risk of complications.

▪ Symptoms suggestive of endometriosis but few clinical signs, where there is a desire for a trial of medical therapy in the period before a laparoscopy or where a laparoscopy is not desired for definitive diagnosis and treatment.

Superficial removal of endometriosis with various ablative techniques has been shown in a randomised trial to produce long-term

11

symptomatic improvement in women with mild and moderate disease [6,7]. Six months after surgery in women with stage I, II or III endometriosis, 62.5 per cent of the treated women had improved compared with 22.6 per cent in the placebo group.

The surgical approach to endometriosis should be the meticulous removal of extrauterine disease, leaving the uterus and ovaries, particularly in women wishing to become pregnant. Excision using either monopolar hook electrode, the carbon dioxide laser or scissors has been shown to be highly effective using both laparotomy and laparoscopy [8].

The 5-year risk of a diagnosis of new endometriosis following laparoscopic excision is approximately 20 per cent. There are significant and sustained improvements in pelvic pain, dyspareunia and painful bowel movements after extensive laparoscopic excision.

Best results are achieved from patients in whom the pain is accurately correlated with specific pelvic pathology (e.g. pain in the pouch of Douglas or uterosacral nodules) [9]. Excision or destruction of the endometriotic tissue, particularly deep infiltrating endometriotic implants, may be of benefit. Ovarian endometriomas should be excised, including the capsule.

Extensive laparoscopic excision

Surgical preparation before laparoscopic clearance includes the necessity for bowel preparation with fluids such as Cleanprep, GoLytely, Picolax. Patients need to be counselled as to the risk of bowel injury, peritonitis and colostomy and the possibility of laparotomy. A four-puncture laparoscopic approach with a 10 mm umbilical trocar for the laparoscope and three 5 mm lower ports for the surgical instruments is used. Excision is done using 5 mm monopolar electrosurgical scissors, either on cut modality or coagulation, depending on the vascularity of the lesion. Additional haemostasis is achieved using bipolar forceps. The endometrial lesion is excised by elevating the peritoneum adjacent to the deposit and opening it. The cut edge is grasped and pulled towards the midline and the excision is extended until the lesion is completely outlined. It is then undercut and freed so that the whole lesion and a surrounding margin of healthy tissue is removed. All tissue is examined histologically.

11

Both uterosacral ligaments are frequently extensively involved and invasive deposits may be found in the rectovaginal septum, the front of the rectum and in the ovaries. The use of vaginal and rectal probes enables definition of the peritoneal surface and the endometriotic deposits project outwards.

Endometriosis is removed by beginning on the left pelvic side wall just cephalic to the last deposit. The excision is extended towards the uterus lateral and parallel to the left uterosacral ligament. The uterosacral ligament is pushed medially and down and healthy tissues including the ureter are pushed upwards and laterally away from the dissection. The incision is then extended across the back of the uterus and healthy tissue above the deposits. It then transects the right uterosacral ligament and is continued along the right pelvic side wall just lateral to and above the right uterosacral ligament until it extends beyond all the visible deposits. It is then taken across the front of the rectum to join with the original incision. This block of tissue is then undercut and freed from the underlying structures. This usually incorporates all of the uterosacral ligaments, the recto-vaginal septum and the prerectal tissues down to the level of the pelvic floor.

Ovarian endometriomata are drained. The cavity is flushed. A biopsy of the wall is taken and then the surface of the cyst is vaporised with a monopolar electrosurgical ball, a carbon dioxide (CO_2) laser or an argon beam coagulator.

Cystoscopy may be done at the end of the procedure by injecting indigo-carmine dye (American Regent Laboratory, New York) to check the integrity of the bladder and ureters. Alternatively, any perforation of the bladder in laparoscopic surgery is indicated by the urinary catheter bag 'ballooning up' due to gas transmission. A rectal integrity test may also be done using methylene blue dye. Prophylactic antibiotics are given intraoperatively.

Laparoscopic excision results in a marked improvement in dysmenorrhoea and lower abdominal pain. With relief of the anatomical distortions perirectally, bowel symptoms improve. With advanced invasive endometriosis there is a large fibromuscular reaction around the endometrial glands and stroma. It is unlikely that hormonal medication removes such fibromuscular deposits. Hormonal suppression does not appear to be of long-term clinical benefit where there is nodular invasive disease.

11

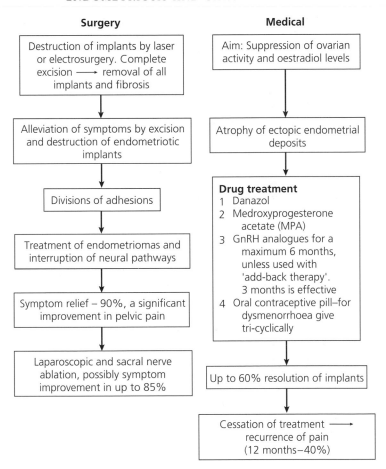

Fig. 11.3 The management of endometriosis.

Surgery and fertility (Fig. 11.3)

With severe endometriosis, fertility is improved by successful lysis of adhesions, removal of endometriomas and restoration of normal anatomy. Other causes of infertility must be excluded or corrected.

Treatment can be by laparoscopy or laparotomy, with microsurgical technique [10].

Destroying all visible lesions does not establish normal fertility [11]. Patients may still need other assisted reproductive techniques such as:

- Controlled ovarian superovulation using low dose fertility drugs to create two to three oocytes with intrauterine insemination (IUI) of partner's sperm.
- *In vitro* fertilisation (IVF).

A systematic review comparing IUI and ovarian hyperstimulation to no treatment in women with subfertility and minimal or mild endometriosis showed significantly better pregnancy rates [12,13]. Outcomes following IVF in women with endometriosis compared to those with tubal infertility showed that pregnancy rates per cycle were significantly lower in the endometriosis group (25 per cent versus 36 per cent, $p < 0.005$) [14].

A meta-analysis of published non-randomised controlled trials suggested that surgical treatment of endometriosis associated with infertility resulted in higher pregnancy rates than medical treatment or expectant management [15].

Following laparoscopic surgery recurrence rates are only of the order of 20 per cent compared to up to 75 per cent for medical treatment. It must be noted that hysterectomy does not always relieve all symptoms of endometriosis, probably because of extrauterine deposits in the lower bowel and around the ureter and in the rectovaginal septum. Radical laparoscopic excision of all areas of advanced invasive endometriosis produces a marked improvement in local and general symptoms, but evaluation is limited to <5 years.

Hysterectomy

Pain due to endometriosis and adenomyosis may be treated by hysterectomy once childbearing is complete. Where the ovaries are normal there is no indication to remove them. All endometriotic tissue is removed from the ovary. Ten per cent of women will require another gynaecological operation following hysterectomy for endometriosis when the ovaries remain in situ [16].

11

Table 11.3 The Rome criteria for irritable bowel syndrome. (With permission from Drossman *et al* (1990) [18].)

At least 3 months of intermittent or constant pain that is relieved by defecation and associated with a change in the frequency or consistency of the stool
And at least two of the following:
Altered stool frequency
Altered stool form (diarrhoea, pellet formation, etc.)
Altered stool passage (straining, urgency, etc.)
Passage of mucus
Bloating

PELVIC PAIN – IRRITABLE BOWEL SYNDROME [17]

Irritable bowel syndrome (IBS) is a common (20 per cent of women), heterogeneous, chronic, relapsing, functional bowel disease (i.e. pain is due to changes in bowel habit from abnormal behaviour of the bowel, or abnormal perception of the physiological process). The agreed criteria (Rome criteria) may be seen in Table 11.3 [18]. IBS is associated with up to 50 per cent of consultations with a gastroenterologist. Forty to sixty per cent of patients have symptoms of depression or anxiety, are more neurotic and less extroverted, and traumatic life events frequently precede the onset of IBS symptoms. Abuse is not uncommonly associated. Stress and enteric infection may result in persistent muscle dysfunction. IBS is a diagnosis of exclusion.

Investigations for IBS

- Haematology
- Laparoscopy (to exclude endometriosis)
- Flexible sigmoidoscopy
- Lactose tolerance test
- Exclude infectious, metabolic and structural disorders of the gastrointestinal tract
- In patients more than 40 years of age, colonoscopy or double-contrast enema.

11

Results not compatible with a diagnosis of IBS

- Elevated erythrocyte sedimentation rate (ESR) (exclude colonic adenocarcinoma, villous adenoma)
- Increased C reactive protein in serum (exclude ulcerative colitis, Crohn's disease)
- Leukocytosis
- Blood, pus or fat in the stools
- Stool volumes above 200 g per day or persistence of diarrhoea during fasting weigh against IBS (exclude parasites, e.g. giardiasis).

Essentially it is a diagnosis of exclusion, diagnosed from the history alone. Women with IBS have an increased incidence of non-bowel symptoms, including bladder dysfunction, dyspareunia and back pain. More than 50 per cent of IBS patients retain their symptoms 1–10 years later. Children with IBS retain the disease as adults.

Management of irritable bowel syndrome

- Reassure the patient of the absence of serious organic disease, but acknowledge the problem. Explain the nature and mechanisms of symptoms and identify aggravating and alleviating factors.
- Dietary and symptoms diary may identify exacerbating factors for IBS.
- Luminal factors (carbohydrates, bile acids, food allergens) may have a role in patients with predominantly diarrhoea symptoms. Observe symptoms after withdrawal of these.
- Lactose, fructose, sorbitol, aspartame and caffeine intake can affect IBS. Abnormal food sensitivity is controversial, but lactose intolerance is well recognised.
- Soluble dietary fibre may improve diarrhoea through stool water absorption, and/or induction of more normal colonic contractility patterns, but the routine use of bran in IBS patients is not recommended because bowel disturbance is often adversely affected.

Pharmacological treatment of symptoms of IBS

1 Diarrhoea

- Loperamide (2 mg b.i.d.; does not cross the blood–brain barrier) or diphenoxylate (2.5–5 mg q.i.d.) or cholestyramine (half to one packet up to twice daily)

11

2 Constipation

- Intensive fibre regimen – wheat bran, $\frac{1}{2}$ cup to 1 bowl per day
- Osmotic laxatives may be added if fibre alone is insufficient
- Prokinetic agents – metoclopramide, dromperidone
- Cisapride (5–10 mg t.d.s.) for constipation as the predominant symptom. It acts through acetylcholine release at the myenteric plexus level and agonism of 5-hydroxytryptamine receptor subtypes, increasing small bowel and colonic transit.

3 Pain, distension and gas

- Cimetropium bromide (50 mg t.d.s.) is a gut-selective agent
- Antidepressants may be helpful through their central analgesic effects, anticholinergic activity or relief of depression
- Amitriptyline, 10–25 mg for every hour of sleep
- Desipramine, 50 mg for every hour of sleep.

Benzodiazepine-like anxiolytics may be used for short periods. The use of other agents such as somatostatin agonists, calcium-channel blockers, GnRH agonists and serotonin-receptor antagonists is experimental.

BLADDER-RELATED PAIN

The principal urological causes of pain are interstitial cystitis and urethral syndrome. Interstitial cystitis is an inflammatory condition of unknown aetiology characterised by pain and bladder symptoms such as urgency, frequency and nocturia. The pain typically increases as the bladder fills and is relieved by passing urine and may be recreated by pressure on the bladder base on vaginal examination. Cystoscopy identifies submucosal oedema and petechiae. A 'Hunner' ulcer is pathognomonic.

Chronic urethral syndrome is characterised by irritative symptoms as well as post-void fullness and incontinence, which is rare in interstitial cystitis. Urethral syndrome is associated with vulvar irritation, vulvodynia, dyspareunia and postcoital voiding difficulties and CPP.

MUSCULOSKELETAL PAIN

Pain arising from the musculoskeletal system characteristically varies with movement and posture and may be exacerbated at the

11

end of the day. Pain can usually be elicited by manoeuvres which stress the affected joints or ligaments. Muscle pain may be due to poor posture. Recently interest has centred on myofascial trigger points, for instance in the abdominal wall (a hyperirritable spot, within a tight band of muscle or fascia).

NERVE-RELATED PAIN

Entrapped nerves in scar tissue or fascia may give rise to pain typically at or beneath a scar in the distribution of the nerve. The pain tends to be sharp or stabbing in nature, or may be a constant dull ache. It is usually highly localised and may be exacerbated by some movements. Diagnosis can be confirmed by injection of local anaesthetic at the site of maximal tenderness, at the level of the fascia, giving complete relief of the pain.

REFERENCES

1 Koninckx, P.R., Lesaffre, E., Meuleman, C., Cornillie, F.J. & Demeyere, S. (1991) Suggestive evidence that pelvic endometriosis is a progressive disease, whereas deeply infiltrating endometriosis is associated with pelvic pain. *Fertility and Sterility*, **55**, 759–765.

2 Buttram, V.C. (1985) American Fertility Society classification of endometriosis. *Fertility and Sterility*, **43**, 347–352.

3 Waller, K.G. & Shaw, R.W. (1993) Gonadotrophin-releasing hormone analogues for the treatment of endometriosis: long-term follow-ups. *Fertility and Sterility*, **59**, 511–515.

4 Moghissi, K.S., Schlaff, W.D., Olive, D.L., Skinner, M.A. & Yin, H. (1998) Goserelin acetate (Zoladex) with or without hormone replacement therapy for the treatment of endometriosis. *Fertility and Sterility*, **69**, 1056–1062.

5 Howell, R., Edmonds, D.K., Dowsett, M., Crook, D., Lees, B. & Stevenson, J.C. (1995) Gonadotrophin-releasing hormone analogue (goserelin) plus hormone replacement therapy for the treatment of endometriosis: a randomised controlled trial. *Fertility and Sterility*, **64**, 474–481.

6 Sutton, C.J., Ewen, S.P., Whitelaw, N. & Haines, P. (1994) Prospective randomised double-blind trial of laser laparoscopy in the treatment of pelvic pain associated with minimal, mild and moderate endometriosis. *Fertility and Sterility*, **62**, 696–700.

7 Sutton, C.J., Pooley, A.S., Ewen, S.P. & Haines, P. (1997) Follow-up report on a randomised controlled trial of laser laparoscopy in the treatment of pelvic pain associated with minimal to moderate endometriosis. *Fertility and Sterility*, **68**, 1070–1074.

11

8 Redwine, D.B. (1991) Conservative laparoscopic excision of endometriosis by sharp dissection: life table analysis of reoperation and persistent or recurrent disease. *Fertility and Sterility*, **56**, 628–634.

9 Garry, R., Clayton, R. & Hawe, J. (2000) The effect of endometriosis and its radical laparoscopic excision on quality of life indicators. *British Journal of Obstetrics and Gynaecology*, **107**, 44–54.

10 Hughes, E.G., Fedorkow, D.M. & Collins, J.A. (1993) A quantitative overview of controlled trials in endometriosis-associated infertility. *Fertility and Sterility*, **59**, 963–970.

11 Adamson, G.D. & Pasta, D.J. (1994) Surgical treatment of endometriosis-associated infertility: meta-analysis compared with survival analysis. *American Journal of Obstetrics and Gynecology*, **171**, 1488–1505.

12 Nulsen J.C., Walsh, S., Dumez, S. & Metzger, D.A. (1993) A randomised and longitudinal study of human menopausal gonadotrophin with intrauterine insemination in the treatment of infertility. *Obstetrics and Gynecology*, **82**, 780–786.

13 Tummon, I.S., Asher, L.J., Martin, J.S.B. & Tulandi, T. (1997) Randomised controlled trial of superovulation and insemination for infertility associated with minimal or mild endometriosis. *Fertility and Sterility*, **68**, 8–12.

14 Landazabal, A., Diaz, I., Valbuena D. *et al.* (1999) Endometriosis and *in vitro* fertilisation: a meta-analysis. *Human Reproduction*, **14** (Abstract book 1), 181–182.

15 Marcoux, S., Maheux, R. & Berube, S. (1997) Canadian Collaborative Group on Endometriosis. Laparoscopic surgery in infertile women with minimal or mild endometriosis. *New England Journal of Medicine*, **337**, 217–222.

16 Namnoum, A.B., Gehlbach, D.L., Hickman, T.N., Rock, J.A. & Goodman, S.B. (1995) Incidence of symptom recurrence after hysterectomy for endometriosis. *Fertility and Sterility*, **64**, 898–902.

17 Lynn, R.B. & Friedman, S.S. (1993) Irritable bowel syndrome. *The Lancet*, **329**, 1940–1945.

18 Drossman, D.A., Thompson, W.G., Talley, N.J., Funch-Jensen, P., Janssens, J. & Whitehead, W.E. (1990) Identification of subgroups of functional gastrointestinal disorders. *Gastroenterology International*, **3**, 159–172.

11

12 Vulval Disease and Gynaecological Dermatology

VULVAL DISEASE

Defining and treating vulval disease can be complex because of the chronicity of conditions and the implications in terms of psychosexual function. Accurate diagnosis is critical rather than merely giving empirical treatment. Vulval pain may be of psychosomatic origin or may be a physical disorder. In addition, there may be a psychosexual response to a physical disease or a physical response (e.g. vaginismus) to an emotional disorder. A history includes physical, psychological and sexual aspects of a woman's health. In particular ask about vulval pain following life stress.

History taking for vulval disease

Dermatology history
Enquire about:
- Atopy, eczema, psoriasis, lichen planus, other skin diseases, allergy
- Family history, personal history of the above
- Use of current and past topical and systemic medications.

Symptoms
- None, irritation, pruritus, soreness, pain, bleeding, lumps, burning, discharge
- Dysuria, dyspareunia
- Genuine contact dermatitis of the vulva is rare.

Time of onset of symptoms
- Relation to life events/stress/other medical conditions
- Duration – less than 1 month, 1–3 months, 3–12 months, 1–5 years, 5–10 years, 10+ years
- Area of discomfort
- Precipitating/exacerbating/alleviating factors

- Any treatment that has been tried
- Sexual consequences
- History of sexual abuse?

Examination of the vulva

- The skin should be examined generally, including the mouth.
- Inspect the vulva under good lighting conditions; ideally, the vulval area should be examined under colposcopic magnification.
- Posterior fourchette fissures may mimic vestibulitis and therefore women should be examined 24–48 hours after sexual intercourse.
- Swabs should be taken when necessary.
- Biopsies should be performed under local anaesthetic. Use 4 mm Keyes disposable punch biopsy forceps or take an ellipse of tissue.
- Refer patients with unusual conditions.
- Record findings in accurate diagrammatic form, accurately annotating the normal anatomy, observing the lesions and measuring them.
- Note typical dermatological descriptions of lesions, e.g. flat, papules, plaques, erosion, ulcers, tumour, excoriation, condyloma, scaling, fissures, other. Multifocal, generalised, other mucosal lesions – check for similar lesions on other parts of the body.
- Send pathology to a pathologist with skills in diagnosing vulval conditions.
- Photographic recording is useful.

Normal vulval anatomy

- The labia majora are two prominent longitudinal folds bounding the urogenital vestibule. They taper posteriorly approaching the anus and blend anteriorly to form the mons pubis. The skin of the outer surface of the labia is pigmented and contains hairs. The inner surfaces are smooth with large sebaceous glands. Within the labial fold is areolar and fatty tissue.
- The labia minora are two small cutaneous folds between the labia majora. The skin is hairless with no fat. Sebaceous glands open onto their surface. They meet anteriorly forming the prepuce of the clitoris.
- The vestibule is the area between the labia minora bounded anteriorly by the clitoris, posteriorly by the fourchette, deeply by the

hymen and extends laterally to Hart's line (usually visible macro-scopically). It represents the junction of the non-keratinised and keratinised skin on the medial surface of the labia minora. On non-keratinised skin perfumes, in particular, are more irritant.

▪ The orifices of the vagina, urethra and the duct of the major vestibu-lar (Bartholin's) and Skene's glands (periurethral) open onto the vestibule. It is supplied by S_3 and S_4 branches of the pudendal nerve.

▪ The lymphatics of the upper vagina join those from the cervix and reach the external iliac and internal iliac nodes. The middle and lower regions drain along the vaginal vessels to the internal iliac groups. The lowest part of the vagina (below the hymen) drains to the superficial inguinal node groups.

Defining vulval pain

Classification of vulval pain

The simplest classification describes vulval pain according to the presence or absence of physical vulval skin changes.

(1) Visible skin changes present
    (a) Lesions confined to the vestibule, e.g. vestibulitis
    (b) Lesions which involve part or all of the vulva and which include the vagina, perianal skin and inner thighs, e.g. infec-tion, dermatoses, trauma, neoplasia, manifestations of sys-temic disease, etc.
(2) Absent skin changes
    (a) Vulvodynia (essential 'dysaesthetic burning')
    (b) Pudendal neuralgia and 'other perineal pain syndromes'
    (c) Vaginismus, which may present as vulval pain and may be primary or secondary to another definable vulvovaginal disorder.

The 'vulval pain syndrome'

The International Society for the Study of Vulval Disease (ISSVD) gave the following definition of vulval dysaesthesia [1,2]: vulval dysaesthesia encompasses all vulval pain syndromes of unknown aetiology:

(1) Localised vulval dysaesthesia corresponding with the current term vestibulitis.
(2) Generalised vulval dysaesthesia corresponding to the current term vulvodynia.

Vulval pain with visible skin changes

- Lesions confined to the vestibule
- Vestibulitis (also termed focal vestibular adenitis and localised vulval dysaesthesia).

Classically vestibulitis (prevalence 1.5 per cent) demonstrates exquisitely tender erythematous areas localised to the major (Bartholin's) or Skene's vestibular gland. 'Allodynia' is innocuous stimuli causing pain. It is severe pain on vestibular touch or attempted vaginal entry, and to pressure, and it is localised within the vestibule with physical findings of erythema confined to the vestibule. Isolating aetiological factors for vestibulitis are not consistent. Infections such as *Candida* and human papillomavirus (HPV) have failed to demonstrate a clear aetiological factor. Iatrogenic factors, such as irritants (including lubricants, soaps and topical steroids), hormones, the early and prolonged use of oral contraceptives, may be risk factors but vestibulitis often occurs in the hypo-oestrogenic postpartum period.

Typically women are between 20 and 40 years of age and present with a history of provoked pain, such as superficial dyspareunia, inability to insert tampons and pain during gynaecological examinations. Women may have had pain from their first attempt at sexual intercourse or there may have been a period of normal sexual activity with the development of pain subsequently.

Vulval vestibulitis is diagnosed by three criteria:

(1) Severe pain on vestibular touch or attempted vaginal entry
(2) Tenderness to pressure localised within the vestibule
(3) The physical findings of erythema confined to the vestibule.

Urogenital sinus syndrome

Vestibulitis occurs in association with symptoms from other tissues derived from the urogenital sinus – the bladder and the urethra. In addition, patients may have other chronic pain syndromes such as low back pain, repetitive strain injury and fibromyalgia. It ought not to be dismissed as due to psychosexual factors just because there is no identifiable physical basis. Neurochemical factors and the release of inflammatory mediators such as prostaglandins, histamines, serotonin and other kinins may actuate the afferent nerve loop by stimulating nociceptive fibres to account for the pain.

Management

In the absence of a known cause, management strategies are inevitably empirical and directed at symptom control. Techniques to cope with pain need to be taught. Disappointment, anger and depression are common to all chronic pain sufferers. Supportive counselling is useful and patient support groups may benefit some. The patient needs to be reassured that it is not psychological in origin just because we do not understand the aetiology.

Treatment

(1) Eliminate potential irritants, especially perfumed products.

(2) Avoid topical therapies generally, but emollients such as aqueous cream or emulsifying ointment may help.

(3) Use lubricants and topical anaesthetic agents (e.g. Emla) for sexual activity. Apply 20 minutes before sexual activity.

(4) Surgical intervention should only be undertaken as a last resort. Best results are obtained where localised areas of pain are demonstrated. It is usually not successful with diffuse areas of erythema or persistent vulval pain unrelated to intercourse.

Visible skin changes which involve all or part of the vulva

(1) Gynaecological
  (a) Infection
      (i) Protozoan, e.g. pediculosis pubis
     (ii) Fungal, e.g. candidiasis (this may be cyclical)
    (iii) Bacterial, e.g. Bartholin's abscess
     (iv) Viral, e.g. herpes virus
      Infection may involve the adjacent skin, e.g. vagina, perianal region, thighs, etc.
  (b) Manifestations of systemic disease, e.g. Crohn's disease
  (c) Neoplasia, e.g. vulval intraepithelial neoplasia, carcinoma
  (d) Trauma
(2) Dermatological
  (a) Acute symptoms – irritation
      (i) Allergic contact dermatitis – fragrance, preservatives, vehicle. There are four types of allergic-mediated responses.
        ▪ Contact urticaria or type 1. This is an IgE-mediated reaction that is immediate (20 minutes).

- Type 4 allergic extrinsic dermatitis that requires a day or two to evolve, mediated by long memory T cells.
- Phytodermatoses – plant-induced. Ask about the application of non-orthodox varieties of unctures.
- Photophytodermatoses, e.g. allergy to chrysanthemums, parsley, celery, bergamot. Light activates the perfume irritant. Type 2 contact urticaria can occur with activation from sunlight. This type of reaction may be relevant with sunbed use.

(ii) Steroid rebound dermatitis

(iii) Irritant dermatitis (including topical medications, physical abrasion or over-zealous cleaning)

(b) Acute or chronic dermatoses – vulvar dermatoses

(i) Lichen sclerosus (see below)

(ii) Lichen planus

(iii) Psoriasis

(iv) Lichen simplex chronicus – epidermal thickening and excoriation are very typical.

Women with vulval pain with absent skin changes

Dysaesthetic vulvodynia [3]

Dysaesthetic vulvodynia is a chronic cutaneous dysaesthesia causing non-localised vulval pain. Unlike vulval vestibulitis where pain is provoked, women with dysaesthetic vulvodynia have a more constant neuralgic-type pain in the region of the vulva, occasionally involving the perianal area. The nature of the pain is often described as burning or aching and is often analogous to other neuralgic pain syndromes such as post-herpetic neuralgia.

The patient complains of burning, stinging, irritation or rawness. Dyspareunia is not a consistent feature. Clinical examination of the vulva is normal. Often it is a diagnosis by exclusion, with the history of negative physical findings in response to therapy defining the condition.

Most sufferers are middle-aged and elderly (peri- and postmenopausal). Symptoms may be aggravated by sitting. There may be other associated pelvic symptoms such as lower back pain, bowel and urinary tract symptoms. Occasionally the pain is localised to the clitoris or vagina.

Treatment – low dose amitriptyline [4]

- Amitriptyline enhances the activity of the descending inhibitory tracts within the central nervous system and therefore modifies activity within the dorsal horn of the spinal cord.

12

- Initiate therapy at a low dose, e.g. 10 mg/day (taken at night). The dose is increased if needed up to 70 mg/day, titrated up for total control of pain.
- Fluoxetine (20 mg) may be used if amitriptyline is not tolerated. Carbamazepine, widely used for trigeminal neuralgia, may help.
- Dothiepin (50–100 mg nocte) has both anticholinergic and antidepressant activity. Imipramine and nortriptyline are alternative drugs to use. Side effects include dry mouth, weight gain and sedation. While it is possible to report a 'hungover effect', many women benefit from improved sleep quality.

Occasionally there is an overlap with vulval pain syndromes and the term vestibulodynia has been coined to describe the features of both vestibulitis and vulvodynia.

Pudendal neuralgia

This defines those patients otherwise included in the dysaesthetic/essential vulvodynia category but who show a true neuropathy of the pudendal nerve or its branches. There is sensory loss over the nerve distribution with burning pain and sometimes intermittent pain radiating into the legs. It may be caused by injury, infection, tumours or organic causes such as sacral meningeal cysts and neurofibromas.

Vaginismus

Vaginismus is involuntary vaginal spasm caused by contraction of the pelvic floor (levator ani) muscles following attempts at introital or vaginal penetration. It may be primary, requiring psychosexual counselling, or secondary, where the underlying pathology needs to be treated, followed by re-education of the pelvic floor muscles.

Iatrogenic

Iatrogenic causes can include, for example, post-laser therapy.

DERMATOLOGICAL VULVAL CONDITIONS

Lichen sclerosus [5]

- This has an incidence of 1 in 300 to 1 in 1000, and presents most likely pre-puberty or peri- or postmenopausally. The aetiology is possibly autoimmune.

- Symptoms are intense pruritus interfering with sleep, pain occurring with excoriation and erosion and bacterial infection and cellulitis. Dyspareunia may occur because of introital narrowing.
- Clinical signs are pallor, excoriation and lichenification with oedema and shrinkage of the labia minora. Later on the skin loses its pigmentation and becomes porcelain white and acquires a thinned texture with wrinkling. Purpura and extensive ecchymoses may be seen. In children telangiectasia are seen. Blistering is an unusual feature. Eventually architectural distortion occurs. The clitoris is buried under the clitoral hood. Resorption of the labia minora occurs with narrowing of the introitus. Lesions of lichen sclerosus often extend from the perianal area forming a figure of eight configuration and they may go into the genitocrural fold. The skin may have a white macerated appearance due to oedema overlying hyperkeratosis. It does not occur on mucosal surfaces and therefore does not occur in the vagina. Squamous cell carcinoma develops in 6 per cent.

Treatment

Treatment comprises very potent topical corticosteroids such as clobetasol propionate 0.05 per cent (Dermovate).

Use of clobetasol propionate: for the average case of lichen sclerosus apply clobetasol propionate nightly for 2–4 months, depending on the severity. Occasionally application will be necessary twice a day where there is severe squamous hyperplasia. Following that, the patient can apply ointment in relation to symptoms, i.e. itching and irritation, and review should be yearly. Alternatively the patient with more severe disease may apply ointment once per fortnight or once a month as prophylaxis. The patient will identify the interval of recurrent symptoms and attempt to prophylactically avoid them by application of the ointment.

Erosive vulvovaginitis

Erosion is the loss of the epidermis and occurs with inflammatory, bullous, infective and neoplastic processes. Ulcers are deeper than erosions.

Erosions may form after loss of a fragile blister roof (pemphigus) or from intertriginous rubbing blisters (bullous pemphigoid). Blisters become eroded and thus are a more serious disorder because of secondary infection.

Excoriation is erosion caused by scratching. It is a secondary feature of pruritic vulval dermatoses.

Types of erosive vulvovaginitis

Erosive lichen planus
- Mucocutaneous lichen planus: itchy, purple, flat-top papules on cutaneous sites. Vulval symptoms are often severe and unremitting.
- Eroded areas may be surrounded by a reticulated white border. Vulval adhesion commonly occurs with labial atrophy, fusion and loss of the clitoris, together with loss of tissue mass.
- The keratinised skin in the perineal and perianal area often shows classic purple papules and plaques of lichen planus.

Differential diagnosis

Bullous pemphigoid
This is the commonest of blistering diseases. It usually affects the elderly, affecting the vagina as this is a mucosal site. Symptoms are of pain, itching and dysuria. Histology of a cutaneous blister shows a subepidermal split at the dermoepidermal junction with a mixed dermal inflammatory infiltrate consisting of numerous eosinophils.

Cicatricial pemphigoid
This is a scarring bullous disease affecting mucosal surfaces. Cicatricial pemphigoid is most like erosive lichen planus. This is a rare form of pemphigus. It affects keratinised skin.

Vulval scarring is often indistinguishable from erosive lichen planus. Erosions can develop on the labia, urethra, vagina, rectum or perianal skin. Scarring with labial fusion is common, with or without clitoral burial, and vaginal introital stenosis is often a complication. Urethral stenosis may require dilatation. Lesions may also be inside the conjunctiva and oral cavity.

Potent corticosteroid treatment and treatment of secondary infection are the essential local therapy for autoimmune bullous diseases.

Pigmented lesions of the vulva

Ten to twelve per cent of women have pigmented vulval lesions. Most of these lesions are benign lentigines, which are histologically a proliferation of melanocytes along the basal layer of the epidermis. Lentigines histologically are a palisade proliferation of melanocytes along the basal layer of the epidermis. Two per cent of women have vulval naevi.

Other discrete lesions that may be pigmented: seborrhoeic keratoses, vascular lesions, genital warts, malignant tumours such as melanoma, basal cell carcinoma, squamous cell carcinoma, vulval intraepithelial neoplasia (VIN) and blue naevi.

Diffuse hyperpigmentation can be seen in inflammatory lesions such as lichen simplex chronicus, lichen planus and discoid lupus erythematosus.

Benign naevi – junctional compound or intradermal

These are typically small, darkly pigmented, slightly raised papules found on the mucosal and keratinising skin. Compound naevi contain both a junctional and intradermal component. They are benign lesions which are small, dome-shaped, hyperpigmented papules. Intradermal naevi are small, soft, skin-coloured papules, not unlike a skin tag.

Vulval melanoma

- Clinically these lesions are deeply pigmented with irregular borders. They occur on mucosa as well as on hair-bearing skin.
- Mucosal melanomas may be flat and they eventually develop a nodular component which indicates a poor prognosis. A nodular component indicates a vertical growth phase.
- Vulval melanomas constitute about 10 per cent of vulval cancer.
- Labia majora lesions are of the superficial spreading type.
- Vulval melanomas tend to be more advanced (i.e. deeper) at the time of diagnosis than melanomas elsewhere.
- Lesions <0.85 mm deep carry a 10-year survival rate of up to 96 per cent, while lesions deeper than 3.6 mm have a 10-year survival rate of just less than 50 per cent. Survival is related to the level or Breslow depth of the melanoma on the vulva.

TOPICAL STEROIDS AND VULVAL DISEASE

Topical steroids are grouped as:
(1) Mild, e.g. hydrocortisone
(2) Moderately potent
(3) Potent
(4) Very potent, e.g. clobetasol propionate.

This classification is based on a standardised vasoconstrictor assay as a measure of potency. This test measures how long blanching persists on the forearm after a measured amount of steroid is applied. The longer blanching (vasoconstriction) persists the more potent the steroid.

Mild topical steroids are relatively safe (e.g. 1 per cent hydrocortisone cream). They are effective anti-inflammatory and emollient agents, are safe to use in intertriginous areas (axillae and groin) as well as the face and have a low risk of *Candida* superinfection.

Moderately potent topical steroids (e.g. clobetasone butyrate 0.05 per cent (Eumovate)) are absorbed well from vulval skin and are the highest strength needed for most vulval conditions. They ought to be prescribed in judicious amounts.

Superpotent topical steroids may produce a significant systemic absorption; 2 g (the size of a sample tube) per day of 0.05 per cent clobetasol propionate can suppress the hypothalamic–pituitary–adrenal axis. Use of clobetasol propionate 0.5 per cent (Dermovate) should not exceed 50 g/week.

Systemic effects can include aseptic necrosis of the femoral head, glaucoma and cataracts. Bruising or petechial (non-blanching) erythema are the first signs of steroid side effects. Long-term side effects include dermal atrophy and striae.

After use for more than 6 weeks, topical steroids with high potency can cause steroid rebound dermatitis when they are discontinued. Loss of steroid vasoconstriction results in rebound vasodilatation of the cutaneous capillaries, often with burning discomfort which can only be relieved with reapplication of the topical steroid. Those with fair skin and a tendency to flush easily are more susceptible. It is recognised as an erythematous pustular eruption.

Other side effects include acute outbreaks of recurrent herpes simplex, HPV and molluscum contagiosum. Other infections may be exacerbated, e.g. candidiasis, tinea, impetigo and infestations such as scabies.

Potency is related to the vehicle in which the steroid is mixed. The vehicle must carry the drug through the skin. When the stratum corneum is hydrated medications penetrate better. That is why cream is effective as a mixture of water in oil since the skin is hydrated with water and the moisture is sealed in with the oil. Ointment-based steroids are more potent than the same preparation in a cream or lotion base because ointments are more occlusive.

Table 12.1 Steroid response of vulvar dermatoses.

Thick scaly lesions (usually pruritic)
Lichen sclerosus (psoriasis)
Lichen simplex chronicus
Blisters and erosions
Lichen planus
Dermatitis/eczema
Bullous diseases

Occlusion keeps the skin moist by retarding evaporation of water. Therefore, medications penetrate for a longer time. A very potent steroid cream applied to a dry dermatosis can be only as effective as a medium strength steroid in an ointment base. Ointments are less likely to contain allergens like preservatives, which are necessary in water-based creams. Unfortunately, many women don't care for the tacky feel of ointments so they don't use them as often as they should.

An oozy wet skin should be treated with a cream because it will dry it out. A dry scaly skin should be treated with an ointment base. If a bit of both is required Locoid Lipocream may be used. In general, creams have very little oil in them and mostly water, so that enables the skin to dry out.

Gels penetrate well because they contain propylene glycol which is excellent for carrying drugs through the skin. However, it can be irritating and particularly to mucosal surfaces, resulting in stinging of the vulva.

In general high dose potent steroids should not be applied for a long time. They should not be used for erythema alone, vulvodynia (burning) or itching in the absence of skin disease (Table 12.1).

Different brands are necessary because some have different preservatives in them, with their potential irritant effects. A history suggestive of preservative sensitivity would imply the need to switch from a cream to an ointment.

CREAMS AND EMOLLIENTS

Emollients have:
- Barriers to transepidermal water loss (TEWL)

12

- Osmotic emollients e.g. aquacare HP with 10 per cent urea holds the water in by osmosis but it is water soluble.
- Emollients include vaseline- and lanolin-based products, such as aqueous cream and emulsifying ointment.

Aqueous cream is often dispensed in large 500 g tubs, but 50 or 100 g tubes are preferred for hygiene and convenience. These are used in place of soap for washing as it is less irritating. It is applied directly to the whole anogenital area before bathing or showering. The cream should be gently but completely rinsed off with hands or a flannel.

How much to prescribe

As 30 g = 1 ounce, therefore multiples of 30 are common; 60 g (2 ounces) will cover the whole body twice. A 30 g tube of cream rubbed in well will be enough for a patient to apply to the entire vulval area three times daily for a week. Twice daily is generally enough and tapering to once daily or even every other day is a good way to decrease usage as the patient improves. If medication has been rubbed well into the vulval area it will be absorbed in about 30 minutes, so that reapplication is not necessary after toileting.

Histopathology of the vulva

The vulva does age. Appearances change with age. The vulva does not have oestrogen receptors beyond the vestibule. Therefore, there is no case for applying oestrogen cream to the vulva. A biopsy of the vulva may often show mild inflammatory reaction in the normal female. Women with organic conditions in addition to the use of steroids may require additional emollient. Soap should be avoided. Soap substitutes include:
- Pinetarsol
- Aqueous cream
- Emulsifying cream.

Some women need a soothing cream such as aqueous cream.

Potassium permanganate solution can be used as a cleansing agent for weeping dermatoses. The solution is antiseptic, destroying bacteria, fungi, viruses and yeasts. It has an astringent drying effect, so therefore must not be continued too long.

Making the solution

Use a 400 mg tablet in 600 ml water or a few crystals or drops of a concentrated 1 per cent solution can be added to the same amount of water so that the solution (or bath water) is just pink. Staining can be a problem.

12

MANAGEMENT OF BARTHOLIN'S SWELLING

A swollen, tender and non-fluctuant Bartholin's gland suggests infection without abscess formation. Genital cultures should be taken including any secretion draining from the Bartholin's ducts and appropriate broad-spectrum antibiotic treatment given. An acutely tender fluctuant gland suggest an abscess has formed. Drainage is required. A non-tender but swollen and fluctuant gland suggests cyst formation without the presence of active infection. Treatment is marsupialisation – a 1 cm incision is made just outside the hymenal ring and the skin edges are sutured to the cyst edges to maintain drainage. Recurrences or abscesses are treated by excision.

EXTRAMAMMARY PAGET'S DISEASE

This is a rare form of intraepithelial carcinoma. It arises in areas containing apocrine glands, possibly from undifferentiated epithelial elements destined to develop into apocrine glands. It is diagnosed on biopsy. Typical features are erythematous eczematous eruption, sometimes with a white-grey crust that is non-responsive to steroids.

Management

Paget's cells frequently extend widely beyond the extent of the visible lesion. Therefore recurrences are common even after vulvectomy. Once the carcinoma has been excluded symptomatic recurrences are best managed by local excision.

Non-neoplastic white vulval skin has historically been difficult to define and classify. Definitions need to comply with clinical descriptions and pathological identity.

SQUAMOUS HYPERPLASIA

Squamous hyperplasia is non-specific hyperplastic epithelial changes which occur only on the vulva. Some believe these hyperplastic lesions, previously called 'leukoplakia', are examples of the latter stages of lichen simplex chronicus (neurodermatitis). The skin is white and usually significantly thickened. A diagnosis should be made by skin biopsy and examined by histopathologists with experience and knowledge of vulval dermatology.

Malignant potential

Lichen sclerosus and hyperplasia may coexist. These cases are at increased risk of developing cellular atypia and progressing to invasive carcinoma. The malignant potential of these lesions is relatively low (up to 5 per cent). The resultant pruritus from lichen sclerosus and squamous hyperplasia leads to scratching with resultant excoriation and secondary skin thickening. Dyspareunia is common.

Management

Potent corticosteroid ointments are the mainstay of initial management. They provide a good early response to the disease. Spontaneous regression or cure is unlikely and lifetime surveillance is advisable.

There is no place for simple vulvectomy since surgery is disfiguring and recurrence of the disease is almost inevitable. Conservative surgery may be necessary if atypia is present or to relieve introital contracture.

VULVAL INTRAEPITHELIAL NEOPLASIA

Vulval intraepithelial neoplasia (VIN) is characterised by loss of epithelial cellular maturation with associated nuclear hyperchromasia, pleomorphism, cellular crowding and abnormal mitoses within the vulval epithelium.

The clinical, colposcopic and histological features of VIN are extremely variable. VIN 1 is difficult to define with certainty. It is represented often by subclinical wart virus. Symptomatic patients generally have evidence of VIN 2 or 3 (previously known as Bowen's disease or carcinoma in situ) (CIS) [6].

12

VIN 3 is characterised by the following features:

- Occurs usually in middle and later life
- Is usually unifocal
- Exhibits a moist erythematous appearance
- Has a sharply defined spreading border.

It usually progresses to invasive cancer within 10 years if untreated.

The dramatic increase in numbers of cases of VIN presenting parallels that of CIN. The increase is seen almost exclusively in younger women with the mean age decreasing from the mid-fifties to the mid-thirties.

Clinical features of lesions

- Unifocal or multifocal
- Pigmented and often papular
- White and sometimes warty or red.

VIN 3 lesions are usually visible macroscopically. Their appearance is enhanced by the application of 5 per cent acetic acid.

Bowenoid papulosis is characterised by multifocal pigmented lesions usually seen in very young women. It is histologically identical with VIN 3, but biologically it may spontaneously regress.

Aetiological factors

These include subclinical wart virus infection, principally HPV type 16. Cigarette smoking is an associative factor in 60 per cent of cases. Cervical intraepithelial neoplasia (CIN) or invasive disease is noted elsewhere in the lower genital tract in up to 50 per cent of cases.

Presentation

VIN usually presents as pruritus or irritation, occasionally visible or palpable skin lesions, which are often asymptomatic. It is important to identify VIN 3 because of its potential to progress to invasive carcinoma. It is frequently misdiagnosed as *Candida* or genital warts. Immunosuppressed patients are at an increased risk of progression to invasion.

12

Table 12.2 Classification of vulval intraepithelial neoplasia (VIN) (International Society for the Study of Vulvovaginal Disease (ISSVD) and the International Society of Gynaecological Pathologists (ISGP)).

Vulval intraepithelial neoplasia
  VIN 1 – mild dysplasia
  VIN 2 – moderate dysplasia
  VIN 3 – severe dysplasia and carcinoma in situ

Non-squamous intraepithelial lesions
  Paget's disease
  Melanoma in situ

Management

Local excision is the best treatment in older women with unifocal disease. Laser treatment has revolutionised the management of multifocal lesions in young women. This avoids extensive and disfiguring surgery.

Classification (Table 12.2)

An important point to note is that the grading of VIN is based on morphological criteria and the risk of invasive disease may not be related to the grade of VIN. Sometimes there is a problem in histological distinction between VIN and vulval condyloma.

Symptoms

- Pruritus – up to 75 per cent
- Vulval pain/soreness
- Lump or lesion noticed in the patient
- Asymptomatic in up to 60 per cent.

Clinical manifestations of VIN are very variable. The lesion is often papular, raised and with a rough surface, not unlike genital warts. Leukoplakia is common. There is no site predilection for VIN. It affects the anus, clitoral glands and the vagina. VIN lesions may be uni- or multifocal.

Diagnosis

Diagnosis requires a histological biopsy. Its incidence is 0.53 per 100 000.

Types of treatment

- Vulvectomy
- Skinning vulvectomy and split skin graft to the denuded site
- Wide local excision
- Topical 5-fluorouracil
- Carbon dioxide laser ablation.

Other treatments (experimental):

- Dinitrochlorobenzene
- Cryosurgery
- Ultrasonic aspiration
- Topical α-interferon gel.

Radical surgery and skin graft are unfavourable because there is up to a 30 per cent incidence of recurrence. Dinitrochlorobenzene is a form of topical immunotherapy that induces a delayed hypersensitivity response, which is believed to reverse vulval atypia. Interferons are cellular proteins which have an inhibitory effect on viral replication. Carbon dioxide laser enables colposcopic assessment with vaporisation of the dysplastic tissue, preserving as much normal tissue as possible.

The risk of laser ablation is that there is a 7 per cent incidence of unsuspected early invasion, which is missed if treated with laser ablation.

Depth of treatment

Excision is indicated for the middle aged and elderly where the risk of invasion may be high. Complete excision enables a definitive diagnosis of the extent of possible invasion. Wide local excision should be done with an 8 mm margin of normal tissue.

VULVAL CARCINOMA

An active approach to the diagnosis and management of vulval lesions may prevent development of cancer in women. Vulval

Table 12.3 Nodal status in T_1 squamous cell carcinoma of the vulva versus depth of stromal invasion and the chance of positive nodes. (Berek and Hacker (1994) [8].)

Depth of invasion (mm)	Percentage of positive nodes
<1	0
1.1–3	8
3.1–5	27
>5	34

symptoms are present for more than 6 months in up to 88 per cent of women and for more than 5 years in up to 28 per cent. Eighty-five per cent of women have clinical evidence of normal skin adjacent to the cancer. Thirty-one per cent of women had three or more medical consultations for vulval symptoms prior to the diagnosis of cancer. Twenty-five per cent of women had had a previous diagnostic vulval biopsy and 27 per cent gave a history of having applied topical oestrogen or corticosteroid to the vulva [7].

Most vulval cancers arise in a background of abnormal skin, most commonly lichen sclerosus and/or squamous hyperplasia (non-neoplastic epithelial disorders) and VIN.

Treatment of VIN significantly reduces the risk of cancer development. Superpotent topical corticosteroids may reduce the small risk of cancer developing in lichen sclerosus. VIN-related carcinoma has increased significantly in young women recently. Often there will be a long history of antecedent symptoms such as pruritus which may relate to precursor lesions. Eighty-five per cent of women have been noted to have clinically abnormal skin adjacent to a vulval malignancy. This, therefore, ought to be subject to biopsy. Therefore if a visible lesion is present referral should be made to a specialist.

Women should be encouraged to self-examine the vulva with a mirror. In addition, symptoms of vulval disease of altered sensation such as pruritus, irritation, rawness and soreness (vulval irritation) should be taken note of and any aberrant skin appearances biopsied [9].

Cigarette smoking and multiple lower genital tract neoplasia is significantly more common in women younger than 50 years of age.

Squamous cell carcinoma of the vulva usually arises in a background of abnormal skin in the older women. Squamous cell carcinoma of the vulva represents at least two different entities: the common keratinising squamous cell cancer, which arises usually in a background of non-neoplastic epithelial disorder and is unrelated to HPV infection; and the less common HPV-related warty or basaloid carcinoma, which arises usually in the corresponding warty or basaloid VIN. The non-neoplastic epithelial disorders – lichen sclerosus and/or squamous cell hyperplasia and 'other' dermatoses – have been reported adjacent to 50–60 per cent of squamous cell vulval carcinomas, whereas VIN has been found adjacent to 20–30 per cent of cancers. The adjacent skin may exhibit mixed epithelial pathology and occasionally it is normal.

VIN is a truly preinvasive disease because of the increase in squamous cell carcinoma of the vulva associated with an increased incidence of VIN, especially in younger women. Nearly all reports of treated and untreated VIN progressing to invasive cancer have occurred within 8 years.

In women of all ages high grade VIN should be considered a lesion with a significant invasive potential. Stopping smoking and long-term follow-up of all patients with VIN is necessary.

Invasive vulval carcinoma developed in 3.8 per cent of patients, and 87.5 per cent of untreated patients progressed to invasive carcinoma within 8 years. The mean time for invasion was 4 years. It is important, therefore, that symptoms should not be attributed to infections such as candidiasis or genital warts. Twenty per cent of women are asymptomatic. VIN 3 is associated with neoplasia elsewhere in the lower genital tract in half of the cases. The vulva therefore should be carefully examined in women with a history of preinvasive or invasive carcinoma of the cervix or vagina. Twenty-five per cent of women have persistent disease or recurrences.

Vulvectomy

This is a historical operation except in the context of cancer, where the entire vulva is covered in a precursor lesion. Women with vulval carcinoma arising in VIN 3 should have radical local excision of the malignancy and a bilateral lymphadenectomy. For a unilateral lesion a unilateral lymphadenectomy is performed. Radical local excision includes a 2 cm margin and excision right down to the deep fascia.

12

Staging of vulval carcinoma is very important. Stage 1 is a lesion in which the stromal invasion is not more than 1 mm, and has a metastatic disease incidence of nil. Local excision may be done without wide margins. If there is >1 mm of stromal invasion there is an increasing risk of nodal involvement. Providing the patient is fit an inguinal lymphadenectomy is recommended. There is an increasing risk of lymphatic spread with increasing depth of invasion.

A simple vulvectomy is a historical procedure. It is an operation in which the skin is excised without the subcutaneous tissue and traditionally is used for treating vulval dermatoses like carcinoma in situ, Bowen's disease, VIN 3 and lichen sclerosus. Now there are more effective methods. A simple vulvectomy should only be used in the older woman in which almost the entire vulva is covered with VIN 3, and the very rare situation of the woman who has long-standing lichen sclerosus with squamous hyperplasia when clobetasol propionate has failed and the patient has been warned that, even if a simple vulvectomy is done, there is a high risk of disease recurrence. The average gynaecologist should not be doing simple vulvectomy. It is a subspeciality procedure. Simple vulvectomy is possible because of good lateral cover. It does not require a skin graft. Normally in both conditions disease does not usually extend beyond the midline of the labia majora. Very occasionally lichen sclerosus can extend onto the inner thigh and buttocks.

ACKNOWLEDGEMENT

Advice from Mr R.W. Jones, Vice President of the ISSVD, is gratefully acknowledged.

REFERENCES

1 Lynch, P.J. (1991) Report of the ISSVD Committee on Vulvodynia. Vulvar vestibulitis and vestibular papillomatosis. *Journal of Reproductive Medicine*, **36**, 413–415.
2 Wilkinson, E.J., Neil, B. & Lynch, P.J. (1986) Report of the ISSVD.
3 McKay, M., Frankman, O., Horowitz, B.J. *et al.* (1991) Vulvar vestibulitis and vestibular papillomatosis. Report of the ISSVD Committee on Vulvodynia. *Journal of Reproductive Medicine*, **36**, 413–415.
4 McKay, M. (1993) Dysesthetic ('Essential') vulvodynia: treatment with amitriptyline. *Journal of Reproductive Medicine*, **38**, 9–13.

5 Powell, J.J. & Wojnarowska, F. (1999) Lichen sclerosus. *The Lancet*, **353**, 1777–1782.

6 Jones, R.W., Baranya, I.J. & Stables, S. (1997) Squamous cell carcinoma of the vulva: the influence of vulvar intraepithelial neoplasia. *Obstetrics and Gynecology*, **90**, 448–452.

7 Jones, R.W. & Joura, E.A. (1999) Analysing prior clinical events at presentation in 102 women with vulval carcinoma: evidence of diagnostic delays. *Journal of Reproductive Medicine*, **44**, 766–768.

8 Berek, J.S. & Hacker, N.F. (1994) *Practical Gynecologic Oncology*, 2nd edn. Hacker, Williams and Wilkins, Baltimore.

9 Jones, R.W. & Rowan, D.M. (1994) Vulvar intraepithelial neoplasia III: a clinical study of the outcome in 113 cases with relation to the later development of invasive vulval carcinoma. *Obstetrics and Gynecology*, **84**, 741–745.

12

13   Gynaecological Surgery

CONSENT FOR SURGERY

Careful consideration should be given to fully informing patients of operative procedure, intention, results and possible complications (Fig. 13.1) [1].

OPERATING THEATRE SET-UP

Operative gynaecology has the usual risks of disease transmission (blood-borne, airborne or contamination of body fluids by direct contact, e.g. human immunodeficiency virus (HIV), hepatitis B and hepatitis C, methicillin-resistant *Staphylococcus aureus* (MRSA)) to operating theatre personnel. Risk is minimised by adopting standard precautions (previously 'universal precautions'). It is not possible to identify all situations of risk of transmission of disease, and even when they are, accidents happen (Tables 13.1 and 13.2).

The risk of seroconversion to HIV is significantly reduced if the needlestick injury is with a solid needle (1 in 5000). If it is through a glove the risk is decreased to 1 in 3000. If there is blood on the glove the risk is increased.

ANATOMICAL CONSIDERATIONS IN GYNAECOLOGICAL SURGERY

Access

- Consideration of Pfannenstiel or midline incision
- Anatomical landmarks – nerves for injection of local anaesthetic
- Characteristics of the sheath
- Peritoneum – healing attachments for mass closure.

Positioning of the patient for operative laparoscopy

Lloyd-Davis

The Lloyd-Davis position is adopted. The hips are at a 15° angle as the basic angle which is adjustable with the leg supports. This position gives good exposure and minimises pressure areas.

The laparoscope is a surgical instrument like a telescope placed through a small incision in the abdomen. Second, third and fourth incisions are also often made for scissors, coagulators or other tools to perform surgery at laparoscopy. These techniques decrease the need for major open surgery.

Pictures or video may be taken during surgery and used to show you what was seen and done. They may be used for teaching other patients and other surgeons these techniques, anonymously. Often visiting nurses or surgeons will be present during your laparoscopy to observe certain laparoscopic procedures. If you object to observation of your surgery by anyone, please make that known. Complaints and/or complications associated with laparoscopy may include, but are not limited to, the following:

Common postoperative complaints	Postoperative complaints	Operative complications
1 Shoulder tip pain	1 Nausea	1 Bowel damage
2 Bloating	2 Haemorrhage	2 Ureter or bowel injury
3 Vaginal bleeding	3 Urinary infection	3 Bleeding
4 Sore throat	4 Infection	4 Anaesthetic problems
5 Painful urination		5 Infections
		6 Unexpected open surgery

Major complications requiring either immediate or delayed further surgery, such as damage to the uterus, tubes, ovaries, bowel, bladder, ureter or other organs are uncommon but do occur. Statistics reveal major complications in fewer than 1 in 1200 patients. Severe complications such as hysterectomy, colostomy or death are rare but may occur. In the event both ovaries are removed or a hysterectomy is performed, this will result in sterilisation.

After careful inspection at the time of laparoscopy, open surgery (laparotomy) may be felt to be more successful operatively. It is generally best to discuss these findings before proceeding as open surgery may mean removing the tubes, ovaries or the uterus and may require additional preparation. In addition, open surgery generally requires 3 to 5 days in hospital and 3 to 6 weeks' recovery.

Successful outcome is not guaranteed.

Fig. 13.1 The International Society of Gynaecological Endoscopy consent form (with adaptation) for gynaecological laparoscopy.

Specific surgery plan (in addition to diagnostic laparoscopy):

___ Hysteroscopy	___ Lysis (cut) of adhesions	___ Appendectomy
___ Remove one tube or ovary	___ Cut uterosacral nerve	___ Vaporisation – endometriosis
___ Remove both tubes/ovaries	___ Remove fibroid uterus	___ Presacral neurectomy
___ Cut adhesions to bowel	___ Hysterectomy	___ Remove ovarian cyst

Other _____

Dr _____ has discussed these procedures with me and given me ample opportunity to ask specific questions. After reading the above information, I understand the benefits and risks involved in these procedures. I also understand that Dr _____ may ask someone else to assist with my surgery and postoperative care.

I realise that during the procedure the above surgeon may become aware of conditions which were not apparent before the start of the procedure and require open surgery. I therefore consent to any additional or different procedure the surgeon deems reasonable and necessary, or appropriate to treat or diagnose such condition.

_____   _____

Date   Signature

_____   _____

Date   Witness

In the event that open surgery is required, I would like the following conditions to apply (please circle one):
I am ready for open surgery / Only for emergency / At doctor's discretion / Only after intraoperative discussion with my family.
Other _____

Date _____ Patient's initials _____ Doctor's initials _____

Fig. 13.1 *Continued.*

Table 13.1 Checklist for HIV counselling.

(1) What an HIV antibody test means (not a test for acquired immune deficiency syndrome (AIDS))
(2) Significance of a negative test ('window period' in relation to recent high risk behaviour)
(3) Significance of a positive test with respect to:
    (a) Medical implications (prognosis and treatment)
    (b) Psychological issues (coping, support, relationships)
    (c) HIV is not noticeable
    (d) Social implications
(4) What are the safeguards with respect to preservation of confidentiality?
(5) Future preventative aspects
(6) If positive – confirmatory test

13

Table 13.2 After a needlestick injury: 'rule of threes' seroconversion.

Virus	Percentage
HIV	0.3
Hepatitis C	3
Hepatitis B	30

Lithotomy

This angles the legs at 90°. This is the position for short procedures and vaginal hysterectomy.

Principles of sterility and draping

Scrubbing should take 3–5 minutes. Commonly 'missed areas' include on top of the thumbs, webs of the fingers and flexor surfaces of the wrists. Hands are less likely to transmit bacteria if they are well dried. The antimicrobial loses its effect after 3–4 hours, so gloves should be changed and consideration given to rescrubbing at 3–4 hours in long cases. Two pairs of gloves should be worn – the smaller ones on second. Goggles or the equivalent should be worn. Drapes for gynaecological surgery should be fluid repellent, non-flammable and non-linting. Only one layer is required providing it has those qualities.

Antimicrobial solutions for patient prepping
- Need to be rapid acting and rapid drying
- Not dependent on cumulative action
- Inhibit rapid regrowth of microbes.

Chlorhexidine (0.5 per cent) and alcohol (70 per cent) – this needs to be used not lavishly because of the risk of fire with the use of the diathermy. Chlorhexidine aqueous is used in the vagina because of the risk of fire in a confined space with hair. The alternative is povidone iodine, which has better anaerobic cover, and covers against yeasts.

Antibiotic prophylaxis in gynaecological surgery

In a meta-analysis of 25 randomised trials of antibiotic prophylaxis [2], it has been established that the use of antibiotics is highly effective in the prevention of serious infections (up to 50 per cent). Suitable antibiotics given as a single intravenous dose are metronidazole, cephazolin and tinidazole.

Risk of venous thrombosis (Table 13.3)

Acquired risk factors
- Surgery
- Trauma
- Increasing age
- Lupus anticoagulant
- Malignant disease
- Oestrogen-containing pills – combined oral contraceptive (COC) and hormone replacement therapy (HRT).

Table 13.3 Risk of thromboembolism (VTE) per 10000.

Risk	Per 10000
Baseline risk for non-carriers and non-users of COC	0.8
Annual risk with factor V Leiden and non-users of COC	5.7 (RR 6.9)
Annual risk for women using COC without factor V Leiden	3.0
Annual risk for women with factor V Leiden and COC use	28.5 (RR 34.7)

RR, relative risk.

Inherited risk factors

- Deficiency of antithrombin III, protein S, protein C – protein C, protein S and antithrombin are the main natural inhibitors of the procoagulant system, so a heterozygous deficiency of these proteins leads to excessive thrombin formation (ten-fold increase in incidence).

- Resistance to activated protein C due to a mutation in clotting factor V (factor V Leiden).

- High concentrations of factor VIII (>1500 IU/l; 150 per cent of normal) are associated with a six-fold increased risk of thrombosis, compared to levels <1000 IU/l.

- Hyperhomocysteinaemia (>18.5 μmol/l) is usually due to impaired methionine metabolism caused by insufficient dietary intake of folic acid and vitamins B_6 or B_{12}, rather than the mutation of cystathionine β-synthase or methylene tetrahydrofolate reductase. It is associated with a 2.5-fold increased risk of thrombosis. At homocysteine levels >20 μmol/l, the risk is increased three- to four-fold.

- A mutation in prothrombin (coagulation factor II) 20210A, found in 2 per cent of the population, increases the risk by two- to three-fold.

Investigate appropriate risk factors for VTE appropriately and treat prophylactically.

Thromboprophylaxis in gynaecological surgery

Give heparin, 5000 units 2 hours before surgery, then every 8–12 hours until the patient is mobile, or give low molecular weight heparins

Low molecular weight heparins:

- Are as effective and safe as heparin
- Have a longer duration of action than unfractionated heparin
- The standard prophylactic regimens do not require monitoring
- Once daily regimen means they are convenient to use.

Regimens are as follows:

- Dalteparin (Fragmin), 2500 units s.c. 1–2 hours before surgery and then 2500 units every 24 hours for 5–7 days, or

- Enoxaparin (Clexane), 20 mg (2000 units) approximately 2 hours before surgery then 20 mg every 24 hours for 7–10 days, or

- Certoparin (Alphaparin), 3000 units 1–2 hours before surgery then 3000 units every 24 hours for 7–10 days.

- Tinzaparin sodium (Innohep).

PRINCIPLES OF LAPAROSCOPIC SURGERY

Basic instrument set (Table 13.4)

Principles of establishing a pneumoperitoneum

13

(1) Method of obtaining the pneumoperitoneum – This is with either a Veress needle or Hassan's technique.

(2) Inflate at a pressure of 15–25 mmHg. Maintain pressure at 12–15 mmHg. Venous pressure in the major intra-abdominal veins is 3–8 mmHg under general anaesthetic. The pneumoperitoneum maintains haemostasis and is the reason for carefully checking the surgical site at deflation and completion of the operation.

(3) Site of entry – umbilicus or Palmer's point.

Caution – use of umbilical entry

Absolute contraindications
- Previous midline incision
- Mass to the umbilicus.

Relative contraindications
- Previous transverse incision
- Known adhesions, e.g. from peritonitis.

With previous abdominal surgery (Fig. 13.2), the safest point to introduce the Veress needle to avoid bowel adhesions is the area of the left hypochondrium (Palmer's point: the midclavicular line immediately below the ninth intercostal space), which statistically is the area of the abdomen with the lowest incidence of adhesions.

Port sites

Visualise the anterior abdominal wall structures – the obliterated umbilical artery (Fig. 13.3) and inferior epigastric vessels (Fig 13.4) and other abdominal wall vessels. Enter under direct vision. Sites depend on operator comfort and access to operative field.

Diathermy

A diathermy unit such as Valleylab (Pfizer, Force 2) may be set on coagulation, cutting and blend. It may be bipolar or monopolar. It

Table 13.4 Standard laparoscopic gynaecology set.

5 black sheaths
5 black handles, 3 ratchet, 2 non-ratchet
1 straight scissor insert
1 curved scissor insert
1 straight dissector insert
1 curved Kelly dissector long insert
1 toothed grasper
1 × 3-piece 10 mm port, blue with topcock
   1 trocar, sharp (check tip)
   1 port cap, blue flap
   1 port cannula, blue band
2 × 3-piece 5 mm port, red without stopcock
   2 trocars, sharp (check tip)
   2 port caps, red flaps
   2 port cannulae, red band
1 × 3-piece 5 mm port, red with stopcock
   1 trocar, sharp (check tip)
   1 port cap, red flap
   1 port cannula, red band
1 reducer sleeve, short black
1 lap pin, silver key
4 red 5 mm sealing caps
1 blue 10 mm sealing cap
1 connection, silver for gas tubing like a luer lock
1 gas tube
1 suction irrigation/dissection probe
Knot pusher
1 monopolar diathermy grey lead, black attachment
1 light lead (grey cable)

4 Carins forceps
1 straight Mayo
1 Metzenbaum scissors
1 needle holder
2 Littlewoods forceps
1 No. 3 BP handle
1 Bonney's toothed forcep
1 Gillies' toothed forcep
1 5 cm Langenbeck retractors
2 scabbards (long)
1 sponge-holding forcep
8 towel clips, ball end
1 TST indicator

13

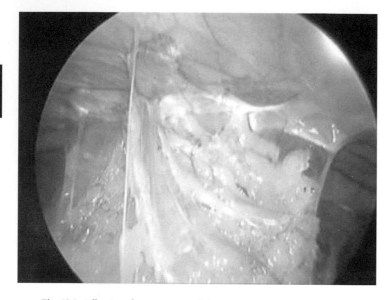

Fig. 13.2 Adhesions from previous abdominal surgery at the umbilicus at risk of trocar trauma at insertion.

should always be used with a smoke evacuator to avoid inhalation of plume which has microscopic tissue particles.

Monopolar

Use at levels of:
Coagulation   40 W.
Cutting   40 W
Blend   40/40
Some use it up to 90 W.

Bipolar

Use at 40 W.

There is a medicolegal requirement (in the USA) to use a device to assess the end-point power. Stray energy can cause unseen burns that manifest only after patient discharge as infection and possible major

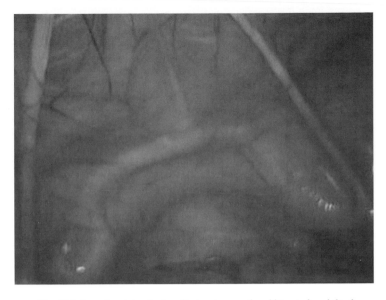

Fig. 13.3 Anterior abdominal wall structures – the obliterated umbilical artery.

complication with damage to bowel, etc. Capacitive coupling can occur. Therefore all plastic or all metal parts should be used, not a combination of both.

Active electrode monitoring using the Electroshield EM 2⁺ searches continuously for insulation failure and capacitive coupling during monopolar electrosurgical procedures. If stray energy is detected the monitor signals the electrosurgical generator to deactivate before patient injury can occur. The EM 2⁺ also offers end-point current monitoring during bipolar electrosurgery. This application informs the operator of the relative end point of complete dessication of tissue during procedures such as laparoscopically assisted vaginal hysterectomy (LAVH). The electroscope AEM is compatible with virtually all electrosurgical generators with quality control monitoring.

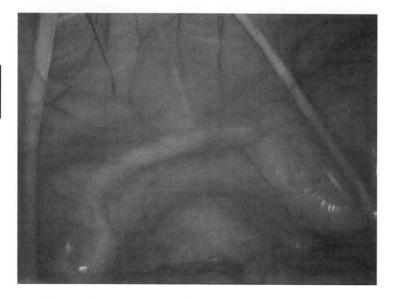

Fig. 13.4 Inferior epigastric vessels.

Haemostasis

Full familiarity with all methods of haemostasis is essential. These include diathermy, clips, ligators and suturing. Principles of managing major haemorrhage include pressure, access, clamping and ligation.

Irrigation

- Use water and not saline because saline can haemolyse red blood cells with long procedures.
- Use the underwater test for haemostasis.
- Insert methylene blue into the bladder to check bladder integrity, although any perforations of the bladder with laparoscopic surgery

will manifest by the urinary bag with catheter attached blowing up with gas from the intraperitoneal space.

- Bowel – air in the rectum visualised with a sigmoidoscope while the pelvis is floated identifies any breaches of integrity in the bowel wall.

13

Complications from laparoscopic surgery

Damage can occur in normally situated structures and/or in structures adherent to the abdominal wall. Overall, the risk of bowel damage is 0.4 in 1000 and for major vessels 0.2 in 1000 (Table 13.5 for figures for more than 350 000 closed laparoscopic procedures reported over 20 years) [3,4]. The overall rate of adhesions is 10 per cent and the rate of severe adhesions containing bowel near the umbilicus is 5 per cent. More than 90 per cent of these occur after previous laparotomy. The incidence of bowel perforation with adherent bowel near the umbilicus is approximately 3 per 1000.

The death rate from laparoscopy is approximately 1 in 36 000. Damage to abnormally adherent bowel accounts for two thirds of the injuries and half the deaths associated with laparoscopy.

Table 13.5 Laparoscopic entry-related major complications. (With permission from Garry (1999) [3].)

Authors	Year of publication	Total number of cases	Bowel injury		Vessel injury	
			n	Rate per 1000	n	Rate per 1000
Mintz	1977	99 204	31	0.3	48	0.5
Loffer & Pent	1975	32 719	22	0.7	NR	
Bergqvist & Bergqvist	1987	75 035	NR		5	0.07
Querleu et al.	1993	17 521	7	0.4	4	0.2
Chapron et al.	1998	29 966	17	0.5	6	0.2
Härkki-Sirén	1999	102 812	29	0.3	6	0.1
Total		357 257	103	0.4	69	0.2

NR, not reported.

Table 13.6 Rates of adhesions related to previous surgical history.
(With permission from Garry (1999) [3].)

Surgical history	n	Adhesions Rate per 1000	n	Severe adhesions Rate per 1000	n
No previous surgery	519	8	4	4	2
Previous laparoscopy	140	14	2	7	1
Previous Pfannenstiel	145	214	31	69	10
Previous midline	96	531	51	255	30

Hasson, in 1971, described an open technique to avoid damaging bladder and bowel [5]. The American Association of Gynecological Laparoscopists reported over 80 000 laparoscopies by an open approach. The rate of bowel injury was 12 per 1000. The rate of bowel damage following closed laparoscopy was eight times less at 1.5 per 1000 (Table 13.6). It therefore identified the open approach to laparoscopy as not avoiding bowel damage.

Open laparoscopy virtually eliminates major vessel damage, but it does not avoid the risk of bowel damage in an aberrant place. Even with an open approach it is still possible to not diagnose bowel damage at the time of the primary procedure. The open approach does not avoid damage to bowel adherent under the site of the primary incision.

Insufflation using a Veress needle

The Veress needle should be sharp with a briskly reacting stylet. It should be inserted carefully and definitively through the first sheath and through the peritoneum, and two clicks should be felt as the needle passes through. The needle should be inserted just far enough to penetrate the layers of the abdominal wall and locate the tip into the peritoneal cavity. The filling pressure is 25 mmHg intra-abdominally which prevents indentation of the abdominal wall during trocar insertion with the patient in a supine position. The gas pressure is reduced immediately the trocars have been inserted (operating pressure of 12–15 mmHg).

Other complications include abdominal wall blood vessel injury. The inferior epigastric vessels are branches of the external iliac vessels, which arise just before the artery enters the canal and then course up on the undersurface of the rectus muscle. These vessels can usually be identified on laparoscopic inspection of the inner aspects of the abdominal wall and thus can be avoided with the insertion of a trocar. The corresponding vessels on the abdominal wall do not always line up with the inferior epigastric vessels.

Incisional hernia has an incidence of 1.7 per 1000. This is related to the size of the trocar incision. Port sites of more than 10 mm should be closed by suturing both the fascia and the sheath, but should be avoided in preference to smaller port sites.

Types of sutures (Table 13.7) [6]

Absorbable

Catgut is now outdated, because it has synthetic equivalents that are cheaper. As a natural product it runs the risk of an unknown potential for disease transmission. The ideal suture is synthetic absorbable monofilament because of less tissue reaction and therefore less of a foreign body reaction, e.g. monocryl.

Braided absorbable sutures include dexon and vicryl. They are very strong in tensile strength, but tensile strength is not related to the time taken for the suture to dissolve.

Sutures are gauged in terms of standard diameters with 0, 1 and 2 being the commonest sizes used in gynaecology. The larger the number the greater the diameter of suture. Smaller sutures are graded downwards in size from 2-0 to 12-0 (microsutures).

Needles are described in terms of a circle. A taper needle, most commonly used for gynaecology, has a sharp point. A reverse cutting needle avoids cutting through. A conventional cutting needle is used for wounds with no tension because it easily cuts through (Fig. 13.5).

The needle is held on an appropriately sized needle holder (for 0, 1 and 2, a Hegar Mayo needle holder). Needles should always be handled with the instruments and not the fingers. To guard the

Table 13.7 Types of sutures and their characteristics. (Adapted and reproduced with permission from Ethicon, Inc. (1999) [6].)

Suture	Coated VICRYL RAPIDE polyglactin 910	MONOCRYL (dyed and undyed) poliglecaprone 25	Coated VICRYL polyglactin 910	PDSII polydioxanone	PANACRYL	Surgical silk
Type	Braided	Monofilament	Braided monofilament	Monofilament	Braided	Braided
Raw material	Copolymer of lactide and glycolide coated with polyglactin 370 and calcium stearate	Copolymer of glycolide and epsilon – caprolactone	Copolymer of lactide and glycolide coated with polyglactin 370 and calcium stearate	Polyester polymer	Copolymer of lactice and glycolide coated with a polymer of caprolactone and glycolide	Organic protein called fibroin
Tensile strength retention *in vivo*	Approximately 50 per cent remains at 5 days. Lost within 10–14 days	Dyed: approximately 60–70 per cent remains at 1 week Approximately 30–40 per cent remains at 2 weeks. Lost within 4 weeks	Approximately 75 per cent remains at 2 weeks. Approximately 50 per cent remains at 3 weeks	Approximately 70 per cent remains at 2 weeks. Approximately 50 per cent remains at 4 weeks. Approximately 25 per cent	Approximately 80 per cent remains at 3 months. Approximately 60 per cent remains at 6 months. Approximately 20 per cent remains at 12 months	Progressive degradation of fibre may result in gradual loss of tensile strength over time. Loses most strength within 1 year

13

Absorption rate	Minimal until about fourteenth day. Essentially complete by 42 days. Absorption by low hydrolysis	Undyed: approximately 50–60 per cent remains at 1 week. Approximately 20–30 per cent remains at 2 weeks. Lost within 4 weeks. Complete at 91–119 days. Absorbed by hydrolysis	Minimal until about the fortieth day. Essentially complete between 56 and 70 days. Absorbed by slow hydrolysis	remains at 6 weeks. Minimal until about the ninetieth day. Essentially complete within 6 months. Absorbed by slow hydrolysis	Essentially complete in 1.5–2.5 years	Gradual encapsulation by fibrous connective tissue. Usually cannot be found after 2 years
Tissue reaction	Minimal	Slight	Minimal	Slight	Minimal	Moderate
Contraindications and warnings	Due to rapid loss of tensile strength, should not be used where extended approximation of tissues under stress is required or where wound support beyond 7 days is required	Being absorbable, should not be used where extended approximation of tissue under stress is required. Undyed is not indicated for use in fascia	Being absorbable, should not be used where prolonged approximation of tissues under stress is required	Being absorbable, should not be used where extended approximation of tissues under stress is required	Being absorbable, should not be used where extended approximation of tissue beyond 6 months is required	Should not be used in patients with known sensitivities or allergies to silk

13

Table 13.7 *Continued*

Suture	Coated VICRYL RAPIDE polyglactin 910	MONOCRYL (dyed and undyed) poliglecaprone 25	Coated VICRYL polyglactin 910	PDSII polydioxanone	PANACRYL	Surgical silk
Frequent uses	Superficial soft tissue approximation of skin and mucosa only	General soft tissue approximation and/or ligation	General soft tissue approximation and/or ligation	All types of soft tissue approximation	General soft tissue approximation and/or ligation	General soft tissue approximation and/or ligation
Colour of material and how supplied	5-0 through 1 with needles	6-0 through 2 with and without needles. 3-0 through 1 with CONTROL RELEASE needles	8-0 through 3 with and without needles, and on LIGAPAK dispensing reels. 4-0 through 2 with CONTROL RELEASE needles	9-0 through 2 with needles (violet). 4-0 through 1 with CONTROL RELEASE needles. 9-0 through 7-0 with needles (blue). 7-0 through 1 with needles (clear)	3-0 through 2	9-0 through 5 with and without needles and on LIGAPAK dispensing reels. 4-0 through 1 with CONTROL RELEASE needles
Colour code of packet	Violet/red stripe	Coral	Violet	Silver	Plum	Light blue

13

13

Suture	ETHILON nylon	NUROLON nylon	ETHIBOND Excel polyester fibre	PROLENE polypropylene	PRONOVA polypropylene	DERMABOND topical skin adhesire
Type	Monofilament	Braided	Braided	Monofilament	Monofilament	Liquid
Raw material	Long-chain aliphatic polymers nylon 6 or nylon 6,6	Long-chain aliphatic polymers nylon 6 or nylon 6,6	Polyester coated with polybutilate	Isotactic crystalline stereolsomer of polypropylene	Polymer blend of poly (vinylidene fluoride) and poly (vinylidene fluoride–cohexafluoropropylene)	2-octyl cyanoacrylate
Tensile (for strength retention *in vivo*	Progressive hydrolysis may result in gradual loss of tensile strength over time	Progressive hydrolysis may result in gradual loss of tensile strength over time	No significant change known to occur *in vivo*	Not subject to degradation or weakening by action of tissue enzymes	Not subject to degradation or weakening of action of tissue enzymes	Strength of approximated healing tissue at 7 days (for topical application only)
Absorption rate	Gradual encapsulation by fibrous connective tissue at a rate of 15–20 per cent per year	Gradual encapsulation by fibrous connective tissue at a rate of 15–20 per cent per year	Gradual encapsulation by fibrous connective tissue	Gradual encapsulation by fibrous connective tissue	Gradual encapsulation by fibrous connective tissue	Sloughs off skin in 7–10 days

13

Table 13.7 *Continued*

Suture	ETHILON nylon	NUROLON nylon	ETHIBOND Excel polyester fibre	PROLENE polypropylene	PRONOVA polypropylene	DERMABOND topical skin adhesive
Tissue reaction	Extremely low	Extremely low	Minimal	Minimal	Minimal	Minimal
Contraindications and warnings	Should not be used where permanent retention of tensile strength is required	Should not be used where permanent retention of tensile strength is required	None known	None known	None known	Should not be used across mucocutaneous junctions, skin that has dense natural hair or skin that is regularly exposed to body fluids. Do not use on patients with a known hypersensitivity to cyanoacrylate or formaldehyde. Should not be used on wounds with evidence of active infection.

13

Frequent uses	General soft tissue approximation and/or ligation	General soft tissue approximation and/or ligation	General soft tissue approximation and/or ligation	General soft tissue approximation and/or ligation	General soft tissue approximation and/or ligation	Intended for topical application only to close easily approximated skin edges of surgical incisions and thoroughly cleanse trauma-induced lacerations. May be used in conjunction with, but not in place of, subcuticular sutures
						Should not be applied to wet wounds. Should not be used in areas of high tension unless the area will be immobilised during the healing period

13

Table 13.7 *Continued*

Suture	ETHILON nylon	NUROLON nylon	ETHIBOND Excel polyester fibre	PROLENE polypropylene	PRONOVA polypropylene	DERMABOND topical skin adhesive
Colour of material and how supplied	11-0 through 2 with and without needles	6-0 through 1 with and without needles. 4-0 through 1 with CONTROL RELEASE needles	7-0 through 5 with and without needles. 4-0 through 1 with CONTROL RELEASE needles – various sizes attached to TFE polymer pledgets	7-0 through 2 (clear) with and without needles. 10-0 through 8-0 and 6-0 through 2 (blue) with and without needles. 0 through 2 with CONTROL RELEASE needles – various sizes attached to TFE polymer pledgets	6-0 through 2 (clear) with needles. 10-0 through 8-0 and 6-0 through 2 (blue) with needles. 0 through 2 with CONTROL RELEASE needles	Violet 0.5 ml of sterile liquid adhesive in a prefilled, single-use vial
Colour code of packet	Mint green	Mint green	Orange	Deep blue	Cranberry	Violet

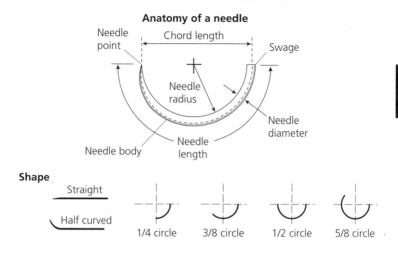

Anatomy of a needle

Shape

Needle points and body shapes with typical applications

Point/body shape	Applications	Point/body shape	Applications
Conventional cutting POINT / BODY	Ligament Skin Tendon	Taper POINT / BODY	Fascia Gastrointestinal tract Muscle Peritoneum Subcutaneous fat Urogenital tract vessels
Reverse cutting POINT / BODY	Fascia Ligament Skin Tendon sheath	Blunt POINT / BODY	Cervix (ligating incompetent cervix) Blunt dissection (friable tissue) Fascia
Precision point cutting POINT / BODY	Skin (plastic or cosmetic)	PC PRIME POINT / BODY	Skin (plastic or cosmetic)
TAPERCUT Surgical needle POINT	Calcified tissue Fascia Ligament Tendon Uterus		

Fig. 13.5 Types of needles and anatomical description.

needle when knot tying, take it from the 90° horizontal position in relation to the tip of the needle holder to facing towards it and rotate 90°. This keeps the point close to the longitudinal axis of the instrument and lessens the risk of needlestick injury to assistants.

HYSTERECTOMY

Alternatives to hysterectomy (see Chapter 7)

Objective assessment of menstrual blood losses confirmed the therapeutic efficacy of minimally invasive techniques. Up to 80 per cent of women are satisfied with improvement in menstruation and the avoidance of hysterectomy. Essentially, hysterectomy is a vaginal operation unless there is an indication to open to inspect the abdomen or to remove bulk.

Indications for hysterectomy

- Dysfunctional uterine bleeding uncontrolled by medical therapy or endometrial ablation or insertion of Mirena intrauterine device (IUD) (see Chapter 7)
- Fibroids causing excessive bleeding, anaemia, pelvic pain and symptoms related to pressure on adjacent organs including compression of the ureter and hydronephrosis
- Uterovaginal prolapse (6.5 per cent)
- Endometriosis and adenomyosis
- Pelvic pain
- Genital tract malignancy (up to 6 per cent)
- Endometrial hyperplasia.

Among uteri weighing >500 g LAVH has a shorter recovery but longer operating time than total abdominal hysterectomy (TAH) with up to a 30 per cent rate of conversion to laparotomy, mostly due to the shape of the uterus rather than the exact uterine size with concomitant distortion of the pelvic anatomy.

GnRH agonists and fibroids

GnRH agonists reduce the size of fibroids and mean uterine volume by up to 70 per cent, with 3 months' treatment, which may enable an abdominal hysterectomy to be converted to a vaginal procedure.

They decrease fibroid vascularity and hence operative blood loss, because they antagonise the effects of oestrogen, which in high concentration cause dilatation, due to oestrogen receptors in the uterine arteries. Vessel calibre is decreased, with a subsequent increase in vascular impedance and decrease in uterine blood flow. The disadvantage of this treatment is the high cost.

13

VAGINAL HYSTERECTOMY

There is much debate as to the indication for LAVH. In general, the ability to perform a vaginal hysterectomy (VH) is greater than what has been traditionally taught.

Contraindications to vaginal hysterectomy

- Uterus >14 weeks' size, >500 g
- Restricted uterine mobility
- Limited vaginal space
- Adnexal mass
- Invasive cancer of the cervix
- VH with an anterior fibroid. The fibroid can obstruct descent of the uterus and is therefore a relative contraindication, unless it can be shelled out.

Common excuses

- The uterus is enlarged
- The need to remove the ovaries
- Nulliparity
- A 'good look' at abdominal organs is essential.

Indications

Indications for VH are broad, depending on the skill of the operator. Absolute size of the uterus is not necessarily a contraindication. Morcellation, bivalving and particularly myomectomy may allow removal of the uterus vaginally. Accessibility may be limited by disease such as endometriosis, adnexal disease, chronic pelvic pain and chronic inflammation, or anatomically due to a narrow vagina or an undescended uterus. Removal of the uterus vaginally is not possible in only 10–20 per cent of cases. A uterus up to 500 g in size can be removed vaginally, but usually up to 280 g (average uterine weight is 70 g). Oophorectomy may be performed in women undergoing vaginal hysterectomy in up to 95 per cent of patients [7,8,9]. Approximately 5 per cent of ovaries remain at the position of the ischial spine. The infundibulopelvic ligament has little or no elasticity without rupture.

VH enables additional procedures to be carried out such as repairing anatomical defects such as cystocele and rectocele. An enterocele should be automatically closed when using appropriate surgical technique for VH.

Technique of vaginal hysterectomy

- The cervix and vaginal mucosa may be injected with Marcain with adrenaline 0.5 per cent (20 ml).
- The circumferential incision is made around the cervix ending in a V-shaped opening pouch of Douglas.
- The bladder is dissected off the anterior aspect of the uterus and displaced anteriorly.
- A throat pack may be inserted to provide traction which displaces the ureter.
- Curved Kocher clamps are inserted into the pouch of Douglas to take the uterosacral pedicles first vertically angled and then horizontally. The tissue is cut and doubly ligated.
- The uterine pedicles are then taken.
- The anterior peritoneum is then opened.
- The uterus is delivered through the vagina.
- The ovarian pedicles are then taken.
- The uterus is removed.
- The peritoneum is then closed in a purse string to include the uterine vessels and uterosacral pedicles and pouch of Douglas peritoneum.
- The vaginal vault is closed, either as an inverted 'Y' or horizontally as a continuous locking suture, securing the uterosacrals into the vaginal mucosa.

PROPHYLACTIC OOPHORECTOMY

Ovarian cancer occurs in 1.4 per cent of female malignancies – 1 in 70 newborn females with a 5-year prognosis unchanged in 30 years of 25 per cent. Ovarian cancer occurs in 7–15 per cent of women who have previously had a hysterectomy. If prophylactic oophorectomy is done at the time of the operation for benign disease, 10–14 per cent of ovarian cancers could be prevented, without additional surgical time, risk or morbidity [10].

Oophorectomy is the only available method to prevent ovarian cancer [11]. It should be considered with risk factors such as:

- Family history of gynaecological cancer
- Past history of breast cancer
- Nulliparity
- Use of the oral contraceptive pill (past and current use of oral contraceptives decreases the risk of ovarian cancer to 1 in 1700)
- Patient request.
  Other complications of conservation of the ovaries:
- Residual ovary syndrome (7–20 per cent)
- Endometriosis requiring further surgery in up to 50 per cent of cases because of pelvic pain
- Premenstrual syndrome (gets worse with age)
- Ovarian failure following hysterectomy at 18 months earlier than the otherwise natural menopause.

Three methods of vaginal oophorectomy

(1) Endoscopic stapler (multi-site endo GIA 30 auto suture, Ascot)
(2) Seitsinger tripolar cutting forceps (Cabot Medical)
(3) Endoloop, using no. 1 polyglactin polymer (vicryl, Ethicon).

The ovary is gently pulled with sponge forceps into the operative field and over to the midline and the mesovarium is clamped, avoiding the fallopian tubes. If a stapler is used it is fired along the full length of the mesovarium. In a few cases a second application is needed.

The Seitsinger tripolar cutting forceps dissect the mesovarium using a standard bipolar generator and precise cutting is achieved by means of a guillotine knife, which is advanced between the jaws of the device. The jaws of the forceps are 20 mm long and 4.5 mm wide and grasp tissue up to 5 mm thick. Further desiccation and cutting are performed until the ovary can be removed.

The endoloop is used with the Sheth clamp or similar. Two loops are usually applied before cutting and removal of the ovary, the endoscopic knot pusher being used to apply the endoloop behind the clamp.

LAPAROSCOPIC HYSTERECTOMY (LH)

Under general anaesthesia, with endotracheal intubation, the patient is placed in the Lloyd-Davis position with 15° flexion at the hips, with both legs and feet supported. The Valtchev uterine mobiliser is inserted into the uterus to antevert it and delineate the posterior vagina.

Three laparoscopic puncture sites are used:

- 10 mm umbilical
- 5 mm lower quadrant on each side, lateral to the rectus abdominis muscle and inferior epigastric vessels. Reduction in wound morbidity and scar integrity as well as cosmesis is enhanced using 5 mm sites.

Retroperitoneal dissection

The anterior broad ligament is stretched out by pulling the fallopian tube medially and scissors are used to incise behind the round ligament for oophorectomy and in front of the round ligament for conservation of the ovaries.

Identification of the position of the ureter

Always start high enough. The ureter is seen most easily where it crosses the pelvic brim at the bifurcation of the iliac vessels. When the uterosacral ligament is thick, the ureter is usually pulled down towards it.

The round ligaments are divided at their midportion using a spoon electrode set at 150 W cutting current. The ovarian pedicles can be taken, using 25–35 W cutting current coagulating until desiccated and then dividing.

Scissors are used to divide the vesicouterine peritoneal fold, with 2–3 cm between it and the bladder dome. The bladder is mobilised off the uterus and upper vagina using scissors, or bluntly with the same spoon electrode or a suction-irrigator, until the anterior vagina is identified.

The uterine arteries are ligated as they ascend the sides of the uterus. The broad ligament on each side is skeletonised down to the uterine vessels. 0-vicryl sutures on a CTB-1 blunt-curved needle (Ethicon JB260) may be introduced into the peritoneal cavity by pulling them through a 5 mm incision. Sutures are tied extracorporeally using a knot pusher. Laparoscopic ligation of the uterine arteries is by either electrosurgery desiccation, suture ligature or staples. All surgical steps after the uterine vessels have been ligated can be done either vaginally or laparoscopically, including anterior and posterior vaginal entry, cardinal and uterosacral ligament division, uterine removal (intact or by morcellation) and vaginal closure.

The cardinal ligaments on each side are divided (either with CO_2 laser at 80 W or with the spoon electrode at 150 W cutting current, or bipolar forceps). The uterosacral ligaments are identified and a 0-Vicryl suture on a CT 1 needle is placed through it, then through the opposite cardinal ligament and underlying posterolateral vaginal fascia just below the uterine vessels, along the posterior vaginal wall fascia over the right posterolateral vaginal fascia, cardinal ligament, and the right uterosacral ligament. This suture is tied extracorporeally and gives excellent support to the vaginal cuff.

A transurethral cystoscopy may be done 10 minutes after injecting 5 ml of indigo carmine dye intravenously to check ureteric function and bladder integrity.

At the end of the procedure, an underwater examination is used to detect bleeding from vessels and viscera tamponaded during the procedure by the increased intraperitoneal pressure of the CO_2 pneumoperitoneum. The pneumoperitoneum is displaced with 2–3 l of Ringer's lactate solution.

The umbilical incision is closed with a single 2-0 Vicryl suture including the deep fascia with the knot buried beneath the fascia.

LAPAROSCOPIC OOPHORECTOMY (Fig. 13.6)

The port sites are introduced as for a laparoscopic hysterectomy using Palmer's point for insertion of the Veress needle if there are previous abdominal scars.

The peritoneum is grasped with forceps at the junction of the bifurcation of the internal iliac artery, which is usually well above any adnexal disease and enables identification of the natural, more bloodless planes for operating in (Fig. 13.6 (a)).

The gonadal vessels are independently ligated after tunnelling beneath them to create a window, ligating each end – the pelvic end

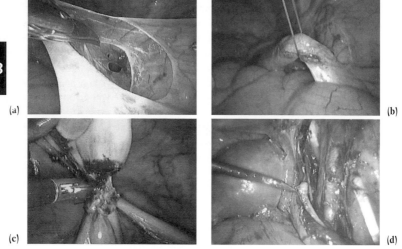

Fig. 13.6 Laparoscopic oophorectomy. (a) Opening the peritoneum. (b) Ligation of the gonadal vessels. (c) Transection of the ovarian pedicle. (d) Identification/dissection of the ureter.

doubly (Fig. 13.6 (b)). This can be done with ties, endoloop or diathermy but beware of vessels retracting retroperitoneally if not ligated. This enables mobilisation of the pedicle and for the ovary to be removed (Fig. 13.6 (c)). If there is any risk of malignancy, the specimen should be 'bagged', i.e. removed intact from one of the port sites to avoid the risk of malignant spread of cells, which can contaminate the port sites.

The ureter may be identified (Fig. 13.6 (d)). The peritoneal cavity is washed out and the port sites removed under direct vision to make sure there is no bleeding. The skin wounds are closed.

SUPRACERVICAL HYSTERECTOMY (CLASSIC INTERSTITIAL SEMM HYSTERECTOMY, CISH)

- Supracervical hysterectomy leaves the cardinal ligaments intact while eliminating the columnar cells of the endocervical canal. After perforating the uterine fundus with a long sound-dilator, a calibrated uterine resection tool (CURT) that fits around this instrument is used to core out the endocervical canal. Then, at laparoscopy, suture techniques are used to ligate the utero-ovarian ligaments. An endoloop is placed around the uterine fundus to the level of the internal os of the cervix and tied. The uterus is divided at its junction with the cervix and removed by laparoscopic morcellation.

- This may have further complications with regard to persistence of bleeding due to endometrial tissue present.
- All smears should be normal.

GENITAL PROLAPSE

- Uterine
- Cystocele
- Rectocele
- Enterocele.

Genital prolapse has an incidence of 2.04 per 1000 woman years. Uterovaginal prolapse affects around 20 per cent of women, requiring major gynaecological surgery.

Vault prolapse

Vaginal vault prolapse occurs in 0.2–50 per cent of women who have had a hysterectomy. It is the result of a combination of intrinsic defects such as weakness of tissue collagen and damage to the pelvic floor and its nerve supply during childbirth. It may occur as a consequence of a hysterectomy (because vascular or nerve damage has occurred). Forty per cent of women present within the first 2 years after hysterectomy, 25 per cent within 10 years and 35 per cent more than 10 years after their hysterectomy.

Symptoms of vaginal vault prolapse

'A bulge'

- Protrusion of the vagina through the introitus
- Pelvic discomfort on standing

- Difficulty with control of micturition, predisposition to urinary tract infections
- Difficulty with intercourse
- When severe, irregular spotting or discharge associated with ulceration
- Increase pelvic pressure 'heaviness' and backache.

Sexual symptoms

- Is the patient sexually active?
- Is dyspareunia a problem?
- Is there any incontinence with sexual activity?

Changed sensations of bladder function with prolapse

- Stress incontinence
- Frequency (diurnal and nocturnal)
- Urgency
- Urgency incontinence
- Hesitancy
- Weak or prolonged urinary stream
- Feeling of incomplete emptying
- Manual reduction of the prolapse to start or complete bladder emptying
- Positional changes to start or complete voiding.

Changed function of the bowel

- Difficulty with defecation
- Incontinence of flatus
- Incontinence of liquid stool
- Incontinence of solid stool
- Faecal staining of underwear
- Urgency of defecation
- Discomfort with defecation
- Digital manipulation of vagina, perineum or anus to complete defecation
- Feeling of incomplete evacuation
- Rectal protrusion during or after defecation.

The nerve supply to the pelvic floor and sphincter mechanism:

- Is derived mainly from the pudendal nerve but there are some fibres passing on the inner surface of the levators to supply some of the sphincter mechanism.
- It passes down on the inferior surface of the levator after passing over the ischial spine and proceeding down to supply the sphincter mechanism as well as some of the anal mucosa.
- Damage to it occurs with difficult and traumatic childbirth because the nerve is relatively fixed at the ischial spine and so stretching occurs with subsequent damage (nerves can only stretch 12 per cent without damage).
- This may lead to denervation of the pelvic floor and sphincter mechanism which reduces the support to the rectum and the function of the sphincter mechanism to maintain continence.
- The extreme cases will lead to rectal prolapse and total incontinence which are obvious at examination, with the rectum folding out of the anal canal. It can be visually seen with the anal canal gaping when examined and a very short canal with poor to no contraction to the palpating finger. There is associated marked perineal descent and a negative clinical reflex. The normal mechanism whereby the pelvic floor and sphincters contract during coughing is lost and so soiling occurs on any increased intra-abdominal pressure.
- A lesser degree of this occurs with less nerve damage and the patient may notice loss of control of flatus or liquid stool.
- Other symptoms which may occur are mucosal prolapse within the anterior wall of the rectum leading to incomplete evacuation and mucous leakage. This usually occurs after defecation and the feeling may necessitate the return to the toilet to further try and evacuate the bowel.
- While these symptoms may be evident the signs are not always clearly seen.
- Defecating proctography is an easy means of detection of these problems and is a good assessment of the degree of loss of function that has occurred. This will demonstrate mucosal prolapse or full-thickness complete prolapse. It would demonstrate leakage of the barium at rest simulating what happens with faeces.

Subclinical damage can occur to the sphincter at childbirth due to direct tearing of the sphincter which is not obvious at examination [12]. This occurs particularly when a third-degree tear occurs during childbirth. A third-degree tear should be considered as very serious sphincter trauma. A high percentage of these women even after repair have faecal incontinence later in life. Detection of this subclinical sphincter damage is best detected by magnetic resonance imaging (MRI) or by transanal ultrasound, 3 months post-delivery.

Symptoms *not* caused by loss of continence or prolapse which can be symptoms of cancer

- Bleeding from the bladder, vagina or bowel
- Vaginal discharge
- Pain in the pelvis or abdomen
- Change in bowel or bladder habit.

Standardisation of terminology of female pelvic organ prolapse and pelvic floor dysfunction [13]

The following is the International Continence Society (ICS) terminology for standardising lower urinary tract function and prolapse. The object is to identify the degree of pelvic organ prolapse to enable comparison of treatment modalities. Figures 13.7 and 13.8 show that the terms 'cystocele', 'rectocele', 'enterocele' or 'urethrovesicle junction' have been replaced by anatomical nomenclature. It is an attempt to quantify the degree of prolapse.

Prolapse is evaluated relative to a fixed anatomical landmark that can be consistently and precisely identified. The hymen is the fixed point of reference used for this system to describe quantitative prolapse.

The anatomical position of the six defined points for measurement are given in centimetres above or proximal to the hymen (negative number) or in centimetres below or distal to the hymen (positive number). The plane of the hymen is defined as zero (Fig. 13.9).

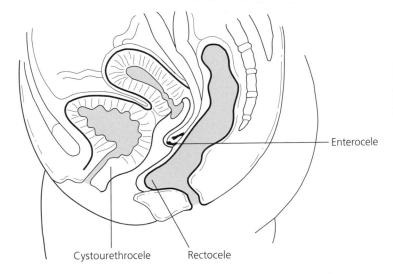

Enterocele

Cystourethrocele   Rectocele

Fig. 13.7 Female genital tract prolapse. Conventional anatomical description of prolapse. (With permission from Jackson and Smith (1997) [14].)

Point Aa: This is located in the midline of the anterior vaginal wall, 3 cm proximal to the external urethral meatus. Aa relative to the hymen is −3 to +3 cm.

Point Ba: This represents the most distal position of any part of the upper anterior vaginal wall from the vaginal cuff or anterior vaginal fornix to point Aa. By definition point Ba is at −3 cm in the absence of prolapse and would have a position value equal to the position of the cuff in women with total post-hysterectomy vaginal eversion.

Two points are on the superior vagina. These points represent the most proximal locations of the normally positioned lower reproductive tract.

Point C: A point that represents either the most distal (i.e. most dependent) edge of the cervix, or the leading edge of the vaginal cuff (hysterectomy scar) after total hysterectomy.

Point D: This represents the location of the posterior fornix (or pouch of Douglas) in women with an intact uterus and cervix. It represents the level of uterosacral ligament attachment to the proximal

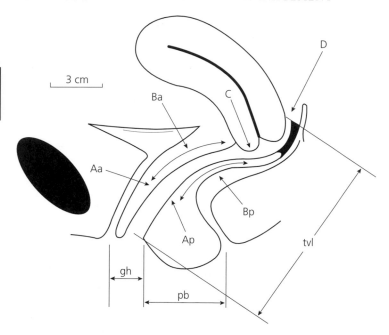

Fig. 13.8 Six sites (points Aa, Ba, C, D, Bp and Ap), genital hiatus (gh) and total vaginal length (tvl) for quantitative description of pelvic organ prolapse quantification (POPQ) (International Continence Society definitions). Aa, point defined as 3 cm from the hymen or the anterior vaginal wall; Ba, most distal point of upper anterior vagina from hymen when compared to point A; C, lowest point of cervix; D, posterior fornix; Bp, most distal point of upper posterior vagina from hymen when compared to point A;
Ap, point defined as 3 cm from the hymen on the posterior vaginal wall; pb, perineal body; gh, genital hiatus; tvl, total vaginal length. (With permission from Bump *et al.* (1996) [13].)

posterior cervix. It is included as a point of measurement to differentiate suspensory failure of the uterosacral cardinal ligament complex from cervical elongation.

There are two points on the posterior vaginal wall:

Point Bp: The point that represents the most distal (i.e. most dependent) position of any part of the upper posterior vaginal wall from the vaginal cuff or posterior vaginal fornix to point Ap. By definition

anterior wall	anterior wall	cervix or cuff
Aa	Ba	C
genital hiatus	perineal body	total vaginal length
gh	pb	tvl
posterior wall	posterior wall	posterior fornix
Ap	Bp	D

Fig. 13.9 Three-by-three grid for recording quantitative description of degree of genital prolapse adopted by the International Continence Society. (With permission from Bump *et al.* (1996) [16].)

point Bp is at least –3 cm in the absence of prolapse and would have a positive value equal to the position of the cuff in a woman with total post-hysterectomy vaginal eversion.

Point Ap: This point is located in the midline of the posterior vaginal wall 3 cm proximal to the hymen. By definition the range of position of point Ap relative to the hymen is –3 to +3 cm.

Point gh: The genital hiatus is measured from the middle of the external urethral meatus to the posterior midline hymen. The perineal body (pb) is measured from the posterior margin of the genital hiatus to the mid-anal opening. Measurements of the genital hiatus and perineal body are given in centimetres.

Objective of surgery

- To restore the abnormal state to its normal anatomic position.
- To restore function.
- To perform the appropriate procedure that results in the least chance of recurrence of the problem.
- To operate when more conservative treatments – such as exercise, oestrogen therapy and the use of pessaries inserted in patients – fail.
- Repair other defects at the same time as surgery.

The aim of a vaginal repair is to replace the vagina in its near-horizontal position above the levator ani [15]:

- If the vaginal apex after anterior colporrhaphy can be pulled towards the introitus with an Allis clamp.
- Similarly if the vault comes down after a hysterectomy.

At hysterectomy the uterosacral and cardinal ligaments should be attached to the angles of the vaginal mucosa and sutured into the vault. This has the effect of:

- Preventing post-hysterectomy prolapse
- Tying the angles of the vagina, which is the common site of post-operative bleeding.

Vaginal repair

Sacrospinous colpopexy

Indications
- Vault prolapse
- Second-degree uterine prolapse
- Proccidentia
- Enterocele with or without uterine prolapse if the vault can be pulled down to the hymenal ring.

Sacrospinous fixation
(1) The posterior vaginal wall is opened to its apex. An ipsilateral triangular incision into the skin is made at the perineum. The vaginal mucosa is dissected from the rectum. The rectovaginal space is dissected to the level of the ischial spine. The right hand index finger is placed on the lower border of the ischial spine.
(2) The right hand third finger feels the top of the sacrospinous ligament.
(3) The Miya needle is introduced horizontally in the same plane and rotated 90°. The right hand is pronated so that the needle is fixed against the third finger.
(4) The Miya hook is pushed with the finger to get it into the sacrospinous ligament. The placing of this suture is crucial in relation to normal anatomical structure.

Repairing the vaginal vault prolapse
(1) The 'dimples' at the vaginal apex indicate the site of the previous lateral cervicovaginal junction and are the landmarks that determine the depth for the newly constructed vagina. The redundant

vaginal mucosa caused by the prolapse in the enterocele sac are excised, usually in a diamond shape. Ideally the depth of the vagina after reconstruction should be 10 cm.

(2) The enterocele sac is isolated by blunt and sharp dissection. It is then excised. The muscular defect is then closed.

(3) The sacrospinous ligament is identified. The sacrospinous ligament is approximately 8 cm in length. The Miya needle is used to place the suture into the sacrospinous ligament. It is imperative that the suture be placed 2–3 cm medially from the sacrospinous ligament and a third of the distance from the apex and through the ligament. The pudendal vessels and nerves course around the ischial spine. In addition the hypogastric plexus of veins superiorly and haemorrhoidal vessels medially are at risk.

(4) The Miya hook is pushed with the third finger to get it into the sacrospinous ligament and then the tissue is pushed down to expose the Miya needle tip between the index and third fingers. A notched speculum is placed into the base of the needle so that it cannot come out.

(5) The rectum is retracted using the Breisky–Navratil retractor. The assistant holds the Miya needle in the closed position once it is through the sacrospinous ligament and the surgeon introduces the notched vaginal speculum to retrieve the suture (1 PDS).

(6) With the nerve hook the threads are pulled through. The Miya hook is then opened from the ligament by dropping it down, opening it and the index and third fingers are kept between the hook to guard it. The Miya hook is withdrawn between the index and third fingers. The two ends of the PDS sutures are brought through the vaginal vault at the apex. One is fixed by grasping a loop and running a suture around twice. A 0.5 cm bite is taken. The mobile suture is on top. When the anterior and posterior colporrhaphy and repair of the enterocele are completed the vaginal apex is fixed in position by pulling on the mobile PDS suture with the other one fixed. This has a pulley effect and the apex of the vaginal vault is closely allied to the sacrospinous ligament.

Complications of sacrospinous colpopexy
- Vault haematoma
- Buttock pain from the perforated cutaneous nerve, S_2, S_3 (normally resolves by 6 weeks)
- Blood transfusion

- Loss of sensation on the posterior aspect of the thigh
- Urinary tract infection
- Pudendal artery and nerve damage
- Sciatic nerve injury
- Recurrent vault prolapse after sacrospinous vault suspension is 2.4 per cent (abdominal colposacropexy 1.3 per cent).

Anatomical landmarks
The pudendal complex and the sciatic nerve travel underneath the lateral third of the sacrospinous ligament. Therefore placement of the stitch must be medial to that portion of the ligament. The stitch must be placed as superficial as possible and never across the entire thickness of the sacrospinous ligament. This should decrease the rate of complications associated with this type of colpopexy.

Abdominal colposacropexy [16]
- The patient is placed in the semilithotomy position. The bladder is immobilised anteriorly. Polypropylene mesh, approximately 2.5–4 cm wide, is attached to the anterior vaginal wall with three rows of interrupted 2/0 prolene sutures. If there was a large defect in the anterior vaginal wall mesh can be fixed in a Y-shaped fashion to both the anterior and posterior surfaces.
- The rectum and sigmoid are retracted from the midline.
- The peritoneum over the sacral promontory is excised longitudinally in the midline.
- The loose areolar tissue overlying the sacrum is dissected to expose the anterior longitudinal ligaments of the bodies of the sacral vertebrae.
- The mesh is attached to the ligaments and periosteum with four or five non-absorbable sutures (usually prolene), so that the vagina is gently elevated but without tension.

Complications of abdominal colposacropexy include haemorrhage from the presacral veins which can be profuse. Resorbable sutures are used. Non-resorbable suture material offers no advantage as it can predispose to abscess formation which causes severe pain.

Ureteric injury
The ureter is at risk when:
- The uterosacrals are clamped without retracting the bladder
- The uterine clamp slips

Table 13.8 Clamps used with open surgery.

Gwilliam	Kocher	Maingot	Bonney	Heany
Longitudinal grooves with teeth at the end	These have horizontal grooves with teeth at the end	A heavy forcep, with longitudinal serrations similar to Gwilliams	Horizontal serrations and toothed at the end	Longitudinal serrations, almost like an atraumatic de Bakey in style
They hold tissue at right angles				There are horizontal sections so that when the tissue is clamped it expands into the minute wide serrations and therefore theoretically is less traumatic to the tissue
They are straight or curved	They are usually straight	They are curved or straight	Like a Kocher, but angled, not straight	They are angled not straight and double toothed

- Too much traction is applied to the cervix without retraction in the uterovesicle space
- Previous Caesarean section
- Proccidentia.

Technique of abdominal hysterectomy (Table 13.8)

- The incision is made – usually a Pfannenstiel incision, unless the upper abdomen needs to be explored.
- A balfour-type self-retaining retractor is inserted.
- The bowel is packed out of the pelvis.
- A steep Trendelenburg position is adopted.

13

- If there are any adhesions the normal anatomical relations are restored.
- Straight Kocher clamps are placed alongside the uterus to include the round ligament, fallopian tube and utero-ovarian ligaments. This prevents back bleeding and allows adequate traction.
- The assistant pulls the uterus up to the patient's left with the right hand.
- The right round ligament is visualised and clamped and divided and tied.
- The broad ligament is opened.
- The fallopian tube and utero-ovarian ligament are doubly clamped and divided and doubly ligated.
- The same procedure is performed on the left.
- The peritoneal incisions from right to left are connected from the broad ligament over the bladder at the point of the vesicouterine reflection.
- The loose connective tissue is pushed down from the bladder to expose the endopelvic fascia over the anterior portion of the cervix. 1–2 cm of the entire anterior vaginal wall below the level of the vaginal transection must be exposed.
- A Kocher (or equivalent) clamp is placed curved side down on the side of the cervix at approximately a 45° angle at the position of the uterine artery.
- A small clip is applied to the uterine side to control back bleeding. Tips are allowed to slide off the cervix.
- The tissue is divided close to the cervix.
- The pedicle is doubly ligated.
- The uterosacral ligaments are stretched to expose them by upward and anterior traction on the uterus.
- The vagina is incised and Maingot clamps applied.
- The uterus is removed.
- The uterosacral ligaments are sutured, making sure the vaginal epithelium is included in the lateral angle.
- The vaginal vault is sutured, either using figure of eight sutures or as a continuous running suture with careful attention to each angle.
- The pelvic peritoneum should be included in the suturing of the vagina to aid haemostasis.
- The pelvis is inspected for haemostasis and irrigated.
- Reperitonealisation is not necessary, but may aid haemostasis.

- The packs are removed and the rectosigmoid colon returned to the pelvis.
- The abdomen is closed.

OPERATING FOR GYNAECOLOCIAL CANCER

13

- Local excision is indicated for diagnosis or treatment when the disease is at an early stage.
- Radical excision is indicated for identifying and staging cancer.
- Disease should be approached anatomically with complete excision as correlates with treatment outcome.

Radical hysterectomy

The cure rates for surgery and radiotherapy were thought to be similar for early stage cervical cancer. However, recently five randomised controlled trials have shown the advantage of chemo-irradiation for cervical cancer (see Chapter 14). Surgery previously was thought to have these advantages, especially in younger patients:

- Disease spread can be assessed accurately.
- Ovarian function can be preserved.
- Treatment time is shorter.
- The preservation of sexual function, because the vagina is more functional, although shortened.
- Surgical complications are treatable, whereas those from radiotherapy are chronic and often progressive.
- Postoperative pelvis is assessed more easily on examination for recurrence than a fibrotic postirradiated pelvis.
- Radiotherapy causes damage to surrounding normal organs.
- Radioresistance is overcome.
- A second pelvic malignancy in the irradiated field is avoided.

Surgical technique for radical hysterectomy

- The abdomen is opened through a lower midline incision. This can be extended toward the xyphoid process if upper abdominal surgery is indicated (para-aortic node dissection).
- Intraperitoneal washings are taken. The best cellular yield is from at least 70 ml of wash sent for cytology.
- The peritoneal cavity is checked – the liver, para-aortic nodes.

- Kocher clamps are placed on either side of the uterus including the round ligament, utero-ovarian ligament, broad ligament and fallopian tubes.
- The right round ligament is grasped with straight Kocher forceps and divided, opening up the retroperitoneal space.
- The incision is extended along the vesicouterine fold caudally and cranially parallel to the ovarian vessels.
- The ureter is identified.
- The paravesical space is dissected between the external iliac vessels laterally and the obliterated hypogastric artery medially.
- The utero-ovarian ligaments in the tube are clamped.
- If the ovaries are not being conserved then the infundibulopelvic ligament is clamped.
- The pedicle is divided and ligated.
- Pelvic lymphadenectomy is performed.
- The peritoneum beneath the inguinal ligament is elevated and a Deaver retractor inserted, exposing the full length of the external iliac vessel.
- A second Deaver retractor retracts the bladder medially where it is inserted into the paravesical space.
- With long scissors and Russian forceps, the fatty tissue lateral to the external iliac vessels along the psoas muscle is divided.
- The circumflex vein is at risk where it courses over the external iliac artery.
- The external iliac nodes are gradually dissected off the vessels up to the bifurcation of the common iliac artery.
- The common iliac nodes are separated from the lateral aspect of the common iliac vessels and from the psoas muscle. They are divided above the aortic bifurcation.
- The psoas muscle is retracted laterally and the common iliac vessels medially and any remaining deep and lateral nodes to the common iliac vessels removed.
- Obturator nodes are taken from the lateral side wall by using a Deaver retractor placed inferiorly into the paravesical space and over the external iliac vessels.
- The obturator nodes are removed.
- The accessory obturator vein is at risk.
- Presacral/internal iliac nodes are removed.

13

- The anterior division of the internal iliac artery is clamped and divided at its origin with right-angled forceps.
- The obliterated hypogastric artery is clamped and ligated near the anterior abdominal wall.
- With traction on the uterus, the surgeon's thumb is inserted into the pararectal space and the index finger into the paravesical space. With fingers beneath the cardinal ligament a tunnel is created in the avascular space.
- The cardinal ligament is double clamped flush with the pelvic side wall using long-curved clamps.
- Node dissection and cardinal ligament transection are repeated on the opposite side.
- The ureter is dissected from its attachment to the broad ligament peritoneum on both sides.
- The cul-de-sac peritoneum between both uterosacral ligaments is divided, and the rectum is dissected away from the upper vagina anteriorly and from the medial aspect of the uterosacral ligaments laterally.
- The uterosacral ligaments are clamped with a right-angled clamp lateral to the rectum and divided, allowing the uterus to be lifted up out of the pelvis.
- Upward traction is placed on the uterus and the vesicouterine fold of peritoneum elevated and divided by incising with scissors.
- With sharp scissor dissection, the avascular space between the bladder and the cervix is opened 3–4 cm below the external os of the cervix.
- The ureter is unroofed from its tunnel right down to its entry into the bladder.
- The ureter is elevated with a vein retractor and freed from the top of the cardinal ligament by sharp dissection.
- The uterus is lifted up out of the pelvis. A large curved clamp is placed across the paracolpium beneath the cardinal ligament at the level where the vagina is transected.
- Tenacula are applied to the vaginal cuff and it is closed in two layers with a submucosal number 1 synthetic absorbable suture.
- The paravaginal pedicles are sutured and ligated into the corners of the vaginal vault, as are the uterosacral pedicles.
- A suprapubic catheter is inserted. The catheter is removed when there is a residual volume of <100 ml on two occasions.

Possible postoperative complications of radical hysterectomy

- Urinary retention and faecal impaction, both due to decreased sensation
- Urinary fistula – ureteric or vesicovaginal, 1–2 per cent
- Lymphocyst.

13

Surgery for ovarian cancer and other pelvic malignancy

- Primary surgery is TAH, bilateral salpingo-oophorectomy, and retroperitoneal lymph node sampling, with peritoneal washings, or ascitic fluid for cytology, except in the case of the younger woman, in whom other non-epithelial tumours are more common, such as germ cell tumours. Conservative surgery may be indicated, depending on pathology, and conservative surgery done with adjuvant chemotherapy to preserve fertility.
- In more advanced disease, the value of surgery is less certain. All macroscopic disease should be removed. 'Debulking' has become an inherent part of treatment of ovarian cancer but chemotherapy may well have a more substantive role than surgical cytoreduction.
- Second-look laparotomy does not alter survival rates and its value prognostically is limited, as women develop recurrent disease at variable times after a second-look procedure.
- Interval debulking, when a response to chemotherapy is identifiable, has recently been advocated after chemotherapy if primary surgical debulking was not possible, but this may only give an additional life expectancy of 6 months.
- Palliative surgery does not have the intention of prolonging survival but aims to alleviate symptoms such as bowel obstruction, which occurs in 10–40 per cent of women with terminal ovarian cancer. The prognosis in this situation is usually about 2 months [17].

Complications of major gynaecological surgery (Tables 13.9–13.11) [18–21]

Complications of hysterectomy

There can be a requirement for blood transfusion – 2–12 per cent for abdominal hysterectomy and 2–8 per cent for vaginal hysterectomy, 1 per cent for laparoscopic surgery.

The risk of injury is shown in Table 13.12.

Table 13.9 Risks of hysterectomy. (Dicker *et al.* (1982) [18].)

	Vaginal (%)	Abdominal (%)
Morbidity (1–2 per 1000)	42.8	24.5
Haemorrhage	8.3	15.4
Damage to bowel	0.3	0.4
Bladder	0.3	1.6
Ureter	0	0.3
Cerebral mortality	15.3	32.3
Life-threatening events	0	0.4
Urinary retention	15	4.8
Other	0	0.2

Table 13.10 Bowel injury after various types of gynaecological surgery. (Krebs (1986) [21].)

Type of surgery	Rate per thousand
Laparotomy	8.4
Vaginal hysterectomy	7.3
Laparoscopy	3.0
Dilatation and curettage/evacuation	1.5

Table 13.11 Morbidity from total abdominal hysterectomy. (Clarke *et al.* (1995) [20].)

Morbidity	Percentage
Wound infection	5.2
Urinary tract infection (UTI)	5.0
Other infections	5.5
Bleeding	3.8
Deep vein thrombosis/pulmonary embolism (DVT/PE)	1.4
At 3 months cumulative wound infection or UTI	40.0

Table 13.12 Risk of injury during hysterectomy.

Injury	Percentage risk
Bowel injury	0.1–1
Bladder injury	1–2 (0.2–1.15)[22]
Ureteric injury	0.1–0.5
Unintended major surgical procedure	1.7

For postoperative infections
- Cefuroxime 750 mg i.v. 8-hourly
- Metronidazole 500 mg i.v. 8-hourly or 1 g p.r. 12-hourly or as soon as fluids are tolerated 400 mg p.o. 8-hourly.

Alternatively, cefoxitin alone (1–2 g 8-hourly) may be used. While metronidazole provides cover for more *Bacteroides* isolates than cefoxitin, it need not be added as a routine to cefoxitin.

Deep vein thrombosis

Diagnosis
- Contrast venography
- Non-invasive methods – venous ultrasonographic imaging used to compress proximal veins with the ultrasound transducer. An inability to compress a vein indicates the presence of a deep vein thrombosis (DVT) (sensitivity 98 per cent, specificity 96 per cent)
- Biochemical assays – D-dimer.

Treatment
Treatment of a DVT (Table 13.13) is adjusted dose, intravenous, unfractionated heparin for 5–10 days, combined with oral anticoag-

Table 13.13 Initial treatment of established venous thrombosis of the legs or pulmonary embolism but without refractory hypotension. (Adapted with permission from Lensing *et al.* (1999) [23].)

Unfractionated heparin
5000 U intravenous bolus followed by 30 000–35 000 units per 24 hours by intravenous infusion or 35 000–40 000 units per 24 hours subcutaneously adjusted to maintain APPT at 1.5–2.5 × control baseline value

Low molecular weight heparins
Any of the following:
Enoxaparin 100 anti-Xa units/kg twice daily
Dalteparin 200 anti-Xa units/kg once daily
Tinzaparin 175 anti-Xa units/kg once daily

Give by subcutaneous injection without bolus injection and laboratory monitoring

Both regimens are continued for 5–10 days with an oral anticoagulant started on day 1, then continued alone

APTT, activated partial thromboplastin time.

ulants for at least 3 months [23]. The dose is adjusted to the international normalised ratio of 2.0–3.0. Unfractionated heparin may be given subcutaneously. It requires daily monitoring of the activated partial thromboplastin time (APTT) and the dose is adjusted to maintain the anticoagulant effect at an APTT at least 1.5 times the control value. The anticoagulant response to heparin varies greatly over time between patients as well as in an individual patient.

Low molecular weight heparins (LMWHs) have a longer plasma half-life and almost complete bioavailability after subcutaneous injection. Once or twice daily regimens may be given without the need for laboratory monitoring. Daily LMWH doses vary between 155 and 200 anti-Xa units/kg. Oral anticoagulants are started within 24–48 hours of presentation. LMWHs have the advantage of a substantially lower risk of heparin-induced thrombocytopenia compared with heparin.

Oral anticoagulation is continued for a period of 3–6 months or longer, depending on risk factors and complications. There is always a risk of major haemorrhage.

Other complications

These include symptoms reported that have worsened after the operation that include dyspareunia, decreased libido, hot flushes, poor appetite, constipation, weight gain, back pain and urinary problems. Although psychiatric disturbance can be enhanced, there is evidence for general mood improvement postoperatively.

REFERENCES

1 ISGE Newsletter. The International Society for Gynaecological Endoscopy.
2 Mittendorf, R., Aronson, M.P., Berry, R.E. *et al.* (1993) Avoiding serious infections associated with abdominal hysterectomy: a meta-analysis of antibiotic prophylaxis. *American Journal of Obstetrics and Gynecology*, **169**, 1119–1124.
3 Garry, R. (1999) Editorial: Towards evidence-based laparoscopic entry techniques: clinical problems and dilemmas. *Gynaecological Endoscopy*, **8**, 315–326.
4 Garry, R. & Phillips, Y. (1995) How safe is the laparoscopic approach to hysterectomy? *Gynecological Endoscopy*, **4**, 77–79.
5 Hasson, H.M. (1971) A modified instrument and method for laparoscopy. *American Journal of Obstetrics and Gynecology*, **110**, 886–887.

6 Ethicon (1999) *Wound closure management.* Ethicon, Somerville, NJ.

7 Kovac, S.R. & Cruikshank, S.H. (1996) Guidelines to determine the route of oophorectomy with hysterectomy. *American Journal of Obstetrics and Gynecology*, **175**, 1483–1488.

8 Hefni, M.A. & Davies, A.E. (1997) Vaginal endoscopic oophorectomy with vaginal hysterectomy: a simple minimal access surgery technique. *British Journal of Obstetrics and Gynaecology*, **104**, 621–622.

9 Sheth, S.F. (1991) The place of oophorectomy at vaginal hysterectomy. *British Journal of Obstetrics and Gynaecology*, **98**, 662–666.

10 Jacobs, I. & Oram, D. (1989) Prevention of ovarian cancer: a survey of the practice of prophylactic oophorectomy by the fellows and members of the Royal College of Obstetricians and Gynaecologists. *British Journal of Obstetrics and Gynaecology*, **96**, 510–515.

11 Sighter, S.E., Boike, G.M., Estape, R.E. & Averette, H.E. (1991) Ovarian cancer in women with prior hysterectomy: a 14-year experience at the University of Miami. *Obstetrics and Gynecology*, **78**, 681–684.

12 Snooks, S.J., Swash, M., Mathers, S.E. & Henry, M.M. (1990) Effect of vaginal delivery on the pelvic floor: a 5-year follow-up. *British Journal of Surgery*, **77**, 1358–1360.

13 Bump, R.C., Mattiasson, A., Bo, K. *et al.* (1996) The standardization of terminology of female pelvic organ prolapse and pelvic floor dysfunction. *American Journal of Obstetrics and Gynecology*, **175**, 10–17.

14 Jackson, S. & Smith, P. (1997) Diagnosing and managing genitourinary prolapse. *British Medical Journal*, **314**, 875–880.

15 Cruickshank, S.H. (1991) Sacrospinous fixation – should this be performed at the time of vaginal hysterectomy? *American Journal of Obstetrics and Gynecology*, **164**, 1072–1076.

16 Hardiman, P.J. & Drutz, H.P. (1996) Sacrospinous vault suspension and abdominal colposacropexy: success rates and complications. *American Journal of Obstetrics and Gynecology*, **175**, 612–616.

17 Hunter, R.W., Alexander, N.D. & Soutter W.P. (1992) Meta-analysis of surgery in advanced ovarian carcinoma: is maximum cytoreductive surgery an independent determinant of prognosis? *American Journal of Obstetrics and Gynecology*, **166**, 504–511.

18 Dicker, R.C., Greenspan, J.R., Strauss, L.T. *et al.* (1982) Complications of abdominal and vaginal hysterectomy among women of reproductive age in the United States. *American Journal of Obstetrics and Gynecology*, **144**, 841–848.

19 Harris, W.J. (1995) Early complications of abdominal and vaginal hysterectomy. *Obstetrical and Gynecological Survey*, **50**, 795–805.

20 Clarke, A., Black, N., Rowe, P., Mott, S. & Howle, K. (1995) Indications for and outcome of total abdominal hysterectomy for benign disease: a prospective cohort study. *British Journal of Obstetrics and Gynaecology*, **102**, 611–620.

21 Krebs, H.B. (1986) Intestinal injury in gynecologic surgery: a 10-year experience. *American Journal of Obstetrics and Gynecology*, **155**, 509–514.

22 Brown, J.S., Sawaya, G., Thom, D.H. & Grady, D. (2000) Hysterectomy and urinary incontinence: a systemic review. *The Lancet*, **356**, 535–539.

23 Lensing, A.W.A., Prandoni, P., Prins, M.H. & Buller, H.R. (1999) Deep vein thrombosis. *The Lancet*, **353**, 479–485.

13

14 Gynaecological Oncology

Cheryl Wright

CERVICAL MALIGNANCIES

The world's most common malignancy in women is declining in incidence, as a result of cervical screening programmes. Earlier detection and treatment of cervical cancer has reduced mortality by over 50 per cent.

Clinical presentation and symptoms

An abnormal cervical cytology smear (Pap smear) may be the only indicator of cervical disease. Pap smears have a higher sensitivity for the more common squamous lesions than glandular lesions. Common early symptoms include:
- Abnormal vaginal bleeding (postcoital, intermenstrual, post-menopausal or menorrhagia)
- Vaginal discharge, sometimes malodorous.

With progression of disease, the bleeding may result in anaemia. Dysuria, severe and complete constipation and rectal bleeding may signal bladder or rectal involvement. Renal obstruction may cause pain and lead to hydronephrosis and renal failure. Abdominal or leg pain may be secondary to lymphadenopathy.

Physical examination

Pelvic examination may show an obvious cervical abnormality, such as ulceration or exophytic mass. Extensive involvement of the endo-cervix may result in an enlarged barrel-shaped cervix. A pelvic mass may be palpated.

General examination may reveal evidence of metastases, perhaps as an abdominal mass due to para-aortic lymphadenopathy, or supraclavicular lymphadenopathy. There may be signs of uraemia, anaemia or jaundice.

Diagnosis

A tissue biopsy is required to confirm malignancy (even though a cervical smear may show malignant cells), and to identify the histological type of tumour. Endocervical curettage (ECC) should be done as well, to detect any lesions that may be in the endocervical canal.

Pathology

14

Most cervical cancers are squamous cell carcinomas (over 80 per cent), but adenocarcinomas are increasing in incidence (15–20 per cent) [1]. Both types of cancer are believed to generally arise from a precursor dysplastic lesion [2,3].

Non-epithelial tumours such as sarcomas, melanomas and lymphomas are rare.

Squamous (epidermoid) neoplasias

Squamous cancers arise from dysplastic squamous epithelium at the transformation zone. Over 85 per cent of cervical squamous cancers and precursor lesions contain DNA of the sexually transmitted virus human papillomavirus (HPV). The three major associated risk factors are early age at first intercourse, multiple sexual partners, and a male partner with multiple previous sexual partners. Other factors may include oral contraceptive use, cigarette smoking, parity, family history, and associated genital infections [3]. Immunosuppressed patients (e.g. transplant or AIDS patients) are also at increased risk.

In invasive carcinoma, the neoplastic cells have breached the basement membrane investing the squamous mucosa, and invaded stroma. The lesion has acquired the potential to metastasise and is regarded as malignant. The tumour may be microinvasive (*superficially invasive*) or frankly invasive.

Microinvasive tumours occur in a younger age group than the frankly invasive tumours (43 versus 51 years old) [3], and account for up to 20 per cent of squamous cancers. Colposcopically the lesion resembles a squamous intraepithelial lesion (SIL).

The tumour may qualify as microinvasive if:
- The tumour is not clinically apparent.
- Using FIGO rules, the maximum depth is no greater than 5 mm, and the maximum width is no greater than 7 mm.

- Using Society of Gynecologic Oncology (SGO) rules, the maximum depth is 3 mm, and no capillary/lymphatic space invasion (CLSI) is present [3].

The entire tumour must be removed before accurate measurements can be made; a diagnosis of microinvasion cannot be made on punch biopsy material alone. If microinvasion is diagnosed in a cone, then the margins must be clear of high grade squamous intraepithelial lesion (HSIL) as well as invasive tumour.

Lymph node metastasis, tumour recurrence and death all correlate directly with depth of invasion. Lesions less than 1 mm deep have a positive node rate of <0.5 per cent, and no deaths or recurrences. This rate climbs to 1.3 per cent for deeper lesions up to 3 mm; 0.5 per cent have recurrences, but still no deaths. The positive node rate climbs more sharply to 6.8 per cent for lesions up to 5 mm deep; recurrence in this group reaches 2.3 per cent, with 1.5 per cent deaths [4].

Classifications of squamous cell carcinoma (SCC) have been based on differentiation or degree of keratinisation. Keratinising tumours are more radioresistant, but not all studies have shown that this affects survival [3]. The classifications are:

- Well differentiated (large cell keratinising carcinoma)
- Moderately differentiated (large cell non-keratinising carcinoma)
- Poorly differentiated (small cell squamous cell carcinoma) – note that small cell squamous carcinoma is a different tumour from small cell carcinoma, which is a neuroendocrine tumour similar to oat cell carcinoma of the lung.

Variants of squamous cell carcinoma are:

(1) Papillary squamous (transitional) cell carcinoma [4]
   (a) Rare; microscopically resembles bladder tumour
   (b) Behaves like conventional squamous cancer
(2) Glassy cell carcinoma
   (a) 1–2 per cent of cancers [4]
   (b) Younger, mean age 30–40 years old
   (c) Usually a bulky mass, yet disproportionately less invasion
   (d) Seems to have worse prognosis than conventional squamous cancer, but published series are small
(3) Verrucous carcinoma
   (a) Extremely rare; a bulky exophytic lesion, identical to those that more characteristically occur on the vulva
   (b) Slow growing and locally invasive, but no reports of metastases.

Glandular neoplasias

Adenocarcinoma in situ

Adenocarcinoma in situ (AIS) is the precursor to most invasive adenocarcinomas [2,3]. Skip lesions are not uncommon, and a negative resection margin of a cone does not assure removal of the lesion. Over one third of these patients with a negative margin may have residual AIS or invasive adenocarcinoma. However, Goldstein and Mani in a study of 61 patients found that if the resection margin in a cone was clear of AIS by at least 10 mm, then none of the patients had residual AIS in the subsequent hysterectomy specimen [5].

Invasive adenocarcinoma

- Most adenocarcinomas arise from the endocervical glands, usually in the region of the squamocolumnar junction [2].
- There is a high frequency (over 80 per cent) of HPV infection (types 18 as well as 16, 31) [1].
- Most recent studies indicate that prognosis for typical adenocarcinomas is no worse than for squamous cancer.
- Most have associated AIS; the average interval between presentation of AIS and invasive carcinoma may be about 5 years [2].

  Types of invasive adenocarcinoma are:
(1) Mucinous adenocarcinoma
  (a) Endocervical type – most common
  (b) Also signet ring and intestinal types
(2) Endometrioid adenocarcinoma
  (a) May be even more common than the endocervical type [1]
  (b) Located higher up in the endocervical canal [2]
(3) Clear cell carcinoma – most have been in young women with history of exposure *in utero* to diethylstilbestrol (DES); decreasing incidence
(4) Villoglandular adenocarcinoma
  (a) Rare, first described in 1989
  (b) Often younger patients, less than 40 years old
  (c) Rarely reported outside the uterus, but can be deeply invasive; cone may be sufficient if margins clear, invasion <3 mm, no vascular space invasion
(5) Minimal deviation adenocarcinoma (adenoma malignum) [1]
  (a) About 10 per cent of adenocarcinomas
  (b) Often in women in their forties; occasionally associated with Peutz–Jeghers syndrome

(c) Extremely bland appearance may be difficult to diagnose as malignant on small biopsies

(d) Most have nodal spread, and die of tumour

(6) Serous carcinoma – a papillary lesion identical to those more commonly found in the ovary or endometrium

(7) Mesonephric adenocarcinoma

    (a) Arise from mesonephric remnants deep in the lateral wall

    (b) Diagnosed if

       (i) deep in lateral wall

       (ii) endocervix mucosa uninvolved

       (iii) no evidence of DES exposure

    (c) Rare; aggressive behaviour

(8) Adenoid basal carcinoma [1]

    (a) Associated with HSIL; contain HPV type 16 [6]

    (b) Often picked up in cytology from asymptomatic post-menopausal women

    (c) Cervix usually not enlarged, and no mass palpated

    (d) Prognosis excellent after hysterectomy; occasional reports of nodal metastases.

Adenosquamous

- This has both adenocarcinoma and squamous carcinoma components.
- It is often associated with pregnancy [4].
- Some but not all investigators have believed it has a worse prognosis.

Small cell undifferentiated carcinoma [3]

- This is a neuroendocrine tumour, not to be confused with the small cell type of squamous cancer; similar to oat cell carcinoma of the lung.
- HPV 18 is present in most.
- It is an infiltrative lesion producing an indurated appearance.
- It is very aggressive, producing distant metastases in 80–90 per cent.
- It is very radiosensitive and chemosensitive. Staging should include a bone marrow biopsy.

Pretreatment and staging investigations

Cervical cancer is clinically staged using the FIGO criteria (Table 14.1) [7]. This is not as accurate as surgical staging, but it permits comparison of results of treatment.

Table 14.1 Carcinoma of the uterine cervix – staging. (With permission from Benedet *et al.* (2000) [7].)

FIGO stages			TNM categories
		Primary tumour cannot be assessed	TX
		No evidence of primary tumour	T0
0		Carcinoma in situ (preinvasive carcinoma)	Tis
1		Cervical carcinoma confined to uterus (extension to corpus should be disregarded)	T1
	1A	Invasive carcinoma diagnosed by microscopy. All macroscopically visible lesions – even with superficial invasion – are stage 1B/T1b	T1a
	1A1	Stromal invasion no greater than 3 mm in depth and 7 mm or less in horizontal spread	T1a1
	1A2	Stromal invasion more than 3 mm and not more than 5 mm with a horizontal spread 7 mm or less[1]	T1a2
	1B	Clinically visible lesion confined to the cervix, or microscopic lesion greater than 1A2/T1a2	T1b
	1B1	Clinically visible lesion 4 cm or less in greatest dimension	T1b1
	1B2	Clinically visible lesion more than 4 cm in greatest dimension	T1b2
2		Tumour invades beyond the uterus but not to pelvic wall or to lower third of the vagina	T2
	2A	Without parametrial invasion	T2a
	2B	With parametrial invasion	T2b
3		Tumour extends to pelvic wall and/or involves lower third of vagina and/or causes hydronephrosis or non-functioning kidney	T3
	3A	Tumour involves lower third of vagina, no extension to pelvic wall	T3a
	3B	Tumour extends to pelvic wall and/or causes hydronephrosis or non-functioning kidney	T3b or N1
	4A	Tumour invades *mucosa* of bladder or rectum and/or extends beyond true pelvis[2]	T4
	4B	Distant metastases	M1

[1] The depth of invasion should not be more than 5 mm taken from the base of the epithelium, either surface or glandular, from which it originates. The depth of invasion is defined as the measurement of the tumour from the epithelial–stromal junction of the adjacent most superficial epithelial papilla to the deepest point of invasion. Vascular space involvement, venous or lymphatic, does not affect classification.

[2] The presence of bullous oedema is not sufficient to classify a tumour as T4.

14

Only results from certain examinations are eligible for FIGO staging purposes. Additional investigations may be used to plan treatment, but information obtained from them should not alter the clinical stage. When there is doubt as to which stage a particular cancer should be allocated, the earlier stage is mandatory. The staging examinations may include:

- Clinical examination under anaesthesia (EUA) of the pelvis, performed by both an oncologist and gynaecologist:
  Bimanual pelvic examination – document relationship of tumour to parametrium, vagina and pelvic side walls. Since a smooth indurated parametrium may be only inflamed, a case should be placed in stage 3 only if it is *nodular* to the pelvic wall or if the growth itself extends to the pelvic wall
  Speculum examination.
- Colposcopy, endocervical curettage, hysteroscopy.
- Conisation or amputation of the cervix is regarded as a clinical examination.
- Cystoscopy or proctoscopy may be indicated in the presence of advanced disease or symptoms; suspected bladder or rectal involvement should be confirmed by biopsy.
- Intravenous urography.
- X-ray examination of the lungs and skeleton.

Other investigations (in addition to complete history and physical examination) to assess general health and extent of disease will be needed, for example full blood count, renal and liver function tests, possibly computerised tomography (CT) to assess liver, kidneys and urinary tract, and to assess lymphadenopathy.

Spread and metastasis [4]

Cervical cancers spread directly into the vaginal fornix, up into uterus, parametrial and paracervical tissues, the pelvic wall, and then to other pelvic structures such as the bladder or rectum.

Lymphatic spread involves hypogastric, external iliac and sacral nodes, and then common iliac, inguinal and para-aortic nodes. One third of those with positive para-aortic nodes will have scalene node involvement.

Haematogenous spread is uncommon, and occurs late in the course of the disease. This is usually to lung, liver and bone.

General principles of treating cervical cancer

Surgery and radiation therapy are equally effective in treating early stage, small volume tumours.

Surgery is the treatment of choice for younger fit patients, if there is a low risk of nodal metastases (Table 14.2).

- Surgical staging is the most accurate way of determining disease extent.
- Surgery alone, without radiation, maintains vaginal anatomy and sexual function.
- The ovaries can be preserved and moved out of the way of the postoperative radiation field. They may still receive low doses of scattered radiation, but usually not enough to stop them from functioning (unless the patient is perimenopausal).
- Surgery without radiation avoids the small risk of radiation-induced malignancy.

Radiotherapy alone is the treatment of choice for older less fit patients, those who may not be medically fit for surgery, and those with advanced disease (Table 14.2). Indications include:

- Bulky tumours (>4 cm, at least stage 1B2)
- High risk of nodal involvement
- Lymphovascular involvement
- Abnormal nodes on radiological studies
- Extension of disease onto vaginal wall
- Multifocal disease.

Recently the use of platinum-based chemotherapy given concurrently with radiation has been shown to decrease deaths from cervical cancer by 30–50 per cent. This was demonstrated in five randomised trials for those with stages 1B2 to 4A cervical cancer [8].

Postoperative radiotherapy after radical hysterectomy is indicated for those at high risk of local recurrence:

- Lymphovascular space invasion
- Deep cervical invasion to outer third
- Positive or close (<3 mm) surgical resection margins
- Parametrial involvement
- Positive pelvic or para-aortic lymph node metastases.

Management of other cancers and special clinical scenarios

(1) Small cell undifferentiated (neuroendocrine) carcinoma
   (a) Chemotherapy (e.g. adriamycin, cyclophosphamide, vincristine and etoposide) and radiotherapy to sites of bulky disease

14

Table 14.2 Management of cervical cancer (squamous carcinomas and adenocarcinomas).

Stage	Surgical treatment	Radiation treatment[1]	Survival
1A1 <1% risk of nodal involvement[2]	Conisation Simple hysterectomy	or Brachytherapy as primary treatment	Cure rate greater than 90%
1A1 higher risk (<10%) of nodal involvement[2] 1A2	Modified radical hysterectomy with pelvic lymph node dissection	Postoperative EBRT and/or brachytherapy	Cure rate 85–90%
1B (15–25% risk of nodal involvement)	Radical hysterectomy and bilateral pelvic lymphadenectomy (plus postoperative radical radiotherapy if high risk factors for recurrence present)	or Radical radiotherapy with platinum-based chemotherapy as primary treatment	As above
1B2	Radical hysterectomy and bilateral pelvic lymphadenectomy, plus postoperative radical radiotherapy	or Preferred option of radical radiotherapy with platinum-based chemotherapy, with radiation to para-aortic nodes	As above

2A	Radical hysterectomy and bilateral pelvic lymphadenectomy (plus postoperative radical radiotherapy if high risk factors for recurrence present)	*or* Radical radiotherapy with platinum-based chemotherapy as primary treatment	75–80%
2B	} Preferred option is radical radiotherapy with platinum-based chemotherapy		60–65%
3			25–50%
4A	Pelvic exenteration Radical radiotherapy with platinum-based chemotherapy Symptomatic care only, especially if organ failure or multiple comorbidities		20–35%
4B	Individualised treatment, usually palliative		As above

EBRT, external beam radiation therapy.

[1] Radical radiotherapy is external beam pelvic irradiation and an intracavitary brachytherapy boost, fractionated over 5 weeks.

[2] There is a risk of lymph node involvement in microinvasive carcinoma if:
- Depth of invasion is 3–5 mm in the cone biopsy
- HSIL or invasive tumour at cone resection margin
- Lymphovascular invasion.

14

(b) May be dramatic responses initially to treatment, but early recurrences and distant metastases common; poor prognosis

(2) Carcinoma during pregnancy – for early invasive disease (1A and early 1B), treatment may be delayed until fetal maturity. The outcome of the disease will not be adversely affected [7]

(3) Unexpected finding of invasive cancer in uterus removed for other reasons (simple hysterectomy) – if margins are clear, vault brachytherapy will improve prognosis

(4) Recurrence – treatment options
- (a) Pelvic exenteration
- (b) Chemoirradiation
- (c) Radiation alone
- (d) Palliation.

Side effects of radiotherapy

Acute
- Skin – irritation, erythema, desquamation
- Bladder – frequency, urgency, dysuria
- Bowel – diarrhoea, tenesmus
- Malaise, lethargy, occasionally mild nausea.

Chronic
- Bladder – frequency, haematuria
- Bowel – frequency, occasionally rectal bleeding
- Sexual – vaginal dryness, stenosis, dyspareunia, infertility, menopausal symptoms (from cessation of ovarian function).

Prognosis [4]

- Most deaths occur in the first 3 years.
- Most recurrences happen in the first 2 years; once the tumour recurs, the 1-year survival is about 10–15 per cent.
- Most recurrences are in the pelvis.
- Almost half of the recurrences will develop ureteric obstruction.

OVARIAN MALIGNANCIES

The incidence of ovarian cancer is 9–17 per 100 000 women per year. The incidence is highest in industrialised countries except for Japan.

The lifetime risk for a woman developing ovarian cancer is 1 in 70, and increases with age.

According to the 'incessant ovulation' theory of ovarian cancer, repeated ovulations increase the risk of cancer. This may be secondary to repeated damage and repair of the ovarian surface epithelium. Therefore higher risk is associated with nulliparity and low parity, and reduced risk is found with early age at first pregnancy, early menopause and the use of the oral contraceptive pill [9]. The risk of ovarian cancer decreases 40 per cent in those who have ever used oral contraceptives. The risk drops even further, to 50 per cent, in those who have used it for at least 5 years, and the protective effect lasts for up to 10–15 years after stopping the drug [10].

Genetic factors are implicated in approximately 5 per cent of all ovarian cancers. Three hereditary syndromes showing autosomal dominant inheritance are:

(1) Breast–ovarian cancer syndrome, linked to an inherited mutation in the BRCA1 gene. Carriers of BRCA1 have a 50 per cent lifetime risk of ovarian cancer.

(2) Site-specific ovarian cancer syndrome.

(3) Hereditary non-polyposis colorectal cancer (HNPCC) syndrome (type II Lynch syndrome), which can include colon, breast, endometrial and prostate cancer in affected individuals and which is usually associated with a history of malignancy appearing before the age of 30.

Screening

No effective screening programme for the general population for the identification of ovarian cancer has been established. Studies using a combination of the tumour marker CA125, pelvic abdominal ultrasound and pelvic examination have not produced an acceptable sensitivity or specificity to be used alone or in combination for screening of ovarian cancer.

Patients with a strong family history of ovarian, endometrial, breast and colon cancers may be candidates for genetic testing, in order to identify BRCA1 mutation carriers and HNPCC individuals. Patients with these inherited cancers usually present about 10 years earlier than the previous generation. They may benefit from earlier screening, using CA125 markers and transvaginal ultrasound on a yearly basis, but so far this is unproven.

Clinical presentation and symptoms

Seventy-five per cent of ovarian cancer cases present late, at stage 3 or 4 at diagnosis.

- Abdominal distention may be due to the tumour, ascites or both. This is the most common symptom.
- Respiratory symptoms may result from the increased intra-abdominal pressure or transudation of fluid into the pleural cavity.
- Abdominal discomfort.
- Feeling of pressure in the pelvis.
- Urinary or gastrointestinal tract symptoms.
- Abnormal vaginal bleeding may be present, particularly if the tumour has functional stroma. Any type of benign or malignant tumour may contain stromal cells that are producing oestrogenic or androgenic hormones; the syndrome is not restricted to sex-cord stromal tumours. The most common oestrogen-associated tumours are mucinous and endometrioid carcinomas, and metastatic colo-rectal cancer. Androgenic tumours are most commonly metastatic gastric cancers, primary benign mucinous tumours, and other miscellaneous types [11].
- Acute pain may result from torsion or rupture. Torsion is more often seen with benign tumours that are not adherent to tissues. The most common examples are dermoid cysts and serous cystadenomas. Rupture is more likely to be a malignant tumour.

Paraendocrine syndromes

A variety of paraendocrine syndromes may be associated with ovarian tumours [11]:

- Human chorionic gonadotropin (hCG) secretion may occur with germ cell tumours containing syncytiotrophoblastic cells.
- Hypercalcaemia – small cell and clear cell carcinomas are most common; also serous carcinoma, dysgerminoma, as well as miscellaneous others.
- Cushing's syndrome – cortisol production by steroid cell tumours. It is also found in a variety of tumours that produce ectopic adreno-corticotrophic hormone (ACTH).
- Zollinger–Ellison syndrome – gastrin secretion in mucinous tumours.
- Hypertension related to renin and aldosterone production is most often in sex-cord stromal tumours.

Paraneoplastic syndromes [11]

- Subacute cerebellar degeneration (SCD) – ovarian cancer is one of the most common malignancies associated with paraneoplastic disorder of the nervous system; up to 16 per cent of ovarian cancer patients may be affected. Up to half of those with SCD have ovarian cancer, usually serous carcinoma. The cerebellar manifestations most commonly precede the diagnosis of the cancer, at times by up to several years.
- Dermatomyositis and polymyositis – over 10 per cent may have or develop ovarian cancer, usually serous carcinoma. The onset of the dermatomyositis usually precedes diagnosis of the tumour, which usually becomes evident within 2 years.
- Autoimmune haemolytic anaemia – most often benign dermoid cysts, but some carcinomas too.

14

Physical examination

- Irregular pelvic mass
- Abdominal distention
- Shifting dullness, indicating ascites.

Pretreatment investigations

- Complete personal and family history, in particular any history of breast, ovarian, endometrial, urothelial and bowel cancer
- Physical examination, including pelvic and rectovaginal examination
- Chest X-ray
- CT scan, ultrasound, and barium enema if indicated
- Full blood count, liver and renal function tests
- Tumour markers including CA125, carcinoembryonic antigen (CEA), α-fetoprotein (αFP), βhCG and lactate dehydrogenase (LDH), inhibin.

Investigation of the pelvic mass in reproductive age group women

If the mass has a high chance of being malignant then laparoscopic investigation should not be used. There is the potential for tumour cells to seed along puncture lines, suture lines and trocar ports. Features associated with increased likelihood of malignancy are:

- Older age – one half of tumours in those older than 45 years are malignant; in patients less than 45 years, less than one eighth of the tumours are malignant
- Bilaterality – bilateral tumours are more likely to be malignant; serous tumours and metastases from an extraovarian tumour are common
- Fixed or solid masses
- Complex masses with excrescences – they may have a typical 'cauliflower' intracystic appearance
- Elevated tumour markers.

Pathology [11]

A bewildering array of benign, borderline and malignant tumours affects the ovaries. About two thirds of all ovarian tumours, and 90 per cent of the malignancies, are surface epithelial tumours (Table 14.3). The remaining major categories are sex cord-stromal tumours and germ cell tumours. Dermoid cysts (benign mature teratomas) are the single most common ovarian tumour, and occur in all age groups.

The surface epithelial tumours are further classified into benign, borderline (also called low malignant potential, or atypically pro-liferative tumours) and malignant tumours. Since most of these tumours are of glandular derivation, 'adeno' is usually a root word. Predominantly cystic lesions may have 'cyst' as a prefix, and those with prominent fibrous stroma may have 'fibroma' as a suffix. For instance, a benign cystic tumour composed of serous (tubal) type epithelium would be called a 'benign serous cystadenoma'.

Serous, mucinous, endometrioid and clear cell tumours frequently have a papillary architecture. Beware of a diagnosis of 'papillary carcinoma'. This term, without the proper designation of serous, etc., is meaningless and only indicates that the tumour is an adenocarcinoma.

Borderline tumours

These show greater epithelial proliferation than benign tumours, but lack evidence of invasion into stroma. However, they may be found with peritoneal implants or lymph node metastases. The border-line designation is based on the morphology of the primary tumour, regardless of presence or absence of metastases.

Table 14.3 Surface epithelial tumours of the ovary.

Type	Percentage of type	Mean age	Percentage bilateral	Comments
Serous (20–50%)				Borderline and malignant serous tumours account for 35–40% of all ovarian cancers. CA125 elevated in >80% of carcinomas
Benign	70	40s	10	
Borderline	5–10	46	35	
Malignant	20–25	56	66	
Mucinous (15%)				Most common epithelial tumour in first two decades. Increased incidence in Peutz–Jeghers syndrome. Largest of all epithelial tumours. 3–5% develop in association with dermoid cysts. CA125 elevated in half to two thirds of carcinomas
Benign	75	20s–40s	<5	
Borderline, intestinal	9	41	6	
Borderline, endocervical	1	34	40	
Malignant	15	54	5–10	
Endometrioid (<5%) (benign and borderline forms rare)		56		5–10% arise in endometriosis. One third associated with independent endometrial cancer. CA125 elevated in >80% of carcinomas.
Clear cell (5%) (benign and borderline forms uncommon)		40s–70s	Rare	Tumour most often associated with endometriosis. Highest association with paraendocrine hypercalcaemia
Transitional cell and Brenner	30–70			98% are incidental findings and are benign. Of the clinically detectable ones, 5% are borderline or malignant
Brenner (2–3%)				
Transitional cell (<1%)				
Squamous cell carcinoma				May arise in dermoid cyst.
Mixed				Tumours with at least two different histological types, each forming at least 10% of the tumour

14

Serous tumours

These usually have a complex cystic component. Papillary excrescences frequently line the cysts.

Borderline serous tumours

- About 10 per cent of these tumours may have microinvasion. Their prognosis is similar to that of borderline, rather than malignant, tumours.
- Peritoneal implants of borderline tumours may be non-invasive or invasive type. This is a histological assessment. Ninety per cent of patients with non-invasive implants are free of disease at 4 years, compared with only 17 per cent of those with invasive implants.

Variants

Rarely, the tumour may grow as minute fine granules on the surface of the ovary and peritoneum ('serous surface carcinoma'). Psammoma bodies, laminated rounded calcifications, are frequently found in these tumours. They represent dystrophic calcifications of the necrotic tips of the papillae. One form of low grade serous carcinoma has such an abundance of these bodies that it is termed 'psammocarcinoma'.

Mucinous tumours

Most mucinous tumours are composed of epithelium resembling that of the intestinal tract. The less common type of mucinous epithelium resembles endocervical glands, or Müllerian type epithelium.

- *Borderline tumours* – endocervical-like mucinous borderline tumours (EMBT), compared with intestinal-type mucinous borderline tumours (IMBT), occur in a younger patient (34 versus 41 years), are more often bilateral (40 versus 6 per cent), are smaller, less often multiloculated (20 versus 72 per cent), and are more often found with endometriosis (30 versus 6 per cent). They have an excellent prognosis, even in the presence of lymph node metastases. In contrast, only IMBT is found in association with pseudomyxoma peritonei.
- *Carcinomas* – mucinous carcinomas frequently have numerous areas of benign, borderline and frankly malignant-appearing areas. The implications of this are that a frozen section may not reveal a malignant component; this may not become apparent until numerous permanent sections have been examined.

The differential diagnosis of mucinous tumours, especially bilateral ones, must always include metastases, especially from the colon.

■ *Pseudomyxoma peritonei* – this is the presence of masses of jelly-like mucus in the pelvis and sometimes abdomen. It has previously been ascribed to ovarian mucinous tumours, but some cases are associated with appendiceal mucinous carcinomas which have metastasised to the ovary. If this entity is encountered at surgery, the appendix should also be removed, regardless of its appearance.

14

Spread

Ovarian cancers spread directly to adjacent pelvic organs, the pelvic wall and peritoneal surfaces, especially the right paracolic gutter, the right undersurface of the diaphragm, and onto the omentum. They metastasise via the broad ligament lymphatics to the iliac, obturator and hypogastric lymph nodes, and spread via the infundibulo-pelvic ligament lymphatics to the para-aortic nodes.

Staging and treatment of ovarian carcinomas

Ovarian carcinomas are surgically staged using the FIGO system (Table 14.4) [7].

A staging laparotomy is the cornerstone of management for ovarian cancer. The goal is to have no gross residual disease after the primary surgery (debulking). FIGO's recommended approach to staging is:

(1) A vertical midline abdominal incision is made, immediate peritoneal washings of pelvis and abdomen are performed, and the fluid is sent for cytology.

(2) Careful exploration of intra-abdominal contents:

    (a) Examine and palpate omentum, diaphragm, liver, peritoneal cul-de-sac, adnexal surfaces, as well as aortic and pelvic lymph nodes.

    (b) Biopsy suspicious areas.

    (c) The omentum is a common site of spread and should ideally be removed, even if it is clinically uninvolved.

    (d) Where there is no obvious extraovarian spread, do random peritoneal biopsies from the peritoneal reflection of the bladder, the posterior cul-de-sac, the right and left paracolic

Table 14.4 Carcinoma of the ovary – staging.[1] (With permission from Benedet *et al.* (2000) [7].)

FIGO stages			TNM categories
		Primary tumour cannot be assessed	TX
		No evidence of primary tumour	T0
1		Tumour limited to the ovaries	T1
	1A	Tumour limited to one ovary; capsule intact, no tumour on ovarian surface; no malignant cells in ascites or peritoneal washings	T1a
	1B	Tumour limited to both ovaries; capsule intact, no tumour on ovarian surface; no malignant cells in ascites or peritoneal washings	T1b
	1C	Tumour limited to one or both ovaries with any of the following: capsule ruptured, tumour on ovarian surface, malignant cells in ascites or peritoneal washings	T1c
2		Tumour involves one or both ovaries with pelvic extension	T2
	2A	Extension and/or implants on uterus and/or tube(s); no malignant cells in ascites or peritoneal washings	T2a
	2B	Extension to other pelvic tissues; no malignant cells in ascites or peritoneal washings	T2b
	2C	Pelvic extension (2A or 2B) with malignant cells in ascites or peritoneal washings	T2c
3		Tumour involves one or both ovaries with microscopically confirmed peritoneal metastasis outside the pelvis and/or regional lymph node metastasis	T3 and/or N1
	3A	Microscopic peritoneal metastasis beyond pelvis	T3a
	3B	Macroscopic peritoneal metastasis beyond pelvis 2 cm or less in greatest dimension	T3b
	3C	Peritoneal metastasis beyond pelvis more than 2 cm in greatest dimension and/or regional lymph node metastasis	T3c and/or N1
4		Distant metastasis (excludes peritoneal metastasis)	M1

[1] Liver capsule metastasis is T3/stage 3, liver parenchymal metastasis M1/stage 4. Pleural effusion must have positive cytology for M1/stage 4.

gutters, the subdiaphragmatic surfaces and pelvic side wall area.

(3) Total hysterectomy and bilateral salpingo-oophorectomy.

(4) Infracolic omentectomy.

(5) Pelvic and para-aortic lymphadenectomy.

(6) Excision of all suspicious masses.

In young women who desire to maintain their fertility, conservative surgery may be done if:

- There is no evidence of extraovarian disease.
- The lesion is low stage and low grade.

14

Management of borderline tumours

Unilateral salpingo-oophorectomy is adequate for these women, particularly if they desire future fertility, providing that the other ovary is clinically normal at the time of laparotomy. For women with stage 2 or 3 borderline tumours, careful histological assessment of the implants is important to determine if they are non-invasive or invasive implants. Invasive implants portend a poor prognosis, and more aggressive surgery is indicated. A second-look operation is generally not indicated. The risk of recurrence may occur for up to 14 years, and is in the range of 10–15 per cent for serous borderline tumours. This raises the question of whether the other ovary should be removed, even when the risk is low, once fertility is complete.

Management of early stage ovarian cancer

- Twenty-five per cent of women diagnosed with epithelial ovarian cancer will be detected at stage 1 or stage 2 levels.
- Patients with stage 1A grade 1 tumours have a high rate of cure with surgery alone and do not require further adjuvant therapy.
- Patients with stages 1A (grade 2 or 3) and 1B or 1C tumours, as well as those with clear cell tumours, should have adjuvant post-operative chemotherapy.
- At present the most effective adjuvant therapy has not been clearly established, but most would recommend a platinum analogue, alone or in combination with paclitaxel. External beam radiotherapy may also be used.

Management of advanced ovarian cancer

- Seventy-five per cent of all women affected by epithelial ovarian cancer are diagnosed at stage 3 or 4.
- Medically fit women should have as much of the tumour removed as possible at laparotomy. Maximal cytoreductive surgery is the key to a good prognosis, independently affecting survival. The amount of residual disease at completion of primary surgery influences prognosis.
- Postoperative chemotherapy, using a combination of platinum-based agents and paclitaxel – the use of paclitaxel instead of cyclophosphamide improves median survival from 24 to 38 months [9].

Prognosis of ovarian carcinomas (Table 14.5)

Features that are independently associated with reduced survival are [10]:

- Advanced stage
- High grade
- Large volume of residual tumour after cytoreduction
- Ascites
- Rupture
- Dense adhesion of tumour
- High serum CA125 preoperatively and/or postoperatively.

Relapse

If relapse occurs after a disease-free interval of more than 12 months, the patient may be considered for repeat surgery and/or chemo-

Table 14.5 5-year survivals (%) of surface epithelial tumours.

	Stage 1	Stage 2	Stage 3	Stage 4
Serous borderline	99	90–95		—
Serous carcinoma	76	56	25	9
Mucinous borderline	92	100	51	—
Mucinous carcinoma	83	55	21	9
Endometrioid carcinoma	78	63	24	6
Clear cell carcinoma	69	55	14	4

therapy. Patients with progressive platinum-refractory ovarian cancer may benefit from other drugs such as doxorubicin, etoposide, topotecan, gemcitabine and vinorelbine.

Sex cord-stromal tumours

This category of tumours accounts for 8 per cent of ovarian neoplasms. It comprises tumours of ovarian-type granulosa and theca stromal cells, tumours of testicular-type Sertoli and Leydig stromal cells, and tumours of stromal fibroblasts. They are usually unilateral. Most tumours in this group are benign fibroma/thecoma types. Granulosa cell tumours account for most of the malignant tumours in this category. Serum inhibin is a tumour marker of sex cord-stromal tumours. The α subunit of inhibin may be more specific for granulosa cell tumours.

Granulosa cell tumours [11,12]

There are two histologic types: the adult and the juvenile forms.

Adult granulosa cell tumours (AGCT)
- Ninety-five per cent of granulosa cell tumours.
- Predominantly in women in their fifties.
- Most common ovarian tumour with oestrogenic effects; 5 per cent have associated endometrial carcinoma.
- Treatment is total abdominal hysterectomy (TAH) with bilateral salpingo-oophorectomy (BSO) in menopausal or postmenopausal women. In young women, unilateral oophorectomy is justified if extraovarian spread is not evident, and the contralateral ovary appears normal. Stage 2–4 disease is best treated with adjuvant chemotherapy.
- Prognosis – the 10-year survival for stage 1 tumours is 85–95 per cent. Stage 1 tumours that have ruptured have only a 60 per cent survival rate. Advanced stages have rates of only 25–49 per cent.
- Recurrences can occur commonly many years later, and are usually fatal. Chemotherapy as for germ cell tumours may be used.

Juvenile granulosa cell tumours (JGCT)
- Most occur in the first three decades of life.
- Those occurring in prepubertal children result in isosexual pseudo-precocity in which development of the sexual organs is accelerated.

- Treatment – for stage 1, unilateral oophorectomy is almost always curative.
- Almost all recurrences are within the first 3 years.

Germ cell tumours

Over 95 per cent of germ cell tumours are benign dermoid cysts (mature teratomas). Most of the remaining tumours are malignant. In patients under 21 years old, 20 per cent of ovarian tumours are malignant germ cell tumours. Most are unilateral except the dysgerminoma.

Dysgerminoma [11,12]

- This is the most common primitive germ cell tumour (1 per cent of all ovarian cancers). It is the counterpart to the testicular seminoma.
- It accounts for 20–30 per cent of ovarian cancers encountered during pregnancy.
- Most occur during the second and third decades.
- There is an elevated LDH in 95 per cent; some also secrete low levels of hCG and αFP.
- Up to 20 per cent are bilateral, half of those only being microscopically detected.
- Treatment – stage 1A is treated with unilateral salpingo-oophorectomy with close follow-up. Higher stages are given cisplatin-based chemotherapy. Although dysgerminomas are particularly radiosensitive, radiotherapy may cause secondary leukaemia and infertility in young patients.
- The prognosis is excellent. The 5-year survival for stage 1 is 100 per cent, and 80–90 per cent for higher stage tumours.

Yolk sac tumour (endodermal sinus tumour)

- This is the second most common primitive germ cell tumour.
- Most occur in the second and third decades.
- There is an elevated αFP in most.
- It is rapidly growing and highly malignant, often with extraovarian spread.
- Treatment is by unilateral salpingo-oophorectomy, cytoreduction of extraovarian tumour and chemotherapy.
- The 5-year survival for stage 1 tumours is 70–90 per cent, and 30–50 per cent for higher stage tumours.

Immature (malignant) teratomas

- These are the third most common primitive germ cell tumour.
- They are most common in young adults and children.
- There is an elevated αFP in 65 per cent.
- Histology is similar to dermoid cysts, but malignancy is determined by the presence of *immature* elements, which is usually predominantly neuroepithelial tissue.
- They are graded according to the amount of immature neuroepithelial tissue present.
- Treatment is by unilateral salpingo-oophorectomy and removal of extraovarian tumour, with adjuvant chemotherapy for grades 2 or 3 tumour or metastases.
- Prognosis – 90 per cent survival.

14

FALLOPIAN TUBE MALIGNANCIES

- Fallopian tube malignancies account for less than 0.3 per cent of gynaecological malignancies.
- The mean age of patients is 57 years.
- The most common presenting symptoms are abnormal vaginal bleeding and abdominal pain.
- 'Hydrops tubae profluens' is a symptom complex occurring in about 10 per cent. It is characterised by intermittent colicky pain, relieved by a sudden vaginal discharge of watery fluid.
- CA125 levels are often elevated.

The carcinomas affecting the tube are similar to those of the ovary. Serous carcinoma is the most common (70 per cent), followed by endometrioid and transitional (10 per cent each), and others. These tumours are surgically staged (Table 14.6) [7].

These tumours spread to the peritoneum, adjacent organs and para-aortic and pelvic lymph nodes. Distant metastases are present in almost half of cases. Treatment is as for ovarian cancers.

ENDOMETRIAL CARCINOMAS

Primary malignancies of the endometrium are the most common gynaecological malignancies, and account for 13 per cent of cancers in women [13]. Almost one third of cases occur in premenopausal women, but most patients are over 40 years old.

Table 14.6 Carcinoma of the fallopian tube – staging. (With permission from Benedet *et al.* (2000) [7].)

FIGO stages		TNM categories
	Primary tumour cannot be assessed	TX
	No evidence of primary tumour	T0
0	Carcinoma in situ (preinvasive carcinoma)	Tis
1	Tumour confined to fallopian tube(s)	T1
1A	Tumour limited to one tube, without penetrating the serosal surface; no ascites	T1a
1B	Tumour limited to both tubes, without penetrating the serosal surface; no ascites	T1b
1C	Tumour limited to one or both tube(s) with extension onto or through the tubal serosa, or with malignant cells in ascites or peritoneal washings	T1c
2	Tumour involves one or both fallopian tube(s) with pelvic extension	T2
2A	Extension and/or metastasis to uterus and/or ovaries	T2a
2B	Extension to other pelvic structures	T2b
2C	Pelvic extension (2A or 2B) with malignant cells in ascites or peritoneal washings	T2c
3	Tumour involves one or both fallopian tube(s) with peritoneal implants outside the pelvis and/or positive regional lymph nodes	T3 and/or N1
3A	Microscopic peritoneal metastasis outside the pelvis	T3a
3B	Macroscopic peritoneal metastasis outside the pelvis 2 cm or less in greatest dimension	T3b
3C	Peritoneal metastasis more than 2 cm in greatest dimension and/or positive regional lymph nodes	T3c and/or N1
4	Distant metastasis (excludes peritoneal metastasis)	M1

Clinical presentation and symptoms

Over 90 per cent of women present with abnormal or post-menopausal vaginal bleeding [13]. The risk of malignancy associated with bleeding increases with age (Table 14.7) [14]. Occasionally, asymptomatic women may present with abnormal endometrial cells on a cervical smear.

Two clinicopathologic groups of patients have been described [14].

Table 14.7 The chance of malignancy with postmenopausal bleeding for each decade of life at presentation.

Decade	Percentage of women with endometrial cancer
50s	9
60s	16
70s	28
80s	60

14

Type 1

- Patients tend to be between 40 and 60 years old, including almost all that are less than 40 years.
- Hyperoestrogenism can be due to:
  Chronic anovulation.
  Oestrogen hormone replacement therapy. There is also an increased risk associated with use of tamoxifen. It is a synthetic anti-oestrogen used for treating breast cancer, but it also has a paradoxical agonist effect on the endometrium. The relative risk ranges from 2.2 to 7.5.
  Rarely, a functioning ovarian tumour or polycystic ovarian disease.
- Tumours are usually well-differentiated, endometrioid type of adenocarcinoma, stage 1, confined to the endometrium, and associated with endometrial hyperplasia.
- There is a favourable prognosis after hysterectomy.

Type 2

- Patients tend to be elderly.
- There is no history of hyperoestrogenism.
- The background endometrium is atrophic.
- Tumours are usually a special variant type of adenocarcinoma (e.g. serous carcinoma), high stage, with deep invasion of myometrium.
- There is often a poor prognosis.

Endometrial cancer is the most common extracolonic malignancy in HNPCC syndrome (Lynch II syndrome). HNPCC might be suspected in a younger woman (<50 years old). One third of tumours in this age group are found to have the characteristic microsatellite instability (MSI), and about 20 per cent of these fulfil clinical criteria for HNPCC. The MSI phenotype of these tumours includes high FIGO stage and grade, mucinous differentiation and necrosis [15].

Diagnosis

A single inexpensive satisfactory screening test for endometrial carcinoma does not exist. Women with high risk factors such as abnormal uterine bleeding over the age of 40, massive obesity, history of endometrial hyperplasia, or unopposed oestrogen or tamoxifen use may benefit from a variety of investigations [7].

- Cervical smear – almost half of endometrial cancers may shed cells which can be identified in a cytology smear.
- Transvaginal ultrasound – the cut-off for maximal normal endometrial thickness is 5 mm. It is very rare for a malignancy to be thinner than 5 mm, so this can be useful in ruling out malignancy [14].
- Office-based endometrial sampling – the diagnostic suitability of samples obtained by biopsy compares favourably with those obtained by dilatation and curettage (D&C) [14].
- Hysteroscopy.

Diagnosis requires a tissue biopsy. The first step is an office endometrial biopsy with ECC. A negative biopsy does not rule out a malignancy in a clinically suspicious case. The biopsy should either be repeated, or a D&C may be necessary. A D&C may also be necessary if there is cervical stenosis or the patient does not tolerate the office procedure. The disadvantages of a D&C are:

- It requires anaesthesia.
- There is a risk, albeit small, of uterine perforation.
- Post-curettage adhesions (Asherman's syndrome) may develop.

Pretreatment investigations

- Full history and physical examination, including bimanual pelvic examination to assess local extension
- Blood work including full blood count, liver and renal function tests
- Chest X-ray to exclude pulmonary metastases
- Serum CA125 may useful for following advanced disease
- Cystoscopy, barium enema, CT or magnetic resonance imaging (MRI) scan, bone scan as needed in those with suspected local or distant spread.

Lymph node drainage

The lymphatics drain from a subserosal network into the pelvic and peri-aortic nodes. Some lymphatics at the fundus accompany the round ligament and drain into the superficial inguinal nodes [16].

Pathology

Most cancers of the endometrium are adenocarcinomas, arising from the glandular component. Over 80 per cent of these are the usual, or **endometrioid**, type. The remaining are special variants of adenocarcinoma (serous papillary, clear cell and the rare mucinous carcinomas), squamous cell carcinomas (rare) and undifferentiated carcinomas [14].

Endometrioid adenocarcinoma

Most are the 'usual' type of endometrioid adenocarcinoma. Variants include villoglandular (papillary) and secretory. Endometrioid adenocarcinomas frequently show squamous differentiation. The squamous component may be a benign metaplastic phenomenon (adenoacanthoma), or may also be malignant (adenosquamous carcinoma). The latter have a similar prognosis to poorly differentiated adenocarcinomas [16].

Serous papillary carcinoma

- About 5–10 per cent of endometrial carcinomas are serous papillary carcinomas.
- It is an aggressive tumour, with a tendency for early deep myometrial invasion, often with extensive lymphatic–vascular space invasion (LVSI).
- There is early dissemination beyond the uterus, typically to the peritoneal surfaces.

Clear cell carcinoma

- About 4 per cent of endometrial carcinomas are clear cell.
- They are often associated with a higher stage and poorer prognosis.

Note about 'papillary' tumours

A designation of 'papillary', without any other descriptors such as 'serous', 'villoglandular' or 'endometrioid', is a meaningless term.

Papillary structures can be found in a variety of types of adenocarcinomas. If the term is used in a pathological diagnostic report, the diagnosis should always clearly state which type of papillary tumour is being diagnosed.

Grading

Two clinically aggressive types of carcinoma, the serous and clear cell carcinomas, do not need to be graded because their subtype dictates outcome. The other carcinomas are graded using the FIGO system. This grades tumours as 1, 2 or 3 (well differentiated, moderately differentiated, and poorly differentiated, respectively), depending on the amount of gland formation and the nuclear characteristics.

About 20 per cent of women with low grade tumours on the biopsy will have their tumours upgraded on evaluation of the resected specimen [13].

Spread and metastases [16]

- Invasion is into the myometrium, through serosa into parametria, and late into the bladder or rectum.
- There is lymphatic drainage into the pelvic and then the para-aortic nodes.
- There are pelvic metastases to the ovaries and vagina. Serous carcinomas have a predilection to metastasise to the peritoneal surfaces.
- Spread downward into the cervix (stage 2 disease) is predictive of distant metastases.
- Pulmonary metastases are seen as a late event.

Staging and treatment of endometrial carcinomas

Endometrial carcinomas are surgically staged using the FIGO staging system (Table 14.8). Meticulous surgical staging can identify up to one third of patients with extrauterine disease who were initially thought to have disease confined to the uterus [13]. FIGO's generally recommended approach to staging is [7]:
(1) Vertical midline abdominal incision, and then immediate peritoneal washings of pelvis and abdomen.

Table 14.8 Carcinoma of the corpus uteri – staging. (With permission from Benedet *et al.* (2000) [7].)

FIGO stages		TNM categories
	Primary tumour cannot be assessed	TX
	No evidence of primary tumour	T0
0	Carcinoma in situ (preinvasive carcinoma)	Tis
1	Tumour confined to corpus uteri	T1
1A	Tumour limited to endometrium	T1a
1B	Tumour invades up to or less than half of myometrium[1]	T1b
1C	Tumour invades more than one half of myometrium[1]	T1c
2	Tumour invades cervix but does not extend beyond uterus	T2
2A	Endocervical glandular involvement only	T2a
2B	Cervical stromal invasion	T2b
3	Local and/or regional spread	T3 and/or N1
3A	Tumour involves serosa and/or adnexa (direct extension or metastasis) and/or cancer cells in ascites or peritoneal washings	T3a
3B	Vaginal involvement (direct extension or metastasis)	T3b
3C	Metastasis to pelvic and/or para-aortic lymph nodes	N1
4A	Tumour invades bladder mucosa and/or bowel mucosa	T4
4B	Distant metastasis (*excluding* metastasis to vagina, pelvic serosa, or adnexa; *including* metastasis to intra-abdominal lymph nodes other than para-aortic and/or inguinal nodes)	M1

[1] Ideally, the width of the myometrium should be measured along with the width of tumor invasion.

(2) Careful exploration of intra-abdominal contents – examine and palpate the omentum, liver, peritoneal cul-de-sac, adnexal surfaces, as well as aortic and pelvic lymph node areas.

(3) Extrafascial total hysterectomy with bilateral salpingo-oophorectomy – ligation or clipping of distal tubes initially, to prevent any possible tumour spillage.

(4) Pelvic and para-aortic lymphadenectomy

(a) Some may just selectively sample nodes, reserving complete dissection for those with high risk features such as deep myoinvasion.

(b) Frozen section may assist in determining depth of invasion.

(c) Frozen section on retroperitoneal nodes may identify positive nodes, in which case further node dissection may be unnecessary.

(d) Indications for aortic node sampling include:

    (i) Serous, clear cell, or carcinosarcoma histology

    (ii) Suspicious aortic or common iliac nodes

    (iii) Grossly positive adnexa

    (iv) Grossly positive pelvic nodes

    (v) Invasion of outer half of myometrium.

Treatment of endometrial carcinomas

Abdominal hysterectomy with bilateral salpingo-oophorectomy and lymphadenectomy (as outlined above) is the basic treatment for all stages.

The role of postoperative pelvic irradiation for stage 1 cancers is controversial. A recent prospective randomised trial found that although locoregional control was improved with postoperative radiotherapy, no survival benefit was achieved when compared with surgery alone [17].

Table 14.9 lists the treatments for each stage [7].

Treatment in special situations

- *Incidental finding of malignancy in hysterectomy specimen* – if the tumour is grade 1 or 2, with minimal myoinvasion and no LVSI, then no further therapy is generally needed. If the tumour has high risk factors such as grade 3 morphology, deep myoinvasion, LVSI invasion, or histologically unfavourable type (e.g. serous or clear cell), then additional surgery is indicated, to remove the adnexa and complete the surgical staging.

- *Positive peritoneal cytology* – if there is no other evidence of extrauterine disease, management is controversial. There are insufficient data regarding recurrence risk and treatment results. The cytology should be reviewed by an experienced cytopathologist, since false-positive interpretations may be made of reactive mesothelial cells.

- *Recurrence* – lesions should be excised if possible; isolated pelvic recurrences are potentially curable if they occur more than 1 or 2 years after the initial therapy. Non-localised tumours may be treated with progestogen therapy. Chemotherapy may play a role for patients

Table 14.9 FIGO guidelines for treatment of endometrial carcinoma.

Stage	Treatment

Stage 1, low risk
  Less than half myometrial invasion
  Grade 1 or 2
	No further treatment after surgical staging

Stage 1, high risk
  More than half myometrial invasion
  Grade 3
  Lymphatic–vascular space invasion
	Postoperative pelvic irradiation

Stage 2 – occult cervical involvement	Postoperative pelvic irradiation
Stage 2 – overt cervical involvement	(a) Pelvic irradiation and intracavitary brachytherapy plus adjunctive TAH/BSO with selective sampling of aortic pelvic nodes (b) Wertheim-type radical hysterectomy and BSO, with bilateral pelvic lymphadenectomy and selective aortic node dissection
Stage 3	(a) Postoperative pelvic irradiation if no macroscopic residual disease (b) Postoperative pelvic irradiation plus chemotherapy (carboplatin/taxol) if macroscopic residual disease If advanced disease, unsuitable for surgery, then chemotherapy with or without radiotherapy
Stage 4	Palliative radiotherapy, with or without chemotherapy, with or without hormonal therapy

14

with advanced disease which is not amenable to surgical or radiation treatment.

Prognosis of endometrial carcinomas

There are three prognostic groups, based on stage, grade and depth of myoinvasion.

(1) Grade 1 tumours confined to the endometrium, without evidence of intraperitoneal disease – <5 per cent risk of nodal involvement.

(2) Grade 2 or 3 tumours, invading inner myometrium, no intraperi-toneal disease – 5–9 per cent chance of pelvic nodal involvement, and 4 per cent chance of positive para-aortic nodes.

(3) Grade 2 or 3 tumours, deeply invading myometrium, and/or intraperitoneal disease – 20–60 per cent chance of spread to pelvic nodes, and 10–30 per cent risk of para-aortic nodal involvement.

Survival is over 90 per cent for stage 1 tumours, and 80 per cent for stage 2. These rates are even higher if the tumour is well differentiated [14].

14

UTERINE SARCOMAS

Less than 5 per cent of uterine malignancies are sarcomas. These include leiomyosarcoma, adenosarcoma, carcinosarcoma (or malignant mixed Müllerian tumour, the most common sarcoma), and endome-trial stromal sarcoma (ESS, the least common sarcoma). The only known aetiological factor is a history of previous pelvic irradiation.

Stromal tumours of the endometrium, benign or malignant, are usually polypoid masses. Patients usually present with abnormal vaginal bleeding.

Adenosarcoma

- Adenosarcoma usually occurs in the postmenopausal age group.
- It is composed of two elements: the benign glandular component ('adeno') and the malignant stromal component ('sarcoma').
- The sarcomatous component is the predominant or exclusive element in the areas of myometrial and vascular invasion, as well as in any metastases.
- The presence of **sarcomatous overgrowth** (in which the sarcoma-tous component comprises at least 25 per cent of the tumour) confers a worse prognosis, with recurrence rates of 45–70 per cent. If stromal overgrowth is absent, the recurrence rate is 15–25 per cent [14].
- Recurrences are initially in the pelvis, and may recur distantly (via haematogenous spread) many years later.

Carcinosarcoma (malignant mixed Müllerian tumour – MMMT) [18]

- Most are in elderly postmenopausal patients, but there is a wide age range.

- It usually presents with abnormal vaginal bleeding, but pelvic or abdominal pain is also a common symptom, because about one third have extensive extrauterine disease at presentation.
- It is composed of two elements: a malignant glandular component and a malignant stromal component. Evidence is accumulating that the stromal portion is probably actually a metaplastic carcinoma. Metastases are composed exclusively of the glandular element.
- Stratification of the stromal element into **homologous** (e.g. fibrosarcoma, leiomyosarcoma) and **heterologous** (e.g. rhabdomyosarcoma, liposarcoma, chondrosarcoma, osteosarcoma) elements is of no clinical usefulness.
- It behaves as an aggressive carcinoma. The most important prognostic factors are stage, carcinoma type (serous or clear cell histology is associated with poor prognosis) and LVSI. The only patients with long-term survival are those with small tumours that are only minimally invasive.
- Adjuvant therapy has not been effective, and chemotherapy and radiation therapy do not help with recurrences.

14

Low grade endometrial stromal sarcomas [19]

- These occur in all ages, with a mean age of 40 years.
- Fifty per cent have extended beyond the uterus at staging.
- Many respond to progestational therapies (in contrast to high grade sarcomas).
- Five-year survival is almost 100 per cent. Metastases occur late, and patients may live many years with disseminated disease.

Undifferentiated uterine sarcomas (high grade endometrial stromal sarcoma)

- These are found in older patients, with a mean age of 61 years.
- They behave in a highly aggressive fashion.

Leiomyosarcoma

- Leiomyosarcoma is a smooth muscle neoplasm arising from the myometrium. It does not arise from leiomyomas.
- The mean age is 50 years.

- The most important prognostic factor is stage. Size is also important – tumours less than 5 cm in diameter have a better prognosis.
- The overall 5-year survival is about 10–30 per cent.

Treatment of uterine sarcomas

The primary treatment for all is total abdominal hysterectomy and bilateral salpingo-oophorectomy, with pelvic and peri-aortic selective lymphadenectomy. Cytology washings should be obtained from the pelvis and abdomen, and the diaphragm, omentum and upper abdomen should be thoroughly examined.

Surgery can be curative if the tumour is confined to the uterus. The value of pelvic irradiation is not established, and adjuvant chemotherapy for stage 1 and 2 tumours has not been shown, in a randomised trial, to be effective.

VULVAL MALIGNANCIES

Primary malignancies of the vulva account for about 3–4 per cent of malignant tumours of the female genital tract [7]. They occur predominantly in elderly women, but there is a wide age range. It is a highly curable disease in the early stages.

Clinical presentation and symptoms

There is often a delay in presentation because of patient embarrassment, or failure of the initial physician to adequately examine the vulva. The patient most commonly complains of pruritus, bleeding or a lump. Other symptoms may include pain, discharge or dysuria.

Physical examination

- Red or white macule, papule or plaque
- Exophytic mass or ulcer
- Nodule, lump or blue/black lesion of melanoma, predominantly on labia majora and clitoris
- Granular, red moist eczematous area of Paget's disease, found predominantly on labia majora, but can extensively involve other areas too, including extension onto abdomen and thighs
- Palpable inguinal or femoral lymph nodes may indicate metas-

tases, but clinical assessment of these nodes is unreliable. Almost half of clinically positive nodes may be clear on histology, and conversely almost half of those clinically negative may turn out to contain tumour [20].

Diagnosis

A tissue biopsy is required to confirm malignancy, and to identify the histological type of tumour.

Any pigmented skin lesion should be excised with a 1–2 cm margin [7]. Punch biopsies should *not* be done for pigmented lesions – if the lesion turns out to be a melanoma, it will be impossible to accurately determine the tumour thickness. Post-biopsy wound repair changes will distort the lesion.

Pretreatment investigations

- Full history and physical examination, including bimanual pelvic examination to assess local extension, and to exclude other genital tract lesions
- Blood work including full blood count, liver and renal function tests
- Chest X-ray to exclude pulmonary metastases
- Cystoscopy, barium enema, CT scan, ultrasound as needed in those with suspected local or distant spread.

Lymph node drainage [20]

The anterior labia majora and minora and clitoris drain into the superficial and deep femoral nodes and inguinal nodes, via the presymphyseal plexus. The posterior vulva skips this plexus, draining into the femoral nodes. These eventually drain into the external iliac nodes. Involvement of the pelvic nodes by vulval malignancies is considered distant metastases in the staging classification.

The midline vulval structures often drain bilaterally. Anastomotic channels mean that there is some lymph drainage to contralateral pelvic nodes. About 15 per cent of unilateral cancers spread to nodes on both sides, and about 5 per cent of cancers spread to contralateral nodes only.

Pathology

As in the vagina and cervix, most of the tumours (about 90 per cent) are squamous cell carcinomas. Melanomas are the second most common malignancy [20]. Basal cell carcinomas and Paget's disease each account for about 2 per cent. Other tumours such as sarcomas and unusual subtypes of carcinomas are quite rare.

Carcinomas – invasive squamous cell carcinoma

14

The most common site of involvement is the labia majora (50 per cent), followed by the labia minora (15–20 per cent). In those patients with concurrent lichen sclerosus, the clitoris is far more likely to be involved (41 per cent versus 3 per cent) [21].

Lichen sclerosus and squamous cell carcinoma
- 15–30 per cent have lichen sclerosus [4].
- The cancers in this group are the keratinising type and occur in older women, are more likely to involve the clitoris, and are not associated with vulval intraepithelial neoplasia (VIN) [21].

Types of squamous cell carcinoma

Keratinising
- About two thirds of squamous cancers
- Elderly (mean age 77 years)
- Only 20 per cent or less have HPV [4]
- Two per cent have cervical neoplasia [20].

Basaloid or warty
- Younger (mean age 54 years)
- Over 80 per cent have HPV, usually type 16
- Most have adjacent VIN
- Forty per cent are synchronous or metachronous squamous tumours of the cervix and vagina [20]
- Behaviour is the same as keratinising [4].

Verrucous
- This is an extremely well-differentiated tumour with an exophytic papillomatous growth.
- It is often associated with HPV type 6.

- There may be local recurrences but metastases are very rare.
- There is an excellent prognosis if the tumour is completely excised [4].

Superficially invasive tumours (microinvasive)
- These measure 1 mm or less in thickness, and not greater than 2 cm diameter.
- Only 3 per cent of these tumours spread to local nodes, compared with 19 per cent of tumours 3 mm thick, and one third of tumours that were 5 mm thick [22].
- The 10-year survival for these early tumours is 95 per cent [23].

14

Spread
Squamous cancers spread locally first, to adjacent sites such as the anus, vagina and urethra. They travel to the femoral and inguinal nodes, then to the deep pelvic nodes.

Staging
Vulval carcinomas are surgically staged using the FIGO staging system (Table 14.10) [7].

General principles of treatment of carcinomas
The standard treatments are surgery, often supplemented with external beam radiation therapy (EBRT) for advanced stages. There is a trend towards vulval conservation, and the role of preoperative chemoradiation is evolving. FIGO has produced clinical guidelines for the management of vulval cancers (Table 14.11) [7]. A groin node dissection should be performed if the tumour is more than 1 mm deep. The status of the inguinal nodes will determine treatment to the pelvis.

Prognosis
Nodal status and tumour diameter determine prognosis. LVSI or perineural invasion are strong predictors of lymph node metastasis.

The 5-year survival for node-negative cancers is 80–95 per cent. This drops to 43–66 per cent for node-positive cancers [20]. One large study that evaluated almost 600 vulval carcinomas reported 5-year survival rates for stage 1 as 98 per cent, stage 2 as 85 per cent, stage 3 as 74 per cent, and stage 4 as 31 per cent [24].

Table 14.10 Carcinoma of the vulva – staging. (With permission from Benedet *et al.* (2000) [7].)

FIGO stages			TNM categories
		Primary tumour cannot be assessed	TX
		No evidence of primary tumour	T0
0		Carcinoma in situ (preinvasive carcinoma)	Tis
1		Tumour confined to vulva, or vulva and perineum, 2 cm or less in greatest dimension	T1
	1A	Stromal invasion no greater than 1 mm[1]	T1a
	1B	Stromal invasion greater than 1 mm[1]	T1b
2		Tumour confined to vulva, or vulva and perineum, more than 2 cm greatest dimension	T2
3		Tumour invades any of: lower urethra, vagina, anus	T3
		and/or unilateral regional lymph node metastasis	N1
4A		Tumour invades any of: bladder or rectal mucosa, upper urethral mucosa, or is fixed to bone	T4
		and/or bilateral regional lymph node metastasis	N2
4B		Distant metastasis, including pelvic lymph nodes	M1

[1] Depth measured from the epithelial–stromal junction of the most adjacent superficial dermal papillae to the deepest point of invasion.

Recurrences

Over one third of patients develop recurrences [25,26]. If margins are less than 8 mm, the recurrence rate is 50 per cent [27].

Risk factors for recurrence include high FIGO stage, positive lymph nodes, LVSI, positive resection margins, tumour multifocality and associated high grade VIN [26].

Over half of the recurrences are perineal. Surgical resection of local recurrences may achieve over a 50 per cent 5-year survival rate. Multiple or distant recurrences have only a 15 per cent 5-year survival rate [25].

Bartholin gland cancer

This lesion is often thought initially to be a persisting Bartholin's cyst. Most women are between 40 and 70 years old [4]. The

Table 14.11 Management of vulval carcinoma.

Tumour	Treatment options
T1a	WLE If associated severe dystrophy or LVSI, then consider more radical excision
T1b, T2 (lateral lesion, clinically node negative)	If clinically node negative, tumour 2 cm or less in diameter and 5 mm or less deep, no LVSI and no associated severe dystrophy, RLE with ipsilateral groin dissection Radical hemivulvectomy with en bloc ipsilateral inguinal–femoral node dissection If patient is unable to tolerate surgery, then radical radiation therapy may result in long-term survival
1b, 2 (midline lesion, or lateral lesions that are clinically node positive)	Radical vulvectomy with en bloc bilateral groin dissection Radical vulvectomy with bilateral groin dissection using triple incision technique Postoperative irradiation, with or without chemotherapy, to groin and pelvic node areas
T3	If minimal involvement of distal vagina, urethra or anus, then extended radical vulvectomy and bilateral groin dissection. Preoperative irradiation and chemotherapy, then conservative resection, has also produced good results If more extensive involvement of local organs, then selective exenterative surgery and bilateral groin dissection. Preoperative chemoradiation may shrink tumours sufficiently to avoid an exenterative procedure
T4	Exenterative surgery and radical vulvectomy and bilateral groin dissection. Preoperative chemoradiation may shrink tumours sufficiently to avoid an exenterative procedure

If two or more groin nodes are positive, then pelvic and groin irradiation should be performed. Adjuvant irradiation to the vulva may be considered in those patients with narrow (<8 mm) margins, with LVSI, or tumour thickness greater than 5 mm

WLE, wide local excision, with 5–10 mm margins; RLE, radical local excision with 2 cm margins; LVSI, lymphatic/vascular space invasion.

histological types include a variety of adenocarcinomas and squamous cell carcinomas.

Standard therapy has been radical vulvectomy and bilateral groin dissection. For early lesions, ipsilateral groin dissection and hemivulvectomy may be equally effective. Radiotherapy may be indicated for large primary tumours or inguinal node metastases [7].

The 5-year survival for node-negative tumours is about 50 per cent. This declines to 18 per cent when two or more nodes are involved [4].

Paget's disease

This is a type of adenocarcinoma of the epidermis. It may occasionally progress to invasion of the dermis, or be associated with invasive adenocarcinomas nearby. It typically occurs in postmenopausal white women. It presents as an eczematous type of weeping lesion, often with small foci of white hyperkeratotic areas [4].

Most cases are primary tumours of the epidermis. Sometimes there may be a nearby primary adenocarcinoma, such as of Bartholin's gland, the rectum or urethra, which is sending tumour cells into the epidermis.

Treatment is wide local resection, but it is often very difficult to get clear margins. The tumour frequently extends microscopically far beyond what can be seen clinically. Recurrences often occur, and are treated with re-excision. As long as the neoplasm remains confined to the epithelium, the prognosis is excellent. With invasion, the prognosis worsens, and is dismal when the tumour reaches the lymph nodes.

Basal cell carcinoma (BCC)

This skin lesion occurs predominantly on the labia majora of elderly white women. It is identical to the BCCs which occur commonly on sun-exposed skin. There may be local recurrences, but metastases are rare [20]. Treatment is local excision.

Melanoma

Vulval melanoma differs from cutaneous melanoma in several ways [28]:

- It affects older women, usually postmenopausal.
- It has a worse prognosis. The 5-year survival is only 47 per cent, compared with 80 per cent for skin melanoma.

- The most common type is the mucosal lentiginous melanoma; superficial spreading melanoma (the most common type in skin) is the least common type of the vulva.
- It is only rarely preceded by a naevus.
- Over one third have a polypoid appearance.
- Almost one third are not pigmented.
- Most involve the clitoris or labia majora.

The tumour thickness is measured from the granular layer of the epithelium to the deepest point of invasion. Most tumours are over 1.5 mm thick. A recent large Swedish study of over 200 vulval melanomas found that half of the tumours were over 4 mm thick, and only 13 per cent were 0.9 mm or less [29].

14

Staging of melanoma

- Clinical stage 1 – tumour confined to the vulva, with any satellites being within 2 cm of the primary tumour
- Clinical stage 2 – regional lymph node metastases
- Clinical stage 3 – distant metastases.

Management

Thin melanomas (less than 0.75 mm) are treated with wide local excision, with a 2 cm margin. Thicker tumours require a larger margin. LVSI may be an indication for considering groin dissection. Generally, lymphadenectomy does not improve prognosis [7].

Prognosis

The overall 5-year survival is 30–40 per cent. It drops from almost 60 per cent for node-negative cases to less than 10 per cent for node-positive cases. The Swedish study found that the strongest predictors of survival were clinical stage, macroscopic amelanosis, tumour thickness and ulceration. Increasing tumour thickness correlates directly with decreased survival (Table 14.12). The 5-year survival for stage 1 tumours, non-ulcerated and ulcerated, was 91 and 48 per cent respectively. The rates for melanotic and amelanotic stage 1 lesions were 65 and 39 per cent respectively [28].

Sarcomas

Sarcomas of the vulva are rare. The smooth muscle tumour leiomyosarcoma is the most common. Wide resection is the

Table 14.12 Clinical stage 1 melanomas – survival according to tumour thickness.

	0.9 mm or less	1.0–1.9 mm	2.0–2.9 mm	3.0–3.9 mm	4.0 mm or more
5-year survival (%)	93	59	79	38	35
10-year survival (%)	84	59	35	30	28

14

treatment for most sarcomas. Chemoradiation may play a role, depending on tumour type.

VAGINAL MALIGNANCIES

Vaginal primary malignancies account for only 1–2 per cent of malignant tumours of the female genital tract [4]. Most tumours of the vagina are secondary, usually involving the vagina by direct extension from another site such as the cervix or vulva.

Clinical presentation and symptoms

- An abnormal vaginal cytology smear may be the only indicator of vaginal disease.
- Abnormal vaginal bleeding is the most common symptom of vaginal malignancy.
- There is a discharge.
- Dysuria, tenesmus and constipation may signal bladder or rectal involvement.

Physical examination

- Most carcinomas are found in the upper vagina. Squamous cell carcinomas are usually in the posterior wall, and clear cell adenocarcinomas are more often in the anterior or lateral wall.
- Melanomas are more likely to be present in the lower vagina.
- The childhood malignancies – embryonal rhabdomyosarcoma (sarcoma botryoides) and endodermal sinus tumour – frequently protrude from the vagina as polypoid masses.

- Palpable inguinal or femoral lymph nodes may indicate metastases, secondary to involvement of the lower vagina.

Diagnosis

A tissue biopsy is required to confirm malignancy, and to identify the histological type of the tumour. A cervical and vulval primary tumour should be ruled out. Multiple biopsies of the cervix are indicated to rule out a primary tumour of that site which has extended into the vagina.

14

Pretreatment investigations

- Full history and physical examination, including speculum examination and bimanual pelvic examination (to detect extravaginal spread)
- Colposcopy with multiple biopsies of the cervix to exclude a cervical primary
- Cystoscopy and sigmoidoscopy if warranted by signs or symptoms
- Blood work including full blood count and biochemical screen
- Urinalysis and urine cytology
- Chest X-ray to exclude pulmonary metastases
- Intravenous urogram, barium studies of rectum, transrectal ultrasound, CT and MRI may be used as needed to define the size and extent of the lesion, and to identify locoregional spread.

Lymph node drainage [4]

Superior groups of lymphatics follow the cervical vessels along the uterine artery, and drain into the external iliac nodes. Middle groups, which drain most of the vagina, drain into the hypogastric nodes. Inferior groups drain the lower third, and into the inguinal nodes. The upper two thirds of the vagina drains to the pelvic nodes, the lower third to the inguinal and femoral nodes.

Pathology

Over 90 per cent of tumours are squamous cell carcinomas occurring in adult women. Germ cell tumours or sarcomas are the predominant vaginal malignancy in young girls [20].

Carcinomas

Almost all of the cancers are squamous cell carcinomas. Glands are not normally found in the vagina, so adenocarcinomas are rare.

1 Invasive squamous cell carcinoma

Most invasive squamous cell cancers arise in a background of vaginal intraepithelial neoplasia (VAIN). Many have coexistent, or a history of, cervical or vulval squamous intraepithelial lesions (SILs). HPV type 16 is frequently present [20].

- They appear in postmenopausal women most commonly, but there is a wide range of ages. The mean age of 64 is about a decade later than the mean age for VAIN 3 [4].
- They are usually in the upper vagina, often on the posterior wall.
- Half are ulcerative lesions; the remainder are exophytic or annular constricting tumours [4].
- Rule out a primary tumour of the cervix or vulva.

Behaviour

- There is no correlation between histological grade of tumour and outcome.
- If the tumour is less than 3 mm deep, and there is no LVSI, then nodal spread is unlikely [4].
- Spread is by direct extension into local tissues, bladder, rectum, rectovaginal septum and broad ligament.
- Lymphatic spread is to the pelvic or inguinal lymph nodes. Distant metastases are to the lungs, liver and brain.
- Stage 1 5-year survival is 70–75 per cent [20].
- Recurrence is usually within the first two years [4].

2 Clear cell adenocarcinoma

Most vaginal adenocarcinomas are clear cell carcinomas. The incidence of these tumours peaked in the 1980s, when they accounted for up to 15 per cent of vaginal cancers. Two thirds occurred in women who were exposed in utero to DES, taken by their mothers to prevent miscarriages. One of the teratogenic effects of DES is the formation of glands in the vagina (adenosis), and these are the precursor to clear cell adenocarcinoma [4]. The tumour derives its name from the 'cleared' appearance of its cytoplasm. The cells contain glycogen which is eliminated during tissue preparation for making histological slides.

- Most women are in their teens or twenties.
- It is frequently asymptomatic.
- The tumour is usually in the upper vagina, anterior or lateral wall (compare with squamous carcinoma which is usually on the posterior wall).
- Most are polypoid or nodular.

Behaviour
- There is a higher risk of nodal metastases, which even occur in 5 per cent of stage 1 tumours which are still quite superficial, i.e. <3 mm. Pelvic metastases are found in half of those with stage 2 disease [4].
- Stage 1 5-year survival is about 90 per cent.
- Most recurrences are within 3 years, but disease-free intervals may be many years. One third of recurrences are distant rather than local; the lungs and supraclavicular nodes are common sites [4].

14

3 Other carcinomas

Other carcinomas, such as small cell carcinoma (oat cell-like) and adenosquamous carcinoma, are extremely rare but aggressive tumours.

Staging

Vaginal carcinoma is surgically staged using the FIGO criteria (Table 14.13) [7]. Cases are classified as vaginal carcinoma when the primary site of the growth is in the vagina. Tumours involving the portio and area of the external os should be categorised as carcinoma of the cervix. Tumours involving the vulva should be classified as vulval carcinoma.

General principles of treating vaginal carcinoma

Multiple factors need to be considered in planning therapy [30].

1 Stage

Surgery and radiation therapy are highly effective in treating **early** stage disease. Radiotherapy is the primary treatment for advanced stages.

2 Size and location of tumour

- The lymphatic drainage may be to the pelvic nodes for upper vaginal tumours, and the inguinal nodes for lower vaginal tumours.

Table 14.13 Carcinoma of the vagina – staging. (With permission from Benedet *et al.* (2000) [7].)

FIGO stages		TNM categories
	Primary tumour cannot be assessed	TX
	No evidence of primary tumour	T0
0	Carcinoma in situ (preinvasive carcinoma)	Tis
1	Tumour confined to vagina	T1
2	Tumour invades paravaginal tissues but does not extend to pelvic wall	T2
3	Tumour extends to pelvic wall	T3
	Metastases to pelvic or inguinal lymph nodes	N1
4A	Tumour invades *mucosa* of bladder or rectum, and/or extends beyond the true pelvis (the presence of bullous oedema is not sufficient evidence to classify a tumour as 4A)	T4
4B	Distant metastases	M1

Some tumours may involve a large enough area that both lymph node areas may be affected.
- The tumour may be close to the bladder or rectum, complicating surgical treatment. Posterior wall involvement may necessitate resection of the anterior wall of the rectum.

3 Presence or absence of uterus
Two thirds of cancers are limited to the upper vagina in those who have had a previous hysterectomy. Only one third are limited to this site in those who still have a uterus.

4 History of previous irradiation
5 Side effects of radiotherapy
These include ovarian failure, vaginal stenosis, mucosal ulceration, and formation of fistulae.

Surgery is the treatment of choice if:
- Preservation of ovarian function is desired.
- The lesion is localised VAIN.
- There is prior pelvic irradiation.

Vaginal reconstruction with the use of skin grafts may allow satisfactory function.

Chemotherapy and radiotherapy are occasionally used for locally advanced disease.

Treatment – stage 1

Surgical management options differ for early squamous carcinomas and adenocarcinomas. Adenocarcinomas spread beneath the surface squamous mucosa, so total radical vaginectomy (rather than wide local excision) is indicated for those tumours.

(1) Squamous cancers, superficial lesions (<5 mm thick)
- (a) Surgery
    - (i) Wide local excision
    - (ii) Total vaginectomy
    - (iii) Postoperative adjuvant irradiation if close or positive surgical margins
- (b) Radiotherapy
    - (i) Brachytherapy
    - (ii) EBRT for bulky lesions
    - (iii) EBRT to the pelvis – inguinal nodes included if tumour in lower third of vagina
(2) Squamous cancers, lesions >5 mm thick
- (a) Surgery
    - (i) Tumours of the upper two thirds of the vagina – radical hysterovaginectomy with pelvic node dissection
    - (ii) Tumours of the lower third of the vagina – radical vulvovaginectomy with bilateral groin node dissection
    - (iii) Postoperative adjuvant EBRT if risk of pelvic nodal involvement, poorly differentiated tumour, close or positive surgical resection margins
- (b) Radiotherapy
    - (i) Brachytherapy (interstitial and intracavitary)
    - (ii) EBRT added for poorly differentiated tumours and those with high chance of lymph node metastasis
    - (iii) If lesion in lower third of vagina, then EBRT to pelvic and inguinal nodes
(3) Adenocarcinomas
- (a) Surgery – Total radical hysterovaginectomy
    - (i) With pelvic node dissection for tumours of the upper vagina

(ii) With inguinal node dissection for tumours of the lower vagina

(iii) Adjuvant radiotherapy for close or positive surgical margins

(b) Radiotherapy

(i) Brachytherapy (interstitial and intracavitary)

(ii) EBRT to the pelvis, inguinal nodes if tumour in lower third of vagina

(c) Combined local therapy – wide local excision, nodal sampling, and interstitial radiotherapy.

Treatment – stage 2

Radiotherapy is the preferred option. This includes EBRT and brachytherapy. If surgery is chosen, then radical vaginectomy or exenteration would be required, possibly with adjuvant postoperative irradiation.

Treatment – stage 3

Radiotherapy is the treatment of choice, using a combination of EBRT and brachytherapy, including radiation to the lateral pelvic wall. Occasionally an exenteration-type surgical procedure may be used.

Treatment – stage 4

Treatment is palliative radiotherapy, and is not curative. Platinum-based chemotherapy may play a role.

Recurrences

Most recurrences of squamous carcinoma occur within the first 2 years. A large series showed only 10 per cent were salvaged with radiation or surgery, and those patients had initially presented with stage 1 or 2 disease [30].

Melanoma

- About 3 per cent of primary vaginal malignancies are melanomas [4].
- The median age is 62 years old.
- Most frequently they are found in the lower third of the vagina.

- There is a better prognosis for tumours less than 3 cm diameter – mean survival of 41 months versus 12 months for larger tumours. The overall 5-year survival is less than 30 per cent [31].
- Radiotherapy may offer results comparable to surgery [31].

Childhood tumours

Both of these rare tumours present with bleeding or discharge, and both may protrude from the vagina as polypoid masses.

1 Endodermal sinus (yolk sac) tumour

- They are rare tumours, found in children less than 2 years old [32].
- Serum α-fetoprotein (αFP) is elevated.
- Relapses occur within 2 years, usually locally and often with pulmonary metastases [33].
- A recent study involving 14 children found 100 per cent survival (median 76 months' follow-up) after receiving primary intensive chemotherapy of cisplatin, etoposide and ifosfamide. This was followed by second-look laparatomy or vaginoscopy with resection of any residual tumour, and then postoperative chemotherapy. The authors believe that extensive surgery is not necessary in these patients [32].

2 Embryonal rhabdomyosarcoma (sarcoma botryoides)

- The most common vaginal sarcoma occurs almost exclusively in children <5 years old.
- It is an aggressive tumour that is locally invasive into the bladder and rectum. Metastases occur later, to the lungs, liver, kidneys and bone [4].
- Recent studies indicate an excellent prognosis with primary chemotherapy, with local surgery and radiation in some cases [34,35].

REFERENCES

1 Zaino, R.J. (2000) Glandular lesions of the uterine cervix. *Modern Pathology*, **13** (3), 261–274.
2 Lee, K.R. & Flynn, C.E. (2000) Early invasive adenocarcinoma of the cervix. *Cancer*, **89**, 1048–1055.
3 Crum, C.P., Nuovo, G.J. & Lee, K.R. (1999) The cervix. In: *Diagnostic Sur-*

gical Pathology (ed. S.S. Sternberg), 3rd edn, pp. 2155–2202. Lippincott, Williams and Wilkins, Philadelphia.

4 Kurman, R., Norris, H. & Wilkinson, E. (1992) *Tumours of the Cervix, Vagina, and Vulva*, Vol. 4. Armed Forces Institute of Pathology, Washington, DC.

5 Goldstein, N.S. & Mani, A. (1998) The status and distance of cone biopsy margins as a predictor of excision adequacy for endocervical adenocarcinoma in situ. *American Journal of Clinical Pathology*, **109** (6), 727–732.

6 Cviko, A., Briem, B., Granter, S.R. *et al.* (2000) Adenoid basal carcinomas of the cervix: a unique morphological evolution with cell cycle correlates. *Human Pathology*, **31** (6), 740–744.

7 Benedet, J.L., Bender, H., Jones, H., Ngan, H.Y.S. & Pecorelli, S. (2000) FIGO staging classifications and clinical practice guidelines in the management of gynaecologic cancers. *International Journal of Gynaecology and Obstetrics*, **70** (2), 209–262.

8 Thomas, G.M. (2000) Concurrent chemotherapy and radiation for locally advanced cervical cancer: the new standard of care. *Seminars in Radiation Oncology*, **10**, 44–50.

9 Kristensen, G.B. & Trope, C. (1997) Epithelial ovarian carcinoma. *The Lancet*, **349**, 113–117.

10 La Vecchia, C. & Franceschi, S. (1999) Oral contraceptives and ovarian cancer. *European Journal of Cancer Prevention*, **8**, 297–304.

11 Scully, R.E., Young, R.H. & Clement, P.B. (1998) *Tumours of the Ovary, Maldeveloped Gonads, Fallopian Tube, and Broad Ligament*. Armed Forces Institute of Pathology, Washington, DC.

12 Sanusi, F.A., Carter, P. & Barton, D.P.J. (2000) Non-epithelial ovarian cancers. *The Obstetrician and Gynaecologist*, **2** (2), 37–39.

13 Society of Gynaecologic Oncologists (2000) Guidelines for referral to a gynaecologic oncologist: rationale and benefits: endometrial cancer. *Gynaecologic Oncology*, **78**, S1–S13.

14 Hendrickson, M.R., Longacre, T.A. & Kempson, R.L. (1999) The uterine corpus. In: *Diagnostic Surgical Pathology* (ed. S.S. Sternberg), 3rd edn, pp. 2203–2305. Lippincott, Williams and Wilkins, Philadelphia.

15 Parc, Y.R., Halling, K.C., Burgart, L.J. *et al.* (2000) Microsatellite instability and hMLH1/hMSH2 expression in young endometrial carcinoma patients: associations with family history and histopathology. *International Journal of Cancer*, **86**, 60–66.

16 Silverberg, S.G. & Kurman, R.J. (1992) *Tumours of the Uterine Corpus and Gestational Trophoblastic Disease*. Armed Forces Institute of Pathology, Washington, DC.

17 Creutzberg, C.L., van Putten, W.L.J., Koper, P.C.M. *et al.* (2000) Surgery and postoperative radiotherapy versus surgery alone for patients with stage 1 endometrial carcinoma: multicentre randomised trial. *The Lancet*, **355** (9213), 1404–1411.

18 Kempson, R.L. & Hendrickson, M.R. (2000) Smooth muscle, endometrial stromal, and mixed Müllerian tumours of the uterus. *Modern Pathology*, **13** (3), 328–342.

19 Silverberg, S.G. (2000) Low grade endometrial stromal sarcoma: a rare but often puzzling diagnostic problem. *Pathology Case Reviews*, **5**, 173–180.

20 Frierson, H.F. & Mills, S.E. (1999) The vulva and vagina. In: *Diagnostic Surgical Pathology* (ed. S.S. Sternberg) 3rd edn, pp. 2111–2153. Lippincott, Williams and Wilkins, Philadelphia.

21 Carlson, J.A., Ambros, R., Malfetano, J. *et al.* (1998) Vulvar lichen sclerosus and squamous cell carcinoma: a cohort, case control, and investigational study with historical perspective; implications for chronic inflammation and sclerosis in the development of neoplasia. *Human Pathology*, **29**, 932–948.

22 Sedlis, A., Homesley, H., Bundy, B.N. *et al.* (1987) Positive groin lymph nodes in superficial squamous cell vulvar cancer. A Gynaecologic Oncology Group study. *American Journal of Obstetrics & Gynaecology*, **156**, 1159–1164.

23 Magrina, J.F., Gonzalez-Bosquet, J., Weaver, A.L. *et al.* (2000) Squamous cell carcinoma of the vulva stage 1A: long-term results. *Gynaecologic Oncology*, **76**, 24–27.

24 Homesley, H.D., Bundy, B.N., Sedlis, A. *et al.* (1991) Assessment of current International Federation of Gynaecology and Obstetrics staging of vulvar carcinoma relative to prognostic factors for survival (a Gynaecologic Oncology Group study). *American Journal of Obstetrics and Gynaecology*, **164** (4), 997–1003.

25 Maggino, T., Landoni, F., Sartori, E. *et al.* (2000) Patterns of recurrence in patients with squamous cell carcinoma of the vulva. A multicentre CTF study. *Cancer*, **89** (1), 116–122.

26 Preti, M., Ronco, G., Ghiringhello, B. & Micheletti, L. (2000) Recurrent squamous cell carcinoma of the vulva: clinicopathologic determinants identifying low risk patients. *Cancer*, **88**, 1869–1876.

27 Heaps, J.M., Fu, Y.S., Montz, F.J., Hacker, N.F. & Berek, J.S. (1990) Surgical-pathologic variables predictive of local recurrence in squamous cell carcinoma of the vulva. *Gynaecologic Oncology*, **38**, 309–314.

28 Ragnarsson-Olding, B.K., Nilsson, B.R., Kanter-Lewensohn, L.R., Lagerlof, B. & Ringborg, U.K. (1999) Malignant melanoma of the vulva in a nationwide, 25-year study of 219 Swedish females: predictors of survival. *Cancer*, **86**, 1285–1293.

29 Ragnarsson-Olding, B.K., Kanter-Lewensohn, L.R., Lagerlof, B., Nilsson, B.R. & Ringborg, U.K. (1999) Malignant melanoma of the vulva in a nationwide, 25-year study of 219 Swedish females: clinical observations and histopathologic features. *Cancer*, **86**, 1273–1284.

30 Stock, R.G., Chen, A.S. & Seski, J. (1995) A 30-year experience in the man-

14

agement of primary carcinoma of the vagina: analysis of prognostic factors and treatment modalities. *Gynaecological Oncology*, **56** (1), 45–52.

31 Buchanan, D.J., Schlaerth, J. & Kurosaki, T. (1998) Primary vaginal melanoma: 13-year disease-free survival after wide local excision and review of recent literature. *American Journal of Obstetrics and Gynaecology*, **178** (6),1177–1184.

32 Mauz-Korholz, C., Harms, D., Calaminus, G. & Gobel, U. (2000) Primary chemotherapy and conservative surgery for vaginal yolk sac tumour. *The Lancet*, **355**, 625.

33 Davidoff, A.M., Hebra, A., Bunin, N., Shochat, S.J. & Schnaufer, L. (1996) Endodermal sinus tumour in children. *Journal of Pediatric Surgery*, **31**,1075–1078.

34 Martelli, H., Oberlin, O., Rey, A. *et al.* (1999) Conservative treatment for girls with non-metastatic rhabdomyosarcoma of the genital tract: a report from the Study Committee of the International Society of Pediatric Oncology. *Journal of Clinical Oncology*, **17**, 2117–2122.

35 Andrassy, R.J., Wiener, E.S., Raney, R.B. *et al.* (1999) Progress in the surgical management of vaginal rhabdomyosarcoma: a 25-year review from the Intergroup Rhabdomyosarcoma Study Group. *Journal of Pediatric Surgery*, **34**, 731–734.

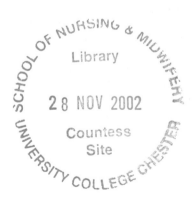

Index

abdominal colposacropexy, 440
abdominal hysterectomy, 441
aciclovir, 341, 342
add-back therapy, 369
adenocarcinoma in situ, 82, 455
adenomyosis, 175
alcohol, 122
amenorrhoea, 101–102, 112
  primary, 101
  secondary, 102
amitriptyline, 385
amphthous ulcers, 343
ampicillin, 334
androstenedione, 246
anorexia nervosa, 104–105
anterior repair, 311
anti-D immunoglobulin, 55, 66
antifibrinolytic agents, 228
antiphospholipid syndrome, 47
aspirin, 50
atrophic vaginitis, 246
atypical glandular cells, 82, 83
atypical squamous cells, 83
augmentin, 337
azithromycin, 332

bacterial vaginosis, 66, 324, 326
  Amsel's criteria, 326
  clue cells, 326
  termination of pregnancy,
    326
Bartholinitis, 333
Bartholin's abscess, 393
Behcet's disease, 343
bethanechol, 318

bisphosphonates, 276
blastocyst, 148
bleeding
  breakthrough, 19
  dysfunctional uterine, 223,
    227
  in early pregnancy, 39
  intermenstrual, 222
  postcoital, 222
  postmenopausal, 177, 222,
    266
body mass index, 122
borderline ovarian tumour, 466
  management, 471
BRCA1, 463
breakthrough bleeding, 19
breast
  cancer, 12, 214, 283
  ultrasound, 212
bromocriptine, 113, 115
bullous pemphigoid, 388
Burch colposuspension, 308

cabergoline, 114
cancer
  breast, 214
    screening for, 211
  cervical, 14, 90, 92, 225
    screening for, 80
  endometrial, 14, 184, 223,
    225, 288, 475
  fallopian tubes, 203, 225
  ovarian, 14, 192–3
    surgery for, 446
  uterine cervix, 457

vaginal, 225
vulval, 225, 397
cancer cell surface antigen 125
    (CA125), 190
Candida, 84, 322, 323, 324
    albicans, 327
    glabrata, 327
candidiasis, 327
    treatment of, 328–9
cefoxitin, 337
ceftriaxone, 334
cervical cancer, 14, 90, 92
    screening for, 80
cervical cytology, 81
cervical dysplasia, 90, 91
cervical incompetence, 50
cervical intra-epithelial
    neoplasia, 82, 83
cervical screening and
    premalignant disease of the
    cervix, 80
cervical smear, 452
cervicitis screen, 324
chemotherapy, 72
chlamydia, 66, 126, 126, 322,
    324, 331, 332, 334, 336
Chlamydia trachomatis, 323,
    330
chlomiphene citrate, 136
choriocarcinoma, 73, 75
chromosomal abnormalities, 45
chronic pelvic pain, 355
cicatricial pemphigoid, 388
ciprofloxacin, 334, 337
clindamycin, 334, 337
clobetasol propionate, 390
clotrimazole, 328
coagulation disorders, 224
colposacropexy, abdominal, 440
colposuspension, ultrasound
    following, 210

combined oral contraceptives,
    7, 364
    contraindications to the use
        of, 15
    examples of, 6
    third generation, 4
computerised tomography (CT),
    110, 112, 115, 159, 175,
    209
condoms, 332, 335
conjugated equine oestrogen,
    228, 253, 262
conjunctivitis, 333
contraception
    emergency postcoital, 21
    first year failure rates, 33
    HRT and, 32
contraindications to the use of
    the COC, 15
corpeus luteum, 165
cryopreservation of oocytes,
    150
cumulative fertility, 122
Cushing's syndrome, 95
cyproterone acetate, 9, 97
cystitis, 334
cystometry, 305
cytology of vaginal discharge,
    324

danazol, 236, 364
DDAVP, 314
deep vein thrombosis, 10, 448
dehiscence, 169
depot-medroxyprogesterone
    acetate (MPA), 23, 24, 25,
    231, 232
    acute bleeding, 228
    hot flushes, 248
    side effects, 24
dermatitis, 350

dermoid cyst, 194
desogestrel, 3, 4, 11
desquamative vaginitis, 330
detrusor hyperreflexia, 316
detrusor instability, 313
diathermy, 408
dihydrotestosterone, 98
disseminated gonococcal
    infection, 333
DNA HPV, 338
dopaminergic agents, 111–12,
    116
doxycycline, 332, 337
ductal carcinoma in situ
    (DCIS), 215
dysfunctional uterine bleeding,
    223
    treatment, 227
dysmenorrhoea, 18, 356
dyspareunia, 351, 352, 357
    endometriosis, 352
    trigonitis, 352

eczema, 327
embryo, freezing of, 149
embryology, 147
emergency postcoital
    contraception, 21
endocervical curettage, 453
endometrial ablation, 237–40,
    242
endometrial biopsy, 223, 266–7,
    478
endometrial cancer, 14, 184,
    223, 288, 475
endometrial hyperplasia, 183,
    266
endometrial thickness, 178
endometriosis, 201, 355
    and chronic pelvic pain, 355
endometritis, 185

endometrium
    anatomy and appearance, 163
    ultrasound assessment of,
        177
erosive lichen planus, 388
erythromycin, 332
ESR, 334
ethinyloestradiol, 1

fallopian tubes
    anatomy and appearance, 164
    carcinoma, 203
    malignancy, 475
famciclovir, 341, 342
fertility, 373
fetal abnormality, 167
fetal maternal haemorrhage, 55
fibroadenomas, 216
fibroids, 173
finasteride, 99
first trimester miscarriage, 39
Fitz–Hugh–Curtis syndrome,
    333, 336
fluconazole, 328
flutamide, 99
follicle-stimulating hormone,
    124, 125, 126, 141, 245,
    246

galactorrhoea, 106, 123
gardnerella, 324
genital herpes
    aseptic meningitis, 340
    cervicitis, 340
    herpes simplex, 339
    incubation period, 340
    lymphadenopathy, 340
    proctitis, 340
    radiculopathy, 340
    recurrence, 340
    serology, 341

genital warts – human papilloma virus, 343
gentamicin, 337
genuine stress incontinence, 305
gestational trophoblastic disease, 69, 76, 171
gestodene, 3, 4, 11
gestrinone (Dimetriose), 236, 366
glucose tolerance, 95
GnRH
    agonists, 141–2, 237, 367, 369, 424
    analogues, 98
gonorrhoea, 324
    complications, 333
granulosa cell tumours, 473
gynaecological endocrinology, 94
gynaecological oncology, 452
gynaecological surgery, 492

hCG, 141
HDL, 4, 10, 251
heat shock proteins, 332
heparin, 50
herpes simplex, 324
HERS study, 179, 252
hirsutism, 96–100
    pharmacological treatment of, 97
HIV, 322, 349
honeymoon cystitis, 334
hormonal contraception and sterilisation, 1
hormone replacement therapy (HRT), 253, 256, 268
    benefits, 270
    breast cancer, 281, 283

coronary heart disease, 279
endometrial cancer, 288
prevention of osteoporosis, 275
triglyceride levels, 288
hot flushes, 246, 247
human papillomavirus, 89, 453
hydatidiform mole, 71
    follow-up, 76
hyperinsulinaemia, 94–5
hyperoestrogenism, 109
hyperprolactinaemia, 105–16, 123, 126
hyperstimulation, 140
hypogonadotrophic hypogonadism, 144
hypothyroidism, 108
hysterectomy, 374, 424
    abdominal, technique of, 441
    complications, 446
    radical, 443
    vaginal, 425

imidazole, 327
imipramine, 314
infertility, 56, 118
    and assisted reproductive techniques, 118
    investigations of, 123
inherited coagulation disorder, 10
intermenstrual bleeding, 222
intraconazole, 328
intracytoplasmic sperm injection, 133
    procedure, 135
intrauterine devices (IUDs)
    advantages, 27
    adverse effects, 27
    benefits, 25

failure rates, 26
mechanism of action, 26
types of, 26
ultrasound identification, 188
intrauterine hyperstimulation,
    374
in vitro fertilisation, 146–51
irritable bowel syndrome, 375

karyotype 45 XO, 45

lactobacilli, 83, 323, 324
Lactobacillus crispatus, 323
laparoscopic ovarian diathermy,
    139
laparoscopic surgery
    complications, 413
    in ectopic pregnancy, 60
large loop excision of the
    transformation zone, 88
LCR chlamydia, 332
LDL, 10, 251
leiomyosarcoma, 485
lesbian bacterial vaginosis, 324
levonorgestrel, 3, 4, 11, 20
lichen planus, 351
lichen sclerosus, 327, 350,
    386–7, 394
lichen simplex chronicus, 350
lupus anticoagulant, 46
luteinising hormone, 94, 95,
    120, 141, 143, 144, 246
lysuride, 114

magnetic resonance imaging
    (MRI), 110, 112, 115, 159,
    162, 175, 208
    cervical abnormalities, 209
    evaluation of pelvis, 202
    ovaries, 199

mammography, 211
mastalgia, 267
menopause, 245
menorrhagia, 221, 222, 226
    medical management, 228
    surgical treatment, 237
menstrual cycle, 222
methotrexate, 58, 59
metronidazole, 325, 337
microinvasive cervical
    squamous cancer, 453
mifepristone (RU486), 23, 64,
    370
Mirena (LNG-IUS), 232, 269
    benefits, 235
    insertion, 233–4
miscarriage, 45, 144
    complete, 41
    incidence, 40
    incomplete, 41
    first trimester, 39
    inevitable, 40
    recurrent, 48, 52
    second trimester, 50
    septic, 40
    threatened or missed, 39, 40,
        42
misoprostol, 64
missed pill, definition, 20
mobiluncus, 324
molluscum contagiosum, 348
multiple pregnancy, 140

Neisseria gonorrhoea, 323,
    333
    cervicitis, 333
    pharyngitis, 333
    proctitis, 333
    urethritis, 333
neonatal conjunctivitis, 331

neonatal pneumonitis, 331
nitroimadazole, 325, 330
non-steroidal anti-
   inflammatory drugs
   (NSAIDs), 230
norethindrone enanthate (NET-
   EN), 23, 25
norethisterone, 4, 231, 262
norgestimate, 3, 4
normal flora, 323
nortestosterone progestogens, 3
   chemical structure of, 5
   in HRT, 260
nuchal translucency, 167

obesity, 94
oestradiol level, 140, 141
oestriol cream, 330
oestrogens, 251
oestrone, 246
oligomenorrhoea, 94
oocytes, cryopreservation of,
   150
oophorectomy
   laparoscopic, 429
   prophylactic, 426
oral contraception, 1
   following trophoblastic
      disease, 76
osteoporosis, 237, 271–8
ovarian cancer, 14, 192–3
   surgery for, 446
ovarian cysts, 188
ovarian hyperstimulation,
   144–6
ovarian tumour, 466
ovaries
   anatomy and appearance,
      164
   polycystic, 196

ovulation, 120, 143
   induction, 136–43
ovulatory follicles, 140
oxybutynin, 314

partner notification, 332
PCR Chlamydia, 332, 334
pelvic floor exercises, 306
pelvic inflammatory disease
   (PID), 200, 335
   actinomycosis, 335
   cervicitis, 335
   chronic pelvic pain, 335
   ectopic pregnancy, 335, 336
   HIV, 335, 348
   infertility, 335
   termination of pregnancy,
      335
   IUCD, 335
pelvic pain, 204
pituitary tumour, 126
polycystic ovary syndrome,
   94–6, 100, 126, 196
polyps, 181
postcoital bleeding, 222
postmenopausal bleeding, 177,
   222, 266
pregnancy
   diagnosing, 37
   early, 37
      bleeding in, 39
      ultrasound imaging of, 38
   ectopic, 55, 56–63, 64, 170
   likelihood, 120
   multiple, 140
   termination of, 63–8
      complications, 67
      mid-trimester, 68
      side effects, 67
   tests, 37

premature ovarian failure, 102–104, 245
premenstrual syndrome, 32
  common complaints, 34
  management, 34
premenstrual tension, 18
progesterone, 125
  types, 259
progestogen-only, 8
progestogens, 3, 9, 260, 262, 364
prolactin, 110, 113, 115, 123
prolapse, 431–8
prophylaxis, 338
psoriasis, 327, 350
pubic lice, 349
pyogenic abscess, 351

quinagolide, 114

radical hysterectomy, 443
Reiter's disease, 331
retained products of conception, 168
rhesus (D) immunoprophylaxis, 54
rubella, 123

sacrospinous colpoplexy, 438
saline infusion sonography (SIS), 174
  for assessment before endometrial ablation, 187
scabies, 349
screening
  cervical cancer, 80
  thrombophilia, 21
second trimester miscarriage, 50
serotonin, 114

serum CA125, 463, 478
sexual assault, 338
sexual health, 321
  examination, 322
  history, 321
  routine screening, 322
sexually transmitted disease, 56
Shirodkar suture, 53
side effects of DMPA, 24
smear, 92
spironolactone, 98
Staphylococcus aureus, 323
Staphylococcus saprophyticus, 323
sterilisation, 56
surgery
  for ovarian cancer, 446
  gynaecological, 402
  tubal, 151
sutures, types of, 415
syphilis (*Treponema pallidum*), 338
  FTA, RPR, VDRL, 338
  Jarisch–Herxheimer, 338
  lymphadenopathy, 338

tamoxifen, 186, 227
TCRE, 237
tension-free vaginal tape, 311
testosterone, 95, 98
third generation COCs, 4
thrombophilia
  investigations for, 250
  screening for, 21
thromboprophylaxis, 407
tinea cruris, 349
topical steroids, 389
total cholesterol, 10
tranexamic acid, 229
transformation zone, 453

transvaginal ultrasound, 156–8
trichomonas, 322, 323, 324, 334
trichomoniasis, 329
    amnionitis, 329
    HIV, 329
    incubation period, 329
    prematurity, 329
triglyceride levels, 10, 251, 288
trisomy 21, 167, 169
tropical sexually transmitted
    infections, 343
tubal surgery, 151
tumours
    germ cell, 474
    granulosa cell, 473

ultrasound
    assessment of the
        endometrium, 177
    bladder neck, 210, 211
    breast, 212
    colposuspension, 210
    imaging of early pregnancy,
        38
    strength of pelvic floor, 210
    stress incontinence, 210
    transvaginal, 156–8
    and the use of imaging in
        gynaecology, 155
    uterovaginal prolapse, 210
urethritis, 333
urinary incontinence,
    definition, 292
urogynaecology, 293
uterine cervix, cancer of, 457
uterine sarcomas, 484
uterovaginal prolapse,
    quantification by
        ultrasound, 210
uterus, anatomy and
    appearance, 162

vaginal discharge, cytology, 324
vaginal hysterectomy, 425
vaginal intra-epithelial
    neoplasia (VIN), 395
vaginismus, 386
vaginitis, 325
    clinical diagnosis, 325
    signs, 325
    symptoms, 325
    treatment, 325
valaciclovir, 341, 342
vasectomy, 134
venous thromboembolism, 12,
    250, 283, 406
Veress needle, 414
vestibular papillomatosis, 345
vestibulitis, 383
von Willebrand's disease, 225
vulval cancer, 397
vulval disease and
    gynaecological
        dermatology, 380
vulval malignancies, 486, 494
vulval pain, 382
vulvar vestibulitis, 351
vulvectomy, 399
vulvodynia, 351
    dysaesthetic, 352, 385
    electromyographic feedback,
        352
    vaginal dilators, 352
    vestibulitis, 351

warts (genital), 343
    cervical cancer, 344
    CIN, 3444, 349
    laryngeal papillomatosis, 344
    VIN, 344
WBC, 336

zona pellucida, 148